INTERNATIONAL ASSOCIATION FOR THE STUDY OF LUNG CANCER

Textbook of Prevention and Detection of Early Lung Cancer

INTERNATIONAL ASSOCIATION FOR THE STUDY OF LUNG CANCER

Textbook of Prevention and Detection of Early Lung Cancer

Edited by

Fred R Hirsch MD PhD

Professor of Medicine & Pathology
University of Colorado Cancer Center
Denver
Colorado
USA

Paul A Bunn Jr MD

Grohne/Stapp Professor and Director
University of Colorado Cancer Center
Denver
Colorado
USA

Harubumi Kato MD PhD

Professor and Chairman
Department of Surgery
Tokyo Medical University
Japan

James L Mulshine MD

Associate Provost of Research
Rush University Medical School
Chicago
Illinois
USA

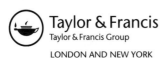

Taylor & Francis
Taylor & Francis Group

LONDON AND NEW YORK

© 2006 Taylor & Francis, an imprint of the Taylor & Francis Group

First published in the United Kingdom in 2006 by Taylor & Francis, an imprint of the Taylor & Francis Group, 2 Park Square, Milton Park, Abingdon, Oxon OX14 4RN

Tel.: +44 (0)20 7017 6000
Fax.: +44 (0)20 7017 6699
E-mail: info.medicine@tandf.co.uk
Website: www.tandf.co.uk/medicine

Every effort has been made to ensure that all owners of copyright material have been acknowledged in this publication, we would be glad to acknowledge in subsequent reprints or editions any omissions brought to our attention.

Although every effort has been made to ensure that drug doses and other information are presented accurately in this publication, the ultimate responsibility rests with the prescribing physician. Neither the publishers nor the authors can be held responsible for errors or for any consequences arising from the use of information contained herein. For detailed prescribing information or instructions on the use of any product or procedure discussed herein, please consult the prescribing information or instructional material issued by the manufacturer.

A CIP record for this book is available from the British Library.

Library of Congress Cataloging-in-Publication Data
Data available on application

ISBN 1-84184-301-6
ISBN 978-1-84184-301-8

Distributed in North and South America by
Taylor & Francis
2000 NW Corporate Blvd
Boca Raton, FL 33431, USA

Within Continental USA
Tel: 800 272 7737; Fax: 800 374 3401
Outside Continental USA
Tel: 561 994 0555; Fax: 561 361 6018
E-mail: orders@crcpress.com

Distributed in the rest of the world by
Thomson Publishing Services
Cheriton House
North Way
Andover, Hampshire SP10 5BE, UK
Tel.: +44 (0)1264 332424
E-mail: salesorder.tandf@thomsonpublishingservices.co.uk

Composition by Wearset Ltd, Boldon, Tyne and Wear, UK
Printed and bound in Great Britain by CPI Bath

Contents

Contributors

Francesca Andriani
Unit of Molecular Cytogenetics
Department of Experimental Oncology
Istituto Nazionale Tumori
Milan
Italy

Erik M Augustson, PhD, MPH
Behavioral Scientist
Tobacco Control Research Branch
Behavioral Research Program
Division of Cancer Control and Population Sciences
National Cancer Institute/SAIC-Frederick
Bethesda, MD
USA

Heinrich D Becker, MD, FCCP
Internal Medicine/Pulmonology
Head Dept. Interdisciplinary Endoscopy
Thoraxklinik
Heidelberg University School of Medicine
Heidelberg
Germany

Christian Brambilla, MD
Department of Pulmonary Medicine
University of Grenoble
Grenoble
France

Elisabeth Brambilla, MD
Albert Bonniot Institute
Hospital Centre
University of Grenoble
France

Paul A Bunn Jr, MD
Grohne/Stapp Professor and Director
University of Colorado Cancer Center
Denver, CO
USA

David M Burns, MD
UCSD School of Medicine
San Diego, CA
USA

David P Carbone, MD
Division of Hematology and Oncology
Vanderbilt University Medical Center
Nashville, TN
USA

David C Christiani, MD, MPH, SM
Harvard School of Public Health
Harvard Medical School/Massachusetts General
Hospital
Boston, MA
USA

Tommaso A Dragani, PhD
Unit of Genetic Susceptibility
Department of Experimental Oncology
Istituto Nazionale Tumori
Milan
Italy

Andinet A Enquobahrie, MS, PhD Student
Cornell University
School of Electrical & Computer Engineering
Ithaca, NY
USA

Manuela Gariboldi, PhD
Unit of Genetic Susceptibility
Department of Experimental Oncology
Istituto Nazionale Tumori
Milan
Italy

Laurie E Gaspar, MD, MBA
Professor & Chair, Department of Radiation
Oncology
University of Colorado
Aurora, CO
USA

Claudia I Henschke, PhD, MD
Department of Radiology
Weill Medical College of Cornell University
New York, NY
USA

Fred R Hirsch, MD, PhD
Professor of Medicine & Pathology
University of Colorado Cancer Center
Denver, CO
USA

James R Jett, MD
Professor of Medicine
Division of Pulmonary and Critical Care Medicine
Mayo Clinic College of Medicine
Rochester, MN
USA

Harubumi Kato, MD, PhD
Professor and Chairman
Department of Surgery
Tokyo Medical University
Shinjuku-ku
Tokyo
Japan

Keith M Kerr, MB, ChB, FRCPath
Department of Pathology
Aberdeen University School of Medicine
Aberdeen Royal Infirmary
Aberdeen
UK

Stephen Lam, MD, FRCPC
Cancer Imaging
BC Cancer Research Center
Vancouver, British Columbia
Canada

Scott J Leischow, PhD
Senior Advisor for Tobacco Policy
Office of the Secretary/ASPE
Department of Health and Human Services
Washington, DC
USA

Kirsten Hall Long, PhD
Assistant Professor, Department of Health Sciences
Research
Mayo Clinic College of Medicine
Rochester, MN
USA

Patricia L Mabry, PhD
Behavioral Scientist
Tobacco Control Research Branch
Behavioral Research Program
Divisional Cancer Control & Population Sciences
National Cancer Institute/SAIC-Frederick
Bethesda, MD
USA

Giacomo Manenti
Unit of Genetic Susceptibility
Department of Experimental Oncology
Istituto Nazionale Tumori
Milan
Italy

Deborah Marshall, PhD
Program for Assessment of Technology in Health
Centre for Evaluation of Medicine
St. Joseph's Hospital and McMaster University
Hamilton, Ontario
Canada

Pierre P Massion, MD
Division of Allergy, Pulmonary and Critical Care
Medicine
Vanderbilt-Ingram Comprehensive Cancer Center
Nashville, TN
USA

David E Midthun, MD
Associate Professor
Division of Pulmonary and Critical Care Medicine
Mayo Clinic College of Medicine
Rochester, MN
USA

Glen D Morgan, PhD
Program Director
Tobacco Control Research Branch
Behavioral Research Program
Division of Cancer Control & Population Sciences
National Cancer Institute
Bethesda, MD
USA

James L Mulshine, MD
Associate Provost for Research
Rush University Medical School
Vice President for Research
Rush University Medical Center
Chicago, IL
USA

Masayuki Noguchi, MD
Department of Pathology
Institute of Basic Medical Sciences
Graduate School of Comprehensive Human Sciences
University of Tsukuba
Japan

D Maxwell Parkin, MD
Descriptive Epidemiology Group
IARC
Lyon
France

Harvey I Pass, MD
Professor of Surgery and Oncology
Wayne State University and Karmanos Cancer
Institute
Detroit, MI
USA

Anthony P Reeves, PhD
Associate Professor
School of Electrical and Computer Engineering
Cornell University
Ithaca, NY
USA

Luca Roz
Unit of Molecular Cytogenetics
Department of Experimental Oncology
Istituto Nazionale Tumori
Milan
Italy

Tracey Schefter, MD
Associate Professor, Department of Radiation
Oncology
University of Colorado
Aurora, CO
USA

Dorith Shaham, MD
Department of Radiology
Hadassah Medical Center
Jerusalem
Israel

Gabriella Sozzi, PhD
Unit of Molecular Cytogenetics
Department of Experimental Oncology
Istituto Nazionale Tumori
Milan
Italy

Shusuke Sone, MD
Director, Azumi General Hospital
Ikeda-machi, Kitaazumi-gun
Nagano
Japan

G Sutedja, MD, PhD
Department of Pulmonary Medicine
Vrije Universiteit Medical Center
Amsterdam
The Netherlands

Stephen J Swensen, MD
Professor of Radiology
Department of Radiology
Mayo Clinic College of Medicine
Rochester, MN
USA

Melvyn S Tockman, MD, PhD
Director, Molecular Screening and Population
Studies
H. Lee Moffitt Cancer Center & Research Institute
Tampa, FL
USA

Jerzy E Tyczynski, PhD
Research Scientist/Epidemiologist
Cancer Prevention Institute
Dayton, OH
USA

J Usuda, MD, PhD
Department of Surgery
Tokyo Medical University
Shinjuku-ku
Tokyo
Japan

Carola A van Iersel, MSc
Department of Public Health
Erasmus Medical Centre
Rotterdam
The Netherlands

Rob J van Klaveren, MD, PhD
Dept of Pulmonology
University Hospital Rotterdam
Rotterdam
The Netherlands

Nico van Zandwijk, MD, PhD
Head of the Department of Thoracic Oncology
The Netherlands Cancer Institute – Antoni van
Leeuwenhoek Ziekenhuis
Amsterdam
The Netherlands

William D Travis, MD
Attending Thoracic Pathologist
Department of Pathology
Memorial Sloan Kettering Cancer Center
New York, NY
USA

David F Yankelevitz, MD
Department of Radiology
Weill Medical College of Cornell University
New York, NY
USA

Pinar B Yildiz, MD
Division of Allergy, Pulmonary and Critical Care
Medicine
Vanderbilt University Medical Center
Nashville, TN
USA

Rowena Yip, MS
Department of Radiology
Weill Medical College of Cornell University
New York, NY
USA

Wei Zhou, MD, PhD
Department of Environmental Health
EH/Occupational Health
Boston, MA
USA

Preface

Lung cancer is the leading cause of cancer death throughout the world. It is estimated that well over a million new cases will be diagnosed per year globally, and despite intensive research efforts the prognosis is still poor. In best case scenarios only about 15% of the patients will survive 5 years after primary diagnosis. The reason for the poor prognosis is late diagnosis and lack of efficient treatment for systemic disease. In two-thirds of the cases, lung cancer has already spread to regional lymph nodes or beyond at the time of initial diagnosis.

Since we know what the carcinogen is that causes most of this disease, it is essential to continue efforts to reduce and ultimately eliminate exposure of people to tobacco in all of its forms. Sustained efforts with tobacco control have been successful and as a result throughout the world, there are millions of people who have overcome their nicotine addiction and stopped smoking. Smoking cessation has an immediate favorable effect on an individual's risk of cardiovascular disease but the risk of developing lung cancer remains elevated throughout many years compared to never smokers. For these former smokers, it is important to consider how to find a potential lung cancer at a time prior to lethal metastatic dissemination.

Many researchers have come to believe that the best chance to improve outcomes with lung cancer is to refocus efforts in finding or preventing early lung cancer, as our success with controlling advanced lung cancer has been limited. Reports are emerging about the use of high resolution spiral CT as a promising tool to find early lung cancer in high-risk populations. This process of lung cancer screening is a new and challenging area for lung cancer research. Recent developments in imaging techniques as well as new developments in endoscopic techniques make the potential of early detection of lung cancer very promising. Furthermore, intensive search for (other) biomarkers to identify risk or to be used for early detection is ongoing. As the field matures, a full range of new tools from risk assessment to minimally invasive intervention tools may be needed to optimally manage early lung cancer because the clinical challenges are quite different from managing metastatic cancer.

Since the health consequences of tobacco exposure are global, lung cancer is a profoundly important public health issue. Issues such as the economic dimensions of this problem emerge as important. Moving to preventive-based care represents a significant challenge since it also implies a major shift in the focus of care. Preventive care requires strategies that move attention from an individual diagnosed with a cancer to a population of individuals at high risk of developing lung cancer. This new dynamic crosses conventional lung cancer research boundaries and requires new types of interdisciplinary alliances to succeed.

The Association is an international forum for the diverse professionals involved in the care of people with lung cancer. In this volume, we have focused on major prevention issues that have general interest throughout the world. Consistent with the mission of the International Association of Lung Cancer (IASLC), we have recruited leading researchers from the Association to discuss the state-of-the-art for a range of issues involved in the prevention and early detection of lung cancer. We have also greatly benefited from the international composition of the Association in recruiting the contributors to this text. Other groups of professionals, which have not previously been integrated in the lung cancer scientific community, such as health economists and behavioral scientists, will assume larger roles in lung cancer research as lung cancer prevention matures as a discipline. Accordingly, we have also reached beyond the Association membership to recruit thought leaders in critical areas to fully cover the broad spectrum of issues within lung cancer prevention.

This volume captures the perspectives of a broad range of research leaders across the various fields in lung cancer prevention. In the IASLC we view the spectrum of research and care, from tobacco control to palliative care, as complementary and support all as essential in meeting different aspects of the needs of patients and the general population. This volume is designed to provide clinicians, as well as research investigators, with a comprehensive, state-of-the-art guide to lung cancer prevention. The goal is not only to have this book served as a teaching tool for the membership of the Association but also to encourage a greater participation of the scientific community in lung cancer prevention research. The spirit of the IASLC is to be inclusive in its lung cancer activities and to engender cooperation among different disciplines and orientations to mitigate the negative health consequences of tobacco exposure. Thus, it is a goal through this book to nurture greater cross-disciplinary efforts to understand how to effectively detect and prevent early lung cancer.

The editors of this book are deeply indebted to the many outstanding contributors to this volume and greatly appreciate the generous efforts in sharing their insights. Many of the chapters of this book represent compilation of emerging information that would be otherwise very hard to find. The efforts of these talented authors in developing this book are an important contribution to the vibrancy of the IASLC.

Finally we would like to thank the talented editorial and production staff of Taylor and Francis in producing such an attractive and timely volume.

Fred R. Hirsch
Paul A. Bunn Jr.
Harubumi Kato
James L. Mulshine

1 Global epidemiology of lung cancer

Jerzy E Tyczyński, D Maxwell Parkin

Contents Introduction • Global (geographical) differences • Epidemiology of lung cancer in particular continents • Lung cancer risk and protective factors • Differences by histology • Time trends • Survival of lung cancer patients

INTRODUCTION

Lung cancer is the commonest cancer in the world today (12.3% of all new cancers, 17.8% of cancer deaths). There were an estimated 1.2 million new cases and 1.1 million deaths in 2000.[1] Approximately half (52%) of all new cases occur in developed countries.[2] Lung cancer is nearly three times more frequent in males than in females (the sex ratio (M:F) is 2.7:1).

GLOBAL (GEOGRAPHICAL) DIFFERENCES

Lung cancer is relatively more important in developed (22% of all cancer deaths) than developing (14.6% of cancer deaths) countries.

In men, the areas with the highest incidence and mortality are Europe, North America and Australia/New Zealand. The rates in China, Japan and South East Asia are moderately high, while the lowest rates are found in southern Asia (India, Pakistan), and sub-Saharan Africa (Figures 1.1, 1.2 and 1.3). In certain population subgroups (e.g. US blacks, New Zealand Maoris), incidence is even higher, and with current incidence rates, men in these two groups have about a 13% chance of developing a lung cancer before the age of 75.

In women, the geographic pattern is a little different, reflecting different historical patterns of tobacco smoking. Thus, the highest incidence rates are observed in North America and north-west Europe (UK, Iceland, Denmark) with moderate incidence rates in Australia/New Zealand and China (Figures 1.1, 1.2 and 1.3).

In general, geographic patterns are very much a reflection of past exposure to tobacco smoking.[3]

EPIDEMIOLOGY OF LUNG CANCER IN PARTICULAR CONTINENTS

Africa

Approximately 18 000 lung cancer deaths were estimated in Africa in the year 2000. The average mortality rates were $7.2/10^5$ in males and $1.9/10^5$ in females.[4] The estimated number of new lung cancer cases in Africa is 19 500 per year, which is 1.9% of the global total.[5] The average estimated incidence rate for Africa is $7.8/10^5$ in men and $2.0/10^5$ in women. The highest incidence rates in males are observed in the European population of Harare, Zimbabwe ($38.4/10^5$), La Reunion, France ($34.4/10^5$), and Sousse, Tunisia ($30.6/10^5$). In females, the highest incidence rates are noted in the European population of Harare, Zimbabwe ($24.5/10^5$), South Africa (white population) ($8.8/10^5$) and the African population of Harare ($5.9/10^5$).[5]

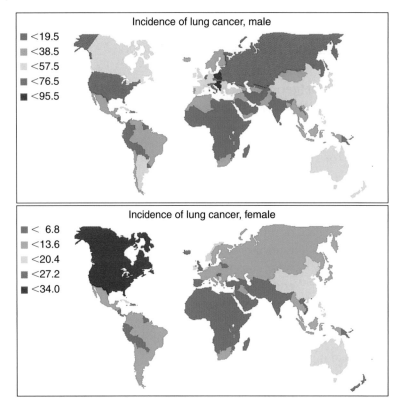

Figure 1.1
Worldwide geographical distribution of lung cancer (based on age-standardized incidence rates, World standard population).[a]

[a] Numbers in key represent lower range of each class. Figure courtesy of Globocan.

Asia

With nearly 0.6 million new lung cancer cases per year, and approximately 0.5 million lung cancer deaths per annum, Asia is the continent with the largest lung cancer burden.[4] The average mortality rate in Asia in the year 2000 was $24.9/10^5$ in men and $8.4/10^5$ in females. Estimated average incidence rates in the year 2000 were $28.4/10^5$ and $9.7/10^5$ for males and females, respectively. The highest incidence rates in males were observed in Hong Kong, China ($67.5/10^5$), Tianjin, China ($59.1/10^5$), Manila, Philippines ($57.0/10^5$), and Lampang, Thailand ($56.5/10^5$). In females, the highest incidence rates were found in Tianjin, China ($36.8/10^5$), Lampang, Thailand ($29.1/10^5$), Hong Kong, China ($26.6/10^5$) and Chiang Mai, Thailand ($25.9/10^5$).[6]

Australia and Oceania

There are nearly 9000 lung cancer deaths per year in the region – 6000 men and 2800 women. The age-adjusted mortality rate in the year 2000 was $33.9/10^5$ in men and $13.6/10^5$ in women.[4] Average age-adjusted incidence rates for the region in the period 1993–1997 were: $42.9/10^5$ for males and $17.8/10^5$ for females.[6] In males, the highest incidence rates in the region were observed in Northern Territory, Australia ($66.4/10^5$), Tasmania, Australia ($47.5/10^5$) and Hawaii, USA ($45.6/10^5$). In females, the highest incidence rates were found in Northern Territory, Australia ($29.4/10^5$) Hawaii, USA ($23.2/10^5$), and New Zealand ($21.5/10^5$).[6]

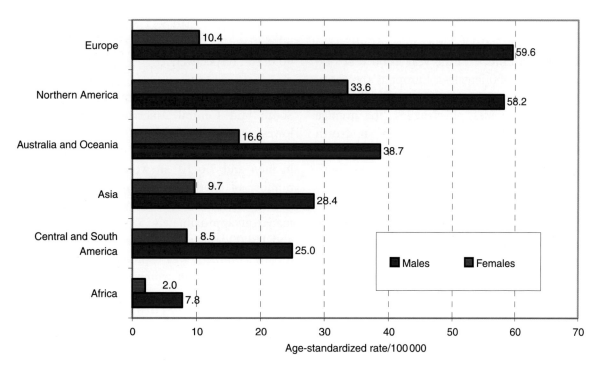

Figure 1.2
Lung cancer incidence, by continents, year 2000.

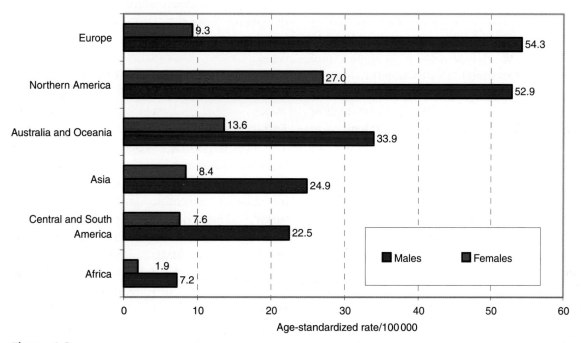

Figure 1.3
Lung cancer mortality, by continents, year 2000.

Europe

Approximately 350 000 lung cancer deaths were estimated in Europe in the year 2000 (280 000 males and 67 000 females). Europe is the continent with the highest average mortality rates $(54.3/10^5)$ in males.[4] In females, the average mortality $(9.3/10^5)$ is lower than in North America $(27.0/10^5)$ and Australia $(13.6/10^5)$, and similar to that observed in Asia and South America (Figure 1.2). The number of new lung cancer cases in 2000 was estimated as 375 000 (303 000 males and 72 000 females).[7] The highest incidence rates in men were observed in Lower Silesia, Poland $(92.3/10^5)$, Vojvodina, Serbia and Montenegro $(78.5/10^5)$, Croatia $(73.6/10^5)$ and Kielce, Poland $(73.4/10^5)$. In females, the highest incidence rates were found in Scotland, UK $(35.4/10^5)$, Merseyside and Cheshire, UK $(32.0/10^5)$, Denmark $(29.7/10^5)$ and north-western England $(28.4/10^5)$.[6]

North America

The annual number of lung cancer deaths in North America has been estimated at 180 000 (110 000 and 70 000 deaths in males and females, respectively).[4] North America has the second highest average mortality rate (after Europe) in males $(52.9/10^5)$ and the highest rate in females $(27.0/10^5)$ – twice as high as in any other continent. The number of new cases per year has been estimated for 205 000 (120 000 in males and 85 000 in females), while the average incidence rates for the whole continent were estimated as $58.2/10^5$ and $33.6/10^5$ in males and females, respectively. The highest incidence rates in males are observed in black populations in the USA, i.e. New Orleans, Louisiana $(107.0/10^5)$, Detroit, Michigan $(94.7/10^5)$ and Central Region, Louisiana $(92.0/10^5)$, as well as in Northwest Territories of Canada $(87.2/10^5)$.[6] In females, the populations with the highest rates are the Northwest Territo-ries, Canada $(72.0/10^5)$, and black and white inhabitants of Detroit, Michigan $(40.8/10^5$ and $40.0/10^5$, respectively).

South and Central America

South and Central America has the second lowest average mortality rate among all continents (higher only than that of Africa), $22.5/10^5$ in men and $7.6/10^5$ in women.[4] The absolute number of deaths from lung cancer in South and Central America in the year 2000 was estimated at approximately 57 000 (41 000 males and 16 000 females). The average incidence rate for the continent was estimated at $25.0/10^5$ in men and $8.5/10^5$ in women.[4] The highest incidence rates in males were observed in Montevideo, Uruguay $(75.9/10^5)$, Bahia Blanca, Argentina $(49.5/10^5)$, Concordia, Argentina $(41.1/10^5)$ and Villa Clara, Cuba $(36.7/10^5)$.[6] In women, the highest incidence rates were found in Villa Clara, Cuba $(15.7/10^5)$, Cali, Colombia $(9.5/10^5)$, Montevideo, Uruguay $(9.2/10^5)$ and in Goiania, Brasil $(8.5/10^5)$.

LUNG CANCER RISK AND PROTECTIVE FACTORS

Tobacco smoking (active)

The most important risk factor for lung cancer is tobacco smoking. The supportive evidence for this association has been reviewed many times by different scientific groups and institutions.[8–13] There is a clear dose–response relationship between lung cancer risk and the duration of smoking, number of cigarettes smoked per day, the degree of inhalation and the age at initiation of smoking.[14–16] The type of cigarettes smoked also influences risk.[17,18]

The proportion of lung cancer cases due to tobacco smoking has been estimated by comparing incidence (or mortality) rates in different areas, with the rates in non-smokers observed in large cohort studies.[19,20] Based on the worldwide incidence rates estimated for 2000, 90–95% of cases of lung cancer in men in Europe and North America are attributable to smoking, and only in the lowest incidence areas of East and West Africa are there no attributable cases. The fractions are lower for women, and several areas (where incidence rates are lower than in non-smoking women in the US and Japan), including south central Asia, have no attributable cases. Worldwide, 85% of lung cancer in men and 47% of lung cancer in women is the consequence of tobacco smoking.

Environmental tobacco smoke (passive smoking)

Environmental tobacco smoke (ETS) is a result of exhaled smoke from smokers and sidestream smoke from burning tobacco products. Sidestream smoke has a higher concentration of carcinogenic compounds than mainstream smoke.[21] It has been shown that passive exposure to tobacco smoke increases the risk of lung cancer.[9] This relationship was shown for the first time at the beginning of the 1980s by several groups.[22–24] It is estimated that exposure to ETS increases risk by 15–25% (even after adjustment for other confounding factors).[25–29] The magnitude of the excess risk was recently confirmed by meta-analysis of several previous studies, showing 25% increased risk caused by the exposure from spouses and 17% increased risk from the exposure at the workplace.[30] Some authors suggest that exposure to ETS in childhood may increase the effect of high doses of ETS exposure in adults.[31–33]

Occupational exposure

There are several types of exposures related to different occupations that are known or suspected to be risk factors for lung cancer. They include exposure to asbestos, some metals (e.g. nickel, arsenic, cadmium, lead), silica, bitumen fumes and ionizing radiation.[34–39]

Asbestos is the main cause of mesothelioma, but it is also reported to increase the risk of lung cancer. Several studies of workers exposed to asbestos employed in mining, cement industry, insulation and textile products showed an elevated risk of lung cancer among exposed compared with unexposed subjects.[40] It has also been suggested that the risk of lung cancer in asbestos workers is elevated only among those who have asbestosis.[34] Exposure to several metals is also known to be responsible for increasing the risk of lung cancer.[41] It has been shown, for instance, that exposure to different forms of nickel may increase the risk of lung cancer from 1.3 to 3.8 times (depending on the type and intensity of exposure).[42] Exposure to arsenic in drinking water may increase lung cancer risk from 1.2 to 2.2 times (depending on sex and intensity of exposure).[43] It is also estimated that exposure to silica may increase the risk of lung cancer by approximately 30%.[40] A small increase of risk (by approximately 15–30%) was found also in workers exposed to bitumen fumes (road paving, asphalt mixing, etc.),[39] although some studies have not confirmed such an association.[44]

Exposure to radon (both occupational and residential) increases the risk of developing lung cancer (see below).

Residential and occupational radon exposure

Radon (^{222}Rn) is a colorless, odorless, radioactive gas that forms from the decay of naturally occurring uranium-238. It issues from uranium-containing rocks and soil into surrounding areas (including homes and underground mines). Hence, people are exposed to radon in both residential and occupational settings. It is estimated that exposure to radon progeny is the second leading cause of lung cancer in developed countries.[45,46]

There is a lot of epidemiological evidence of a relationship between radon exposure and lung cancer, coming from cohort studies of underground miners, case-control studies, as well as from ecologic studies comparing lung cancer incidence (or mortality) across areas with different levels of radon exposure.[47] It has been estimated based on the pooled analysis of 11 cohort studies of radon-exposed underground miners that in smokers 10% of lung cancer cases in males and 12% in females were attributed to radon exposure. In non-smoking men and women the attributable fraction was 28% and 31%, respectively.[45] In addition, studies on residential radon exposure carried out in different countries showed an increasing risk of lung cancer related to an increasing radon exposure in both smokers and non-smokers.[48–52]

Interaction (synergy) between tobacco smoke and other risk factors

The essence of synergism is that when exposure occurs to two agents simultaneously, the risk is greater than if their individual effects were merely additive. Tobacco smoking is a lung cancer risk factor for which epidemiology has provided a large set of evidence of the interactions with other exogenous agents (for both the causation and the protection against causation). It concerns agents, such as asbestos, ionizing radiation, arsenic, silica and dietary factors.[35,53]

Several studies have investigated the interaction between tobacco smoke and asbestos. Most of the studies showed the multiplicative nature of that interaction.[35,54,55] However, a recent study by Gustavsson and colleagues[56] seems to suggest that the effect, although greater than additive, may be less than multiplicative. The 'multiplicative theory' is also questioned by other authors.[57,58]

An interaction between tobacco smoking and exposure to radon has been investigated among uranium and non-uranium miners,[35] as well as among individuals exposed to residential radon.[53] Most of the studies among miners seem to support the multiplicative nature of the association.[35] Also, a study on residential radon exposure and lung cancer suggests that the interaction with tobacco smoking exceeded additivity and was close to a multiplicative effect.[59] These findings have been confirmed by the Committee on the Biological Effects of Ionizing Radiation (BEIR VI).[60]

Exposure to arsenic also interacts with tobacco smoking in lung cancer causation. It has been shown for both occupational exposure to arsenic, and for exposure from drinking contaminated water.[61–64] There is no convincing evidence for a synergistic effect of tobacco smoke on other occupational exposures, or with urban air pollution in the existing literature;[35] however, some authors have suggested that there is a multiplicative effect of nickel exposure and tobacco.[65,66] It is also suggested, based on animal models, that there is synergy between polycyclic aromatic hydrocarbons (PAH) and tobacco smoke.[67]

Diet

It is believed that diet influences the risk of lung cancer.[68] Several studies have investigated the possible role of different dietary items in the etiology of lung cancer. No relation was found between lung cancer risk and the intake of fat or cholesterol.[69] It has been suggested that the consumption of fruits and vegetables reduces the risk of lung cancer.[70] However, evidence of the protective effects of fruit and vegetable consumption are inconsistent.[71–75] In addition, results differ for males and females, smokers and non-smokers, as well as for different histological types of lung cancer. No conclusive evidence was found for any relationship between lung cancer and alcohol consumption.[76]

Ethnicity (race)

Most of the studies on the impact of race (ethnicity) on lung cancer have been done in US populations. The US black population has higher incidence rates than the white population,[77] and they develop lung cancer at a much earlier age.[78] Although incidence and mortality rates in the black population are higher than among whites, it is not clear whether this is entirely due to differences in tobacco exposure, since the prevalence of smoking among African Americans is higher that in the US general population. On the other hand, African Americans have a later age of smoking initiation, and they also tend to smoke less cigarettes per day.[78] Hence, it is unlikely that the difference is entirely due to smoking prevalence. Some authors reported a higher risk at equivalent exposure to tobacco smoke in black populations,[79–81] while others reported no difference in risk.[82] It has been suggested that ethnic difference in smoking menthol cigarettes may play a role, since 75–90% of African Americans smoke menthol cigarettes, and only 20–30% of white smokers do. Some authors suggested that mentholated cigarettes increase risk more than 'normal' cigarettes,[83] however, others questioned this hypothesis.[84,85]

Socio-economic status (social class)

A limited number of studies has investigated the relationship between lung cancer and socio-economic status. In Europe, socio-economic status influences the risk of lung cancer, and this applies to both educational level and the type of occupation.[86–89] Similar observations have been made in Canada, where the risk of lung cancer in males was significantly related to both education and social class.[90] There are clear differences in smoking status in different social groups; in general people with a lower educational level and in manual or unskilled occupations tend to smoke more frequently than better-educated people from higher social classes. Although most studies of social status and lung cancer attempt some sort of adjustment for smoking, it is possible that this is incomplete, and residual confounding explains some of the observed results.

Genetic susceptibility

Although smoking is a major cause of lung cancer, only a proportion of smokers develop lung cancer, suggesting a genetic predisposition in some individuals.[91] Lung cancer susceptibility could be thought of as susceptibility to tobacco smoke exposure through differential carcinogen metabolism, and susceptibility to lung carcinogenesis from polymorphism of oncogenes or tumor suppressor genes.[92] In the late 1950s, Fisher[93] suggested that an association between smoking and lung cancer could be explained by shared genes that predisposed people to start smoking and to develop lung cancer later on. Fisher's hypothesis assumed that the same genes cause both smoking dependence and lung cancer. More recent studies showed, however, that genes that predispose to smoking are different from those that increase the risk of lung cancer.[94]

The study of Gauderman et al[95] showed that heavy smokers have a high lung cancer risk, with or without an inherited major gene mutation. However, the same study indicated that persons inheriting a mutation are at increased risk, whether or not they smoke.

It has been shown that mutations of the tumor suppressor gene *p53* are significantly more frequent in the tumors of subjects who had been exposed to tobacco smoke compared with those non-exposed.[96] Seifart et al[97] showed that intron 4 variation of the surfactant protein B gene was significantly more frequent among patients with squamous cell carcinoma of the lung than in controls. This finding may be important for future prevention activities, since pulmonary surfactant mediates the response to inhaled carcinogenic substances.

DIFFERENCES BY HISTOLOGY

Almost all lung cancers are carcinomas (other histologies comprise less than 1% of cases). In the combined data from the series published in

Cancer Incidence in Five Continents[6] small cell carcinomas comprise about 20% of cases and large cell/undifferentiated carcinomas about 9%. But for the other histological types, the proportions differ by sex: squamous cell carcinomas comprise 44% of lung cancers in men, and 25% in women, while adenocarcinomas comprise 28% of cases in men and 42% in women. Figure 1.4 shows overall incidence rates, and the estimated rates by histological subtype for 30 populations for which a relatively high proportion of cases had a clear morphological diagnosis.[6] Among men, with the exception of certain Asian populations (Chinese, Japanese), only in North

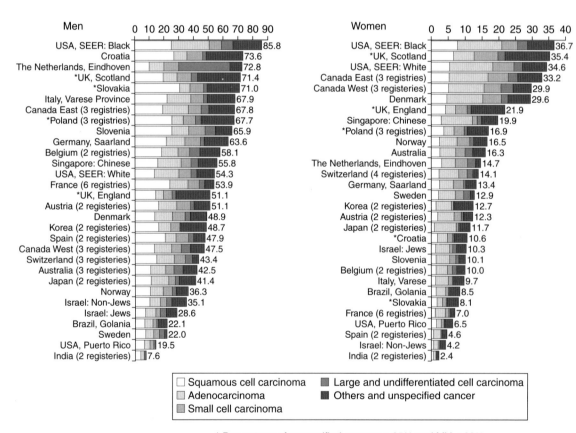

* Percentage of unspecified cancers >25% and MV <80%

Figure 1.4
Age-standardized incidence rates of lung cancer by cell type (around 1995), per 100 000.

America (USA, Canada) does the incidence of adenocarcinoma exceed that of squamous cell carcinoma. In women, however, adenocarcinoma is the dominant histological type almost everywhere, except for Poland and England where squamous cell carcinomas predominate, and Scotland where small-cell carcinoma is the most frequent subtype.[6] Adenocarcinomas are particularly predominant in Asian females (72% of cancers in Japan, 65% in Korea, 61% in Singapore Chinese). The differences in histological profiles are strongly influenced by the evolution of the epidemic of smoking-related lung cancer over time (see below).

TIME TRENDS

Because tobacco smoking is a powerful determinant of risk, trends in lung cancer incidence and mortality are a reflection of population-level changes in smoking behavior, including dose, duration and type of tobacco used.[98,99] Study of time trends in lung cancer incidence or mortality by age group shows that the level of risk is closely related to birth cohort; in the UK and US cohort-specific incidence is related to the smoking habits of the same generation.[100,101] Thus, in men, the countries where smoking was first established were the first to see a diminution in smoking prevalence, followed, in the same generations of men, by a decline in risk. Changes are first seen among younger age groups,[102] and as these generations of men reach the older age groups, where lung cancer is most common, a decline in overall incidence and mortality is seen. The UK was the first to show this (incidence/mortality falling since 1970–74), followed by Finland, Australia, Netherlands, New Zealand, the USA, Singapore and, more recently, Denmark, Germany, Italy and Sweden.[103] In most other countries there is

a continuing rise in rates, and this is most dramatic in some countries of Eastern and Southern Europe (i.e. Hungary, Spain) (Figure 1.5).[7,104] In women, the tobacco habit has usually been acquired recently, or not at all. Thus, the most common picture in Western populations is of rising rates (Figure 1.6), while in many developing countries (where female smoking generally remains rare), lung cancer rates remain very low. A few countries, where the prevalence of smoking in women is declining, already show decreasing rates in younger women; in the UK, where this trend is longest established, there is already a decline in overall incidence and mortality since about 1990 (Figure 1.6).[7,103]

There are, however, clear differences in time trends by histological type. In the US squamous cell carcinoma reached maximum incidence in men in 1981, but the incidence of adenocarcinoma continued to rise (until about 1987 in black males, around 1991 in whites).[105,106] As a result, adenocarcinoma is now the most frequent form of lung cancer in men in the USA (Figure 1.4), while it had only constituted a small minority of cases (around 5%) in the 1950s.[107] In contrast, the incidence of both histological types has continued to increase in females, though there is a suggestion that the incidence of squamous cell carcinomas had reached its maximum by 1990. These changes were related to specific birth cohorts, with maximum incidence in men in the 1925–29 cohort for squamous cell carcinomas and 1935–39 for adenocarcinomas, and in women some 10–20 years later.[105,108] Somewhat similar observations (increasing adenocarcinoma and decreasing squamous cell carcinoma) have been reported from the Netherlands, Japan and UK.[109–111] Possibly part of this differential trend may be due to artefact (changes in classification and coding, improved diagnostic methods for

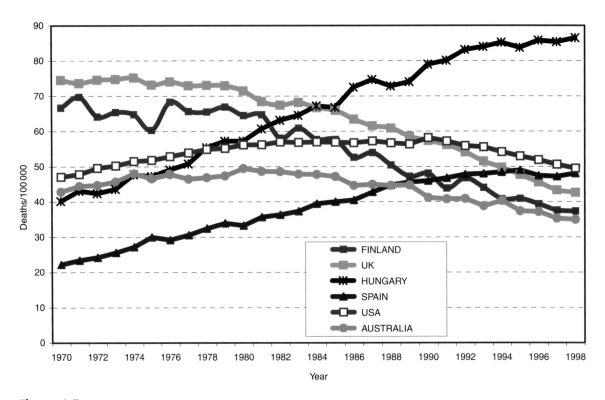

Figure 1.5
Time trends of lung cancer mortality, males (age-standardized rates, World standard population).

peripheral tumors). In part, it may be due to an ever-increasing proportion of ex-smokers in the population, since the decline in risk of lung cancer on smoking cessation is faster for squamous cell tumors than for small-cell carcinomas and adenocarcinomas.[17,112] It seems probable, too, that changes in cigarette composition, to low-tar, low-nicotine, filtered cigarettes, are also responsible, as switching to these 'safer' brands results (in addicted smokers) to more intense smoking (more puffs, deeper inhalation), and hence greater exposure to tobacco-related carcinogens.[113,114]

SURVIVAL OF LUNG CANCER PATIENTS

Patients diagnosed with lung cancer have a poor prognosis. There are some differences between the survival of lung cancer patients in Europe and the United States. In Europe, the average 5-year survival proportion is about 10%, and has not changed significantly over time.[115,116]

Estimates for the United States indicate the average 5-year survival is at about 15%.[117,118] In the US, survival is higher in the white (15%) than in the black population (12%).[118] Also, in Europe, there is a large variability in the survival of lung cancer patients. In the EUROCARE-2 study, the highest lung-cancer survivals were reported in Slovakia (12.8%), Iceland (12.2%) and France (11.9%), whilst the lowest values

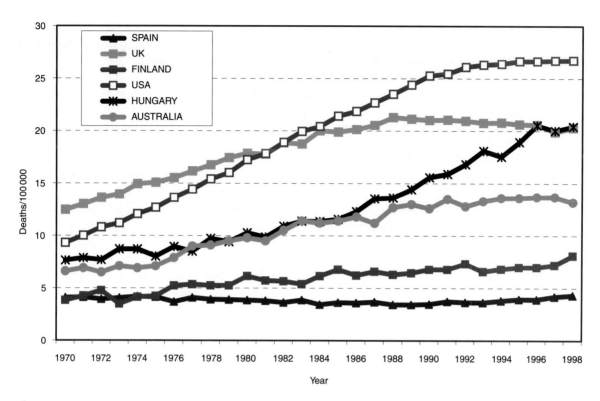

Figure 1.6
Time trends of lung cancer mortality, females (age-standardized rates, World standard population).

were found in Denmark (5.7%), Scotland (6.2%) and Slovenia (6.3%).[119]

The interpretation of survival differences is not, however, straightforward, and longer survival does not necessarily mean lower mortality. There are several possible reasons for differences in survival: quality of data from registries may differ, differences in classifications used and in coding practices, different registration coverage of the populations analyzed (some nationwide registries and some regional registries, not necessarily representative for the whole country). In addition, several early-detection programs may lead to increased survival in particular populations, without impact on mortality rates. It has been shown in randomized controlled trials of lung cancer screening, that

early detection programs based on radiology improved survival but did not reduce mortality from that disease.[120]

REFERENCES

1. Parkin DM, Bray FI, Devesa SS, Cancer burden in the year 2000. The global picture. Eur J Cancer 2001; 37:S4–66.
2. Parkin DM, Global cancer statistics in the year 2000. Lancet Oncology 2001; 2:533–43.
3. Doll R, Peto R, The causes of cancer: quantitative estimates of avoidable risks of cancer in the United States today. J Natl Cancer Inst 1981; 66:1191–308.
4. Ferlay J, Bray F, Pisani P, Parkin DM, GLOBO-CAN 2000: Cancer Incidence, Mortality and

Prevalence Worldwide, Version 1.0, IARC CancerBase No. 5. Lyon, IARC Press, 2001.

5. Parkin DM, Ferlay J, Hamdi-Cherif M, et al, Cancer in Africa. Epidemiology and Prevention, IARC Scientific Publication No. 153. IARC Press, Lyon, 2003.

6. Parkin DM, Whelan SL, Ferlay J, Teppo L, Thomas DB (eds), Cancer Incidence in Five Continents, Vol. VIII, IARC Scientific Publication No. 155. IARC, Lyon, 2002.

7. Tyczyński JE, Bray F, Parkin DM, Lung cancer in Europe in 2000: epidemiology, prevention, and early detection. Lancet Oncology 2003; 4:45–55.

8. International Agency for Research on Cancer (IARC), Tobacco Smoking. Evaluation of Carcinogenic Risk to Humans. IARC monographs on the evaluation of carcinogenic risk to humans. Volume 38. IARC, Lyon, 1986.

9. International Agency for Research on Cancer (IARC), Tobacco smoke and involuntary smoking. Evaluation of Carcinogenic Risks to Humans, Volume 83. IARC, Lyon, 2004.

10. US DHHS. The health consequences of smoking. Cancer. A report of the Surgeon General. US DHHS Publ., Rockville, 1982.

11. US DHHS, Reducing the Health Consequences of Smoking. 25 years of progress. A report of the Surgeon General. USDHHS Pub. 89–8411, Washington, 1989.

12. Royal College of Physicians, Smoking and health now: a new report and summary on smoking and its effect on health, from the Royal College of Physicians of London. Pitman Medical, London, 1971.

13. Royal College of Physicians, Smoking or health: the third report from the Royal College of Physicians of London. Pitman Medical, London, 1977.

14. Engeland A, Haldorsen T, Andersen A, Tretli S, The impact of smoking habits on lung cancer risk: 28 years' observation of 26,000 Norwegian men and women. Cancer Causes Control 1996; 7:366–76.

15. Agudo A, Ahrens W, Benhamou E, et al, Lung cancer and cigarette smoking in women: a multicenter case-control study in Europe. Int J Cancer 2000; 88:820–7.

16. Flanders WD, Lally CA, Zhu B-P, Henley SJ, Thun MJ, Lung cancer mortality in relation to age, duration of smoking, and daily cigarette consumption: results from Cancer Prevention Study II. Cancer Research 2003; 63:6556–62.

17. Lubin JH, Blot WJ, Assessment of lung cancer risk factors by histologic category. J Natl Cancer Inst 1984; 73:383–9.

18. Benhamou E, Benhamou S, Black (air-cured) and blond (flue-cured) tobacco and cancer risk VI: lung cancer. Eur J Cancer 1993; 29A:1778–80.

19. Parkin DM, Pisani P, Lopez AD, Masuyer E, At least one in seven cases of cancer is caused by smoking. Global estimates for 1985. Int J Cancer 1994; 59:494–504.

20. Peto R, Lopez AD, Boreham J, Thun M, Heath C Jr, Doll R, Mortality from smoking in developed countries 1950–2000. Oxford University Press, Oxford, 1994.

21. Jenkins RA, Guerin MR, Tomkins BA, The chemistry of environmental tobacco smoke: composition and measurement. CRC Press LLC, Boca Raton, 2000.

22. Hirayama T, Non-smoking wives of heavy smokers have a higher risk of lung cancer: a study from Japan. BMJ 1981; 282:183–5.

23. Trichopoulos D, Kalandidi A, Sparros L, MacMahon B, Lung cancer and passive smoking. Int J Cancer 1981; 27:1–4.

24. Garfinkel L, Time trends in lung cancer mortality among nonsmokers and a note on passive smoking. J Natl Cancer Inst 1981; 66:1061–6.

25. Fontham ETH, Correa P, Reynolds P, et al, Environmental tobacco smoke and lung cancer in nonsmoking women: a multicenter study. JAMA 1994; 271:1752–9.

26. Cardenas VM, Thun MJ, Austin H, et al, Environmental tobacco smoke and lung cancer mortality in the American Cancer Society's Cancer Prevention Study II. Cancer Causes Control 1996; 8:57–64.

27. Dockery DW, Trichopoulos D, Risk of lung cancer from environmental exposures to tobacco smoke. Cancer Causes and Control 1997; 8:333–45.

28. Boffetta P, Agudo A, Ahrens W, et al, Multicenter case-control study of exposure to environmental tobacco smoke and lung cancer. J Natl Cancer Inst 1998; 90:1440–50.

29. Zhong L, Goldberg MS, Parent M-E, Hanley JA, Exposure to environmental tobacco smoke and the risk of lung cancer: a meta-analysis. Lung Cancer 2000; 27:3–18.

30. Boffetta P, Involuntary smoking and lung cancer. Scand J Work Environ Health 2002; 28 (suppl 2):30–40.

31. Janerich DT, Thompson WD, Varela LR, et al, Lung cancer and exposure to tobacco smoke in the household. N Engl J Med 1990; 323:632–6.

32. Stockwell HG, Goldman AL, Lyman GH, et al, Environmental tobacco smoke and lung cancer risk in nonsmoking women. J Natl Cancer Inst 1992; 84:1417–22.

33. Lee C-H, Ko Y-C, Goggins W, et al, Lifetime environmental exposure to tobacco smoke and primary lung cancer of non-smoking Taiwanese women. Int J Epidemiol 2000; 29:224–31.

34. Churg A, Lung cancer cell type and occupational exposure, In: Samet JM (ed.) Epidemiology of lung cancer. Marcel Dekker Inc., New York, 1994.

35. Saracci R, Boffetta P, Interactions of tobacco smoking with other causes of lung cancer. In: Samet J (ed.) Epidemiology of Lung Cancer. Marcel Dekker Inc., New York, 1994, pp. 465–93.

36. Steenland K, Loomis D, Shy C, Simonsen N, Review of occupational lung carcinogenesis. Am J Ind Med 1996; 29:474–90.

37. Steenland K, Boffetta P, Lead and cancer in humans: where are we now? Am J Ind Med 2000; 38:295–9.

38. Tsuda T, Mino Y, Babazono A, et al, A case-control study of lung cancer in relation to silica exposure and silicosis in a rural area in Japan. Ann Epidemiol 2002; 12:288–94.

39. Boffetta P, Burstyn I, Partanen T, et al, Cancer mortality among European asphalt workers: an international epidemiological study, I. Results of the analysis based on job titles. Am J Ind Med 2003; 43:18–27.

40. Steenland K, Stayner L, Silica, asbestos, man-made mineral fibers, and cancer. Cancer Causes Control 1997; 8:491–503.

41. International Agency for Research on Cancer (IARC), Chromium, nickel and welding. IARC Monographs on the evaluation of carcinogenic risk to humans, Volume 49. IARC, Lyon, 1990.

42. Grimsrud TK, Berge SR, Haldorsen T, Andersen A, Exposure to different forms of nickel and risk of lung cancer. Am J Epidemiol 2002; 156:1123–32.

43. Hopenhayn-Rich C, Biggs ML, Smith AH, Lung and kidney cancer mortality associated with arsenic in drinking water in Cordoba, Argentina. Int J Epidemiol 1998; 27:561–9.

44. Bergdahl IA, Järvholm B, Cancer morbidity in Swedish asphalt workers. Am J Ind Med 2003; 43:104–8.

45. Lubin JH, Boice JD, Edling C, et al, Lung cancer in radon-exposed miners and estimation of risk from indoor exposure. J Natl Cancer Inst 1995; 87:817–27.

46. Alavanja MCR, Biologic damage resulting from exposure to tobacco smoke and from radon: implication for preventive interventions. Oncogene 2002; 21:7365–75.

47. Frumkin H, Samet JM, Radon. Environmental carcinogens. CA Cancer J Clin 2001; 51:337–44.

48. Kreienbrock L, Kreuzer M, Gerken M, et al, Case-control study on lung cancer and residential radon in Western Germany. Am J Epidemiol 2001; 153:42–52.

49. Lagarde F, Axelsson G, Damber L, et al, Residential radon and lung cancer among never-smokers in Sweden. Epidemiology 2001; 12:396–404.

50. Barros-Dios JM, Amparo Barreiro M, Ruano-Ravina A, Figueiras A, Exposure to residential

radon and lung cancer in Spain: a population-based case-control study. Am J Epidemiol 2002; 156:548–55.

51. Wang Z, Lubin JH, Wang L, et al, Residential radon and lung cancer risk in a high-exposure area of Gansu Province, China. Am J Epidemiol 2002; 155:554–64.

52. Kreuzer M, Heinrich J, Wolke G, et al, Residential radon and risk of lung cancer in Eastern Germany. Epidemiology 2003; 14:559–68.

53. Reif AE, Heeren T, Consensus on synergism between cigarette smoke and other environmental carcinogens in the causation of lung cancer. Adv Cancer Res 1999; 76:161–86.

54. Erren TC, Jacobsen M, Piekarski C, Synergy between asbestos and smoking on lung cancer risk. Epidemiology 1999; 10:405–11.

55. Lee PN, Relation between exposure to asbestos and smoking jointly and the risk of lung cancer. Occup Environ Med 2001; 58:145–53.

56. Gustavsoon P, Nyberg F, Pershagen G, et al, Low-dose exposure to asbestos and lung cancer: dose–response relations and interaction with smoking in a population-based case-referent study in Stockholm, Sweden. Am J Epidemiol 2002; 155:1016–22.

57. Liddell FDK, The interaction of asbestos and smoking in lung cancer. Ann Occup Hyg 2001; 45:341–56.

58. Liddell FDK, Joint action of smoking and asbestos exposure on lung cancer. Occup Environ Med 2002; 59:494–5.

59. Pershagen G, Akerblom G, Axelson O, Clavensjo B, Damber L, Residential radon exposure and lung cancer in Sweden. N Engl J Med 1994; 330:159–64.

60. Committee of the Biological Effects of Ionizing Radiation, Health effects on exposure to low levels of radon. BEIR VI. National Academy Press, Washington, 1998.

61. Hertz-Picciotto I, Smith AH, Holtzman D, Lipsett M, Alexeeff G, Synergism between occupational arsenic exposure and smoking in the induction of lung cancer. Epidemiology 1992; 3:23–31.

62. Hertz-Picciotto I, Smith AH, Observations on the dose–response curve for arsenic exposure and lung cancer. Scand J Work Environ Health 1993; 19:217–26.

63. Tsuda T, Babazono A, Yamamoto E, et al, Ingested arsenic and internal cancer: a historical cohort study followed for 33 years. Am J Epidemiol 1995; 141:198–209.

64. Ferreccio C, Gonzales C, Milosavjlevic V, et al, Lung cancer and arsenic concentrations in drinking water in Chile. Epidemiology 2000; 11:673–9.

65. Andersen A, Berge SR, Engeland A, Norseth T, Exposure to nickel compounds and smoking in relation to incidence of lung and nasal cancer among nickel refinery workers. Occup Environ Med 1996; 53:708–13.

66. Grimsrud TK, Berge SR, Martinsen JI, Andersen A, Lung cancer incidence among Norwegian nickel-refinery workers 1953–2000. J Environ Monit 2003; 5:190–7.

67. Rubin H, Synergistic mechanism in carcinogenesis by polycyclic aromatic hydrocarbons and by tobacco smoke: a bio-historical perspective with updates. Carcinogenesis 2001; 22:1903–30.

68. World Cancer Research Fund (WCRF), American Institute for Cancer Research Expert Panel. Food, Nutrition, and the Prevention of Cancer: A Global Perspective. American Institute for Cancer Res., Washington DC, 1997.

69. Smith-Warner SA, Ritz J, Hunter DJ, et al, Dietary fat and risk of lung cancer in a pooled analysis of prospective studies. Cancer Epidemiol Biomarkers Prev 2002; 11:987–92.

70. International Agency for Research on Cancer (IARC), Fruits and vegetables. IARC Handbooks of Cancer Prevention, Volume 8. IARC Press, Lyon, 2003.

71. Feskanich D, Ziegler RG, Michaud DS, et al, Prospective study of fruit and vegetable consumption and risk of lung cancer among men and women. J Natl Cancer Inst 2000; 92:1812–23.

72. Darby S, Whitley E, Doll R, Key T, Silcocks P, Diet, smoking and lung cancer: a case-control

study of 1000 cases and 1500 controls in South-West England. Br J Cancer 2001; 84:728–35.

73. Jansen MCJF, Bueno-de-Mesquita HB, Räsänen L, et al, Cohort analysis of fruit and vegetable consumption and lung cancer mortality in European men. Int J Cancer 2001; 92:913–18.

74. Axelsson G, Rylander R, Diet as risk for lung cancer: a Swedish case-control study. Nutrition and Cancer 2002; 44:145–51.

75. Ruano-Ravina A, Figueiras A, Dosil-Diaz O, Barreiro-Carracedo A, Barros-Dios JM, A population-based case-control study on fruit and vegetable intake and lung cancer: a paradox effect? Nutrition and Cancer 2002; 43:47–51.

76. Bandera EV, Freudenheim JL, Vena JE, Alcohol consumption and lung cancer: a review of the epidemiologic evidence. Cancer Epidemiol Biomarkers Prev 2001; 10:813–21.

77. Wingo PA, Ries LAG, Giovino GA, et al, Annual report to the nation on the status of cancer, 1973–1996, with a special section on lung cancer and tobacco smoking. J Natl Cancer Inst 1999; 91:675–90.

78. Stewart JH IV, Lung carcinoma in African Americans. A review of the current literature. Cancer 2001; 91:2476–82.

79. Harris RE, Zang EA, Anderson JI, Wynder EL, Race and sex differences in lung cancer risk associated with cigarette smoking. Int J Epidemiol 1993; 22:592–9.

80. Krieger N, Quesenberry C Jr, Peng T, et al, Social class, race/ethnicity, and incidence of breast, cervix, colon, lung, and prostate cancer among Asian, black, Hispanic, and white residents of the San Francisco Bay Area, 1988–1992 (United States). Cancer Causes Control 1999; 10:525–37.

81. Gadgeel SM, Severson RK, Kau Y, et al, Impact of race in lung cancer. Analysis of temporal trends from Surveillance, Epidemiology, and End Results database. Chest 2001; 120:55–63.

82. Stellman SD, Chen Y, Muscat JE, et al, Lung cancer risk in white and black Americans. Ann Epidemiol 2003; 13:294–302.

83. Sidney S, Tekawa IS, Friedman GD, Sadler MC, Tashkin DP, Mentholated cigarette use and lung cancer. Arch Intern Med 1995; 155:727–32.

84. Carpenter CL, Jarvik ME, Morgenstern H, McCarthy WJ, London SJ, Mentholated cigarette smoking and lung-cancer risk. Ann Epidemiol 1999; 9:114–20.

85. Brooks DR, Palmer JR, Strom BL, Rosenberg L, Menthol cigarettes and risk of lung cancer. Am J Epidemiol 2003; 158:609–16.

86. Loom AJM van, Goldbohm RA, Brandt PA van den, Lung cancer: is there an association with socioeconomic status in The Netherlands. J Epidemiol Community Health 1995; 49:65–9.

87. Engholm G, Palmgren F, Lynge E, Lung cancer, smoking, and environment: a cohort study of the Danish population. BMJ 1996; 312:1259–63.

88. Martikainen P, Lahelma E, Ripatti S, Albanes D, Virtamo J, Educational differences in lung cancer mortality in male smokers. Int J Epidemiol 2000; 29:264–7.

89. Hart CL, Hole DJ, Gillis CR, et al, Social class differences in lung cancer mortality: risk factor explanations using two Scottish cohort studies. Int J Epidemiol 2001; 30:268–74.

90. Mao Y, Hu J, Ugnat A-M, Semenciw R, Fincham S, Socioeconomic status and lung cancer risk in Canada. Int J Epidemiol 2001; 30:809–17.

91. Paz-Elizur T, Krupsky M, Blumenstein S, et al, DNA repair activity for oxidative damage and risk of lung cancer. J Natl Cancer Inst 2003; 95:1312–19.

92. Caporaso N, DeBaun MR, Rothman N, Lung cancer and CYP2D6 (the debrisoquine polymorphism): Sources of heterogeneity in the proposed association. Pharmacogenetics 1995; 5:S129–34.

93. Fisher RA, Cigarettes, cancer and statistics. Centennial Review 1958; 2:151–66.

94. Hall W, Madden P, Lynskey M, The genetics of tobacco use: methods, findings and policy implications. Tobacco Control 2002; 11:119–24.

95. Gauderman WJ, Morrison JL, Carpenter CL, Thomas DC, Analysis of gene-smoking interaction in lung cancer. Genet Epidemiol 1997; 14:199–214.

96. Husgafvel-Pursiainen K, Boffetta P, Kannio A, et al, p53 mutations and exposure to environmental tobacco smoke in a multicenter study on lung cancer. Cancer Research 2000; 60:2906–11.

97. Seifart C, Seifart U, Plagens A, Wolf M, von Wichert P, Surfactant protein B gene variations enhance susceptibility to squamous cell carcinoma of the lung in German patients. Br J Cancer 2002; 87:212–17.

98. Gilliland FD, Samet JM, Lung cancer. Cancer Surv 1994; 19/20:175–95.

99. Lopez-Abente G, Pollan M, de la Iglesia P, Ruiz M, Characterization of the lung cancer epidemic in the European Union (1970–1990). Cancer Epidemiol Biomarkers Prev 1995; 4:813–20.

100. Brown CC, Kessler LG, Projections of lung cancer mortality in the United States: 1985–2025. J Natl Cancer Inst 1988; 80:43–51.

101. Lee PN, Fry JS, Forey BA, Trends in lung cancer, chronic obstructive lung disease, and emphysema death rates for England and Wales 1941–85 and their relation to trends in cigarette smoking. Thorax 1990; 45:657–65.

102. Muir CS, Fraumeni JF, Doll R, The interpretation of time trends. Cancer Surv 1994; 19/20:519–61.

103. Bray F, Tyczyński JE, Parkin DM, Going up or coming down? The changing phases of the lung cancer epidemic in the 15 European Union countries 1967–1999. Eur J Cancer 2004; 40:96–125.

104. Brennan P, Bray I, Recent trends and future directions for lung cancer mortality in Europe. Br J Cancer 2002; 87:43–8.

105. Devesa SS, Shaw GL, Blot WJ, Changing patterns of lung cancer incidence by histological type. Cancer Epidemiol Biomarkers Prev 1991; 1:29–34.

106. Travis WD, Lubin J, Ries L, Devesa S, United States lung carcinoma incidence trends: declining for most histologic types among males, increasing among females. Cancer 1996; 77:2464–70.

107. Wynder EL, Graham EA, Tobacco smoking as a possible etiologic factor in brochiogenus carcinoma. A study of six hundred and eighty four proved cases. JAMA 1950; 143:328–36.

108. Zheng T, Holford TR, Boyle P, et al, Time trend and the age-period-cohort effect on the incidence of histologic types of lung cancer in Connecticut, 1960–1989. Cancer 1994; 74:1556–67.

109. Janssen-Heijnen ML, Nab HW, van Reek J, et al, Striking changes in smoking behaviour and lung cancer incidence by histological type in south-east Netherlands, 1960–1991. Eur J Cancer 1995; 31A:949–52.

110. Sobue T, Ajiki W, Tsukuma H, et al, Trends of lung cancer incidence by histologic type: a population-based study in Osaka, Japan. Jpn J Cancer Res 1999; 90:6–15.

111. Harkness EF, Brewster DH, Kerr KM, Fergusson RJ, MacFarlane GJ, Changing trends in incidence of lung cancer by histologic type in Scotland. Int J Cancer 2002; 102:179–83.

112. Jedrychowski W, Becher H, Wahrendorf J, Basa-Cierpialek Z, Gomola K, Effect of tobacco smoking on various histological types of lung cancer. J Cancer Res Clin Oncol 1992; 118:276–82.

113. Wynder EL, Muscat JE, The changing epidemiology of smoking and lung cancer histology. Environ Health Perspect 1995; 103(Suppl 8):143–8.

114. Charloux A, Quoix E, Wolkove N, et al, The increasing incidence of lung adenocarcinoma: reality or artefact? A review of the epidemiology of lung adenocarcinoma. Int J Epidemiol 1997; 26:14–23.

115. Sant M, Capocaccia R, Coleman MP, et al, Cancer survival increases in Europe, but international differences remain wide. Eur J Cancer 2001; 37:1659–67.

116. Sant M, Aareleid T, Berrino F, et al, EURO-CARE-3: survival of cancer patients diagnosed 1990–94 – results and commentary. Ann Oncol 2003; 14(Suppl 5):v61–v118.

117. Brenner H, Long-term survival rates of cancer patients achieved by the end of the 20th century: a period analysis. Lancet 2002; 360:1131–5.

118. Jemal A, Murray T, Samuels A, et al, Cancer Statistics, 2003. CA Cancer J Clin 2003; 53:5–26.

119. Berrino F, Capocaccia R, Esteve J, et al (eds) Survival of Cancer Patients in Europe: the EUROCARE-2 Study. IARC Scientific Publication No. 151. IARC, Lyon, 1999.

120. Parkin DM, Moss SM, Lung cancer screening. Improved survival but no reduction in deaths – the role of 'overdiagnosis'. Cancer 2000; 89:2369–76.

2 The molecular epidemiology of lung cancer

David C Christiani, Wei Zhou

Contents Introduction • Tobacco smoking • Tobacco-induced lung carcinogenesis • Genetic aspects of lung cancer risk • Molecular markers of carcinogen dose • Smoking and occupational/environmental exposure interactions • Metabolic gene polymorphisms and variability in lung cancer risk • Conclusions

INTRODUCTION

Lung cancer is one of the most common cancers and has the highest mortality rate among all cancers. Worldwide, lung cancer kills over one million people each year.[1] In the US, lung cancer accounts for 15% of all cancer incidence and approximately 28% of cancer deaths. It was estimated that in 2004 approximately 174 000 new cases of lung cancer would be diagnosed in the US, and an estimated 160 440 men and women would die from the disease.[2]

Lung carcinogenesis in humans requires exposure to environmental agents, including the inhalation of tobacco smoke, radioactive compounds, asbestos, heavy metals and polycyclic aromatic compounds. Overall, about 87% of lung cancer cases are caused by cigarette smoking.[3] Chemical constituents of tobacco smoke have been described,[4] but the specific constituents that most influence carcinogenesis remain poorly understood. Increasing evidence shows that genetic factors are also important determinants of risk. Studies of host–environment interactions can identify groups of individuals who are at greatest risk, and may help in identifying oncogenic pathways. With advances in molecular biology and genetics, it is now possible to assess the role of gene–environment interaction in tobacco-related lung carcinogenesis. Studies that incorporate the use of different biologic markers of susceptibility in human populations are referred to often as molecular epidemiologic studies. The ultimate goal of molecular epidemiology is to fulfill the potential of preventive medicine: prevention and control of diseases.[5] A conceptual approach to the applications of biologic markers to human populations is shown in Figure 2.1.

TOBACCO SMOKING

Tobacco use in the Americas predates the arrival of Columbus, but the social context of its use among Native Americans was largely ceremonial and religious in contrast to the regular and continuous use that characterizes current cigarette smoking.[6] In the United States during 1870, 102 million pounds were used in producing tobacco and snuff and 1.18 million cigars were manufactured, in contrast to 16 million cigarettes. By the turn of the century, some 30 years later, the production of chewing tobacco and snuff had tripled and the production of cigars increased fivefold, whereas the production of cigarettes increased 30-fold. The development of machine-made cigarettes in the 1880s, along with the development of safety matches, provided the technical means for introduction of

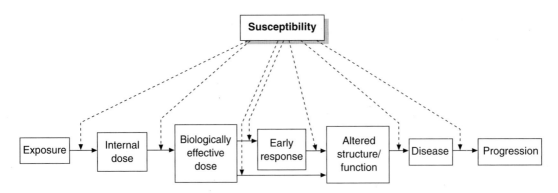

Figure 2.1
Relationship of biomarkers to exposure, susceptibility, and disease. Adapted from[80] with permission.

cigarettes into the main market. Then, introduction of main marketing techniques on a large scale in the first two decades of the century led to a dramatic rise in consumption.[7]

Although mass manufacturing of cigarettes started in the 19th century, the widespread use of tobacco is a relatively recent phenomenon, particularly in low- and middle-income countries which have only taken up this habit in the last 30 years.[8] Globally, about 1.1 billion people (one in three adults) smoke today, of whom approximately 80% live in low- and middle-income countries, and the total number of smokers is expected to reach 1.6 billion by 2025.[9]

The idea that lung cancer might be caused by tobacco was suggested by Rottman in 1898[10] to account for a cluster of cases that he had observed among tobacco workers in Leipzig, and it was mentioned again a decade later in Ader's monograph on the disease.[11] Over the next three decades, several case studies were reported by physicians and surgeons, but solid evidence to support the hypothesis was lacking. In Argentina, Roffo had produced cancers on rabbit skin with tobacco tar as early as 1931,[12] and had shown subsequently that tar contained

benzo[a]pyrene.[13] Little notice was taken of these early epidemiologic findings and it was not until 1950, when five more case-control studies were reported in the UK and the US, that the possibility that cigarette smoking might cause a substantial proportion of all lung cancers became a serious scientific issue. One study started by Wynder, still a medical student, led to the conclusion that 'excessive and prolonged use of tobacco, especially cigarettes, seems to be an important factor in the induction of bronchogenic carcinoma'.[14] The other 1950 study by the British Medical Research Council led to a similar conclusion.[15]

Many of the studies conducted in the subsequent decades have refined further the description of the relationship between tobacco smoking and lung cancer, at the same time reaffirming the causal nature of the association.

TOBACCO-INDUCED LUNG CARCINOGENESIS

Understanding the molecular epidemiology of lung cancer requires appreciation of the process of lung carcinogenesis. Carcinogenesis is a complex process driven by the accumulation of DNA changes within a population of cells, and is typically broken into three stages: initiation, promotion and progression. These heritable genomic alterations, called mutations, result in phenotypic changes that manifest as neoplastic growth. Initiation refers to the fixed genetic change occurring within one cell that confers a growth advantage. This initiated cell then undergoes clonal expansion during the promotion stage. During this period, there may be the further accumulation of mutations and the growth of the emerging cell population becomes unregulated. The final phase of cancer development is termed progression, and induces additional genetic changes that render the tumor aggressive, leading to the metastatic state. Histologic changes, from preneoplasia to carcinoma, accompany the promotion and progression phases.

Lung cancer is a particularly complex disease, inducing mutations after at least 10–20 years.[16] Not all of the genes induced in lung cancer development have been identified, nor is it clear whether mutations must occur in a specific order for carcinoma to develop. It is clear, however, that cancer is a mutation-driven process, and that lung cancer is determined by environmental mutagen exposure. Based on currently available data, the most likely pathway by which tobacco use causes cancer is outlined in Figure 2.2.[17]

Typically, carcinogens have most often been discovered and confirmed as human cancer-causing agents by epidemiologic studies. These data have been the basis of subsequential experimental work that has attempted to understand the mechanism of action of carcinogens, including their metabolism and the DNA structural alteration associated with carcinogen–DNA binding.

Carcinogen metabolism has been well studied and includes a series of experiments to evaluate carcinogens using animal tissues to activate chemical carcinogens to reactive, electron-deficient intermediates.[18] The production of electrophilic metabolic intermediates of polyaromatic compounds that are found in tobacco smoke have been used as a model for investigation of carcinogenic metabolism in humans. Activation of these compounds via multiple forms of the cytochrome P450 enzymes leads to DNA adduct-forming intermediates (e.g., epoxides) that are detoxified further by additional steps in metabolism.[19]

This model of carcinogen metabolism has led to the supposition that understanding the precise balance between activation of procarcinogens and detoxification of reactive intermediates is critical to the estimation of individual

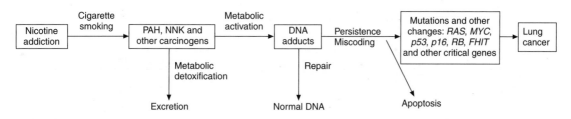

Figure 2.2
Scheme linking nicotine addiction and lung cancer via tobacco smoke carcinogens and their induction of multiple mutations in critical genes. Adapted from[17] with permission.

risk of cancer from exposure to xenobiotic agents. Complicating the process, however, is the fact that these enzyme systems have overlapping substrate specificity and many are inducible by a wide variety of exposures.

In addition to the polycyclic aromatic compounds (PACs), N-nitroso compounds in tobacco smoke have been shown to be potent lung carcinogens. Nitrosamines are direct-acting carcinogens that do not require activation, whereas PAHs are P450 activated to become carcinogens. Tobacco-specific nitrosamines, derived from nicotine and nicotine-like tobacco constituents, are particularly important tobacco carcinogens.[20]

As the genes that code for these metabolic enzymes are cloned, large studies have been undertaken to investigate the role of functional polymorphisms in these genes in lung cancer development (discussed subsequently).

Reactive metabolic intermediates are generated and bind to DNA, and the production of chemically relevant mutations induces processing of the lesion. When the cell encounters these DNA lesions, including covalently bound adducts generated by carcinogen metabolism, they are repaired, generally in cells in which mitosis must occur. Epithelial tissue, such as bronchial epithelium, is actively replicating. The lesions of the DNA therefore are subject to enzymatic DNA repair that occurs with remarkable fidelity before replication. This process of DNA repair is highly complex, but recently has become more amenable to mechanistic study.

Several human clinical conditions, such as xeroderma pigmentosa, Bloom's syndrome and ataxia telangiectasia are well-known examples of disease that arise as a result of DNA repair defects.[21–23] The genes that are responsible for these and other similar diseases are rapidly being cloned and disease-associated genetic alterations are being described.[24,25] Recently,

multiple classes of enzymes that catalyze the repair of specific types of DNA lesions have been discovered. The genetics and biochemistry of other enzymes such as glycosylases, helicases, and exo- and endonucleases are being examined.[26,27] As these systems are described, more information will be given about the nature of mutagenic and carcinogenic lesions, including identification of those that are most difficult to repair, and most associated with error-prone repair, and therefore the most carcinogenic. Polymorphisms of DNA repair genes *OGG1* (8-oxoguanine glycosylase I), *XRCC1* (X-ray repair cross complementing group 1), *XPC* (xeroderma pigmentosum C), *XPD*, *XPF* and *XRCC3* have been identified recently. Studies have suggested that polymorphisms of different DNA repair genes were associated with lower DNA repair capacity and higher risk of lung cancer including gene–smoking interaction associations, although inconsistent results were reported in different studies.[28–33]

If DNA adducts escape cellular repair mechanisms they could persist and may lead to miscoding, resulting in a mutation. Certain mutation could trigger the activation of an oncogene or the deactivation of a tumor suppressor gene, and may allow a cell to begin dividing uncontrollably, potentially resulting in cancer causation.[8]

GENETIC ASPECTS OF LUNG CANCER RISK

Familial aggregation

Familiality of lung cancer has been examined in case-control studies, in genealogy-based searches and in segregation analysis. In establishing familiality, measures of smoking and environmental exposure must be included because these exposures tend to be correlated among family members.[34] Failure to adjust for these possibly correlated environmental exposures severely limits genealogy-based studies.

Familiality of lung cancer has been examined in case-control studies by comparing the recurrence risk (i.e., the probability that a relative is affected by the same cancer) among first-degree relatives in case families to that observed in control families. Tokuhata and Lillienfeld[34] demonstrated excess lung cancer mortality among the relatives of lung cancer patients. In their study, measures of smoking status were obtained for parents and siblings of 270 incident lung cancer patients and 270 age, race, gender and location-matched controls. In men, the association with smoking appeared to be stronger than that which could be attributed to familial factors, but in women the familial association appeared to dominate. The combination of smoking and lung cancer in a relative was synergistic in risk for lung cancer. Smoking relatives of cases had 2–2.5 relative risk for mortality from lung cancer compared with smoking relatives of controls. Although some of the risk attributed to familial aggregation may be related to correlation in the level of smoking, beyond smoking status, non-smoking relatives of lung cancer cases were also at higher risk for lung cancer than non-smoking relatives of controls. In addition, compared with controls, a significant excess of non-cancer respiratory illnesses was observed among case relatives, but this excess was not correlated with smoking status in the relatives.

More recent studies have used a retrospective case-control design to access the association between smoking and familial aggregation of lung cancer. Ooi et al[35] studied first-degree relatives of 336 deceased lung cancer cases and first-degree relatives of 307 of their spouses in Louisiana, an area of high lung cancer incidence. In addition to obtaining quantitative measures of smoking behavior, measures of environmental and occupational exposure were obtained. After adjusting for these exposures, case relatives had a relative risk of 2.4 for lung cancer compared with control relatives. Familial aggregation was more strongly observed among female relatives than among male relatives. Using the same data, Sellers et al[36] reported a relative risk of 1.5 for mortality from any other cancer.

In a smaller study conducted in a geographically and ethnically different region of Louisiana, Sellers et al[37] reported a relative risk of 2.5 for lung cancer among siblings of lung cancer cases compared with siblings of spouse controls.

Shaw et al[38] studied families from south Texas and reported a younger age of onset among probands with relatives who had lung cancer, consistent with Knudson's hypothesis[39] that genetically influenced forms of cancer should have an earlier age-at-onset than sporadic forms.

Sellers et al[40] reported the results of a segregation analysis performed on the Ooi et al data.[35] The results were consistent with a Mendelian segregation of a single codominant locus when a model was fitted that allowed for a genetic component that affects the age of onset of lung cancer. In addition to modeling putative major gene effects, the model simultaneously estimated effects attributed to pack years of cigarette smoking. Using their model, different profiles of genetic and environmental exposure characterize lung cancer cases at various ages. Seventy-one percent of lung cancer cases younger than 50 years of age were at least partially attributable to an underlying genetic susceptibility; by age 70, 72% of lung cancers are attributable to smoking alone.

In a recent population-based family study conducted in metropolitan Detroit, which included 257 non-smoking lung cancer cases and their 2252 relatives, and 277 non-smoking controls and their 2408 relatives, lung cancer in a first-degree relative was associated with a 7.2-fold (95% confidence interval 1.3–39.7) increased risk in the 40- to 59-year-old age group. A positive family history did not increase lung cancer risk among non-smokers 60–84 years of age or their relatives. The results suggest that susceptibility to lung cancer in families of non-smoking cases may be evident only in a subset of relatives of early-onset non-smoking cases.[41]

In another population-based case-control study which included 437 non-smoking lung cancer cases and 437 matched non-smoking population controls, cases were significantly more likely than controls to report having a paternal history of any cancer (odds ratio (OR), 1.67) and aerodigestive tract cancers (OR, 2.78); a maternal history of breast cancer (OR, 2.00); a history of any cancer in brothers (OR, 1.58) and sisters (OR, 1.66); and a nearly significant excess of lung cancer (OR, 4.14; $P = 0.07$), aerodigestive tract cancer (OR, 3.50; $P = 0.06$), and breast cancer (OR, 2.07; $P = 0.053$) in sisters. These results support the hypothesis of a genetic susceptibility to various cancers in families with lung cancer in non-smokers.[42]

MOLECULAR MARKERS OF CARCINOGEN DOSE

Individual variability in carcinogen metabolism and DNA repair may explain differential susceptibility to lung cancer. In recent years, molecular techniques have been applied in epidemiologic studies of cancer. These biologic markers have been used in the following topic areas: determination of internal and biologically effective doses of carcinogen, detection of early pathobiologic effects, especially mutations and somatic cytogenetic alterations, and assessment of variations in individual susceptibility to carcinogens, mainly via metabolic and DNA repair polymorphisms.

Among the 3500 chemicals that have been identified in tobacco smoke, a large number are biologically active compounds. The most important families of carcinogens are PACs, aromatic amines, nitroso compounds, volatile organic compounds (e.g., benzene, formaldehyde), and radioactive elements such as polonium-210. Chemical compounds derived from tobacco smoke have been measured in biological specimens of smokers and non-smokers. DNA adducts, covalently bonded carcinogen–DNA compounds, are formed when chemical carcinogens react with DNA. Several methods of detecting adducts in lung and surrogate tissue, including a sensitive ^{32}P-post-labeling procedure for PACs, have been described. Among the classes of pulmonary carcinogen known as PACs, benzo-[a]-pyrene forms DNA adducts in the lung that are associated with smoking. Recent research indicates that surrogate tissue (blood mononuclear cells) adducts are correlated with lung adducts in cancer patients.[43] Such validation of surrogate markers will permit accurate assessment of interventions such as smoking cessation, chemo-prevention, and elimination of passive-smoking exposure by examining PAC–DNA adducts in the peripheral blood mononuclear cells of relevant populations. Additionally, surrogate tissue (blood) adducts will permit epidemiologic study of large populations exposed to PACs in air pollution or environmental tobacco smoke.

Although the presence of PAC–DNA adducts has not been definitely associated with lung cancer, these adducts appear to be important in the pathway leading to cancer,[44] and interventions aimed at reducing their presence in high-risk individuals are on the horizon. Focusing on 'upstream' markers of dose and early biological effect is particularly important in the prevention of lung cancer, a condition for which there is no effective early detection marker and for which treatment is an ineffective means of control.

SMOKING AND OCCUPATIONAL/ENVIRONMENTAL EXPOSURE INTERACTIONS

There are a number of known occupational/environmental carcinogens, including asbestos, arsenic, coal gas, chromates, nickel and silica.[45] Some have been shown to interact with tobacco smoking in a way that increases the risk of lung cancer multiplicatively. In other words, the risk of lung cancer, when both the occupational exposure and tobacco use are combined, is the product of their individual risk contributions. The best-described example of such synergism is asbestos.[46] Ionizing radiation from inhalation of radon progeny has also been described to act synergistically with smoking, but the data are somewhat conflicting. The overall conclusion from the available evidence appears to be that radon and smoking act more than additively, but less than multiplicatively. In the US large-scale residential radon case-control studies performed in New Jersey, Iowa and Missouri showed that after cigarette smoking, prolonged residential radon exposure is the second leading cause of lung cancer in the general population.[47] Besides the above-mentioned carcinogens, dietary factors including carotenoid, vitamins, fruit, vegetables and meat have also been proposed as potential risk modulators of lung cancer, with contradictory effect across studies.[48–54]

METABOLIC GENE POLYMORPHISMS AND VARIABILITY IN LUNG CANCER RISK

Genetic susceptibility to lung cancer has been examined in many epidemiologic studies that incorporate molecular markers of carcinogen metabolism. Metabolic polymorphisms, leading to different ability to metabolize carcinogens either through activation or detoxification stages, appear to be an important set of genetically influenced traits associated with variability in the risk of lung cancer. Both phase I and phase II metabolizing enzymes may be under the control of polymorphic genes (Figure 2.3, Table 2.1).

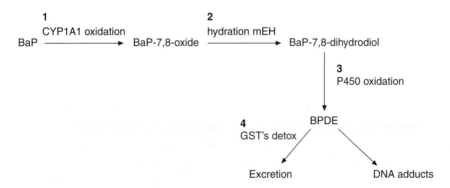

Figure 2.3
Metabolism of benzo[a]pyrene.

Table 2.1 Polymorphic human enzymes and substrates

Polymorphic human enzyme system	Typical substrate	Carcinogens or substrate
Phase I function		
CYP1A1	Benzo-[a]-pyrene	PAHs
CYP3A5	Paclitaxel, docetaxel	Taxanes
NQO1	Diaziquone	Quinoids
MnSOD	O_2^- (oxygen radical)	Superoxides
GPX1	Hydrogen peroxide	Oxygen species
Phase II function		
GST family (e.g. GST-mu, GST-pi, GST-theta)	Epoxide metabolites Cisplatin, carboplatin	Areneoxides Platinum compounds
Dual phase functions		
mEH	Benzo-[a]-pyrene epoxides	PAHs
NAT2	Sulfamethazine	Arylamines

CYP, cytochrome P450; PACs, polycyclic aromatic compounds; NQO1, NAD(P)H:quinone oxidoreductase-1; MnSOD, manganese superoxide dismutase; GPX1, glutathione peroxidase 1; GST, glutathione transferase; mEH, microsomal epoxide hydrolase; NAT2, N-acetyltransferase-2.

Discussion regarding a representative number of candidate gene polymorphisms follows.

Both PACs and nitrosamines, important tobacco carcinogens, require metabolic activation by cytochrome P450 enzyme to exert their genotoxic effects. CYP1A1 and CYP2E1 are important for the activation of PAHs and nitrosamines, and GSTmu plays a major role in the detoxification of PAC-activated intermediates.[55–57] Some other enzymes such as microsomal epoxide hydrolase (mEH) and N-acetylation 2 (NAT2) play dual roles in the activation and detoxification for different substrates.[58–60] These enzymes exhibit wide interindividual variability in their activity. Genetic polymorphisms thought to be linked to functional changes in these enzymes have been associated with lung cancer, but with great inconsistency across studies.[56,57,61–70]

Activation of PACs and arylamines by cytochrome P450s (i.e., CYP1A1) leads to the formation of reactive chemical species that can bind covalently to DNA to form carcinogen–DNA adducts.[55,56] PAC such as benzo[a]pyrene is first oxidized via *CYP1A1* (the structural gene for P4501A1), resulting in the formation of an arene oxide. This metabolite can be activated further to form a dihydrodiol by the action of an epoxide hydratase.[58] Dihydrodiol can then be metabolized across the olefinic double bond by both cytochrome P450 (CYP3A4) and other oxidation systems,[71] thereby forming a diol-epoxide. Diol-epoxides are unstable and rearrange to form carbonations, which are highly reactive. For example, benzo[a]pyrene-7,8-diol-9,10-epoxide forms covalent bonds primarily with the exocyclic amino group of guanosine. This reaction has been shown responsible for activating mutations in the Harvey *ras* (*HRAS-1*) proto-oncogene in several experimental systems.[72,73]

Alternate (and competing) routes of metabolism may lead to inactivation of carcinogens (e.g., PACs), although the formation of conjugates (glutathiones, glucuronides, and sulfate esters) or phenols and tetrahydrotetrol, which facilitate excretion. The balance between metabolic activation and metabolic detoxification, as well as the efficiency of DNA repair pathways, may define cancer risk in an individual exposed to PACs. A positive association between development of lung cancer and the mutant homozygous genotype of *CYP1A1 Msp I* or *CYP1A1 Ile-Val* polymorphism has been reported in several Japanese populations but such an association has not been observed in either Caucasians nor American Africans.[54,55,56,69] On the detoxification side, individuals with the homozygous trait for *GSTM1* (i.e., deletion-no GSTmu product) are at 1.2–1.6-fold increased risk in different populations.[57,67–69] Inconsistent results have been reported on the associations between the polymorphisms of *mEH*, *NQO1* (NAD(P)H:quinone oxidoreductase-1), myeloperoxidase, *NAT2*, *p53* and *GSTP1* and the risk of lung cancer,[62–66,74–79] with gene–gene and gene–smoking interaction associations suggested in some studies.[74,75] Because the current and ex-smoking populations in the United States are large, their traits may be responsible for a considerable, attributable fraction of lung cancer.

These molecular epidemiologic investigations of metabolic gene polymorphisms in lung cancer may lead to new methods of disease control in former smokers who remain at very high risk of diseases. For example, antioxidant chemoprevention may be a reasonable, second-level prevention strategy in ex-smokers with high-risk polymorphisms.

CONCLUSIONS

Epidemiologic research has provided enough information to prevent 85–90% of lung cancer in the world, if societies are prepared to act on the knowledge obtained thus far. In addition, tobacco-induced lung cancer is an excellent model of an environmentally induced cancer, and represents a research opportunity to examine gene–environment interactions.

ACKNOWLEDGMENTS

Supported by NIH grants CA74386, CA92824, ES/CA 06409 and ES00002.

REFERENCES

1. World Cancer Research Fund/American Institute for Cancer Research, Food, nutrition and the prevention of cancer: a global perspective. Washington, DC, American Institute for Cancer Research, p. 37, 1997.
2. American Cancer Society, http://www.cancer.org/docroot/home/index.asp.
3. American Cancer Society, Tobacco use. In: American Cancer Society (ed) Cancer Facts & Figures. Atlanta, GA, American Cancer Society, pp. 29–32, 2001.
4. US Department of Health and Human Services, The health consequences of smoking: 25 years of progress. Washington, DC, US Department of Health and Human Services, Public Health Service, Centers for Disease Control, Office of Smoking and Health. DHHS Publication No. (CDC) 89–8411, 1989.
5. Christiani DC, Utilization of biomarker data for clinical and environmental intervention. Environ Health Perspect 1996; 104 (suppl 5):921–5.
6. US Department of Health and Human Services, Smoking and Health in the Americas. Washington, DC, US Department of Health and Human

Services, Public Health Service, Centers for Disease Control, Office of Smoking and Health. DHHS Publication No. (CDC) 92–8419, 1992.

7. Burrough B, Helyar J, Barbarians at the Gate: The Fall of RJR Nabisco. New York, Harper and Row, 1990.

8. Kuper H, Adami HO, Boffetta P, Tobacco use, cancer causation and public health impact. J Intern Med 2002; 251:455–66.

9. Chaloupka FJ, Development in Practice. Curbing the Epidemic: Governments and the Economics of Tobacco Control. Washington, DC, The World Bank, 1999.

10. Rottman H, Uber primare Lungencarcinoma. Inaugural dissertation. Universitat Wurzburg, 1898.

11. Adler I, Primary malignant growths of the lung and bronchi. London, Longmans Green & Co, 1912.

12. Roffo AH, Der Tabak als Krebserzeugende agens. Dtsch Med Wochnschr 1937; 63:1267–71.

13. Muller FH, Tabakmissbrauch und lungencarcinom 2. Z Krebsforsch 1939; 49:57–85.

14. Wynder EL, Graham EA, Tobacco smoking as a possible etiologic factor in bronchogenic carcinoma. JAMA 1950; 143:329–36.

15. Doll R, Hill AB, Smoking and carcinoma of the lung. Br Med J 1950; 2:739.

16. Harlow E, An introduction to the puzzle. Cold Spring Harb Symp Quant Bio 1994; LIX:709–23.

17. Hecht SS, Tobacco smoke carcinogens and lung cancer. J Natl Cancer Inst 1999; 91:1194–210.

18. Miller CW, Simon K, Aslo A, et al, Mutations in human lung tumors. Cancer Res 1992; 52:1695–8.

19. Law MR, Genetic predisposition to lung cancer. Br J Cancer 1990; 61:195–206.

20. Hoffmann D, Hecht SS, Nicotine-derived N-nitrosamines and tobacco-related cancer: Current status and future directions. Cancer Res 1985; 45:935–44.

21. Gatti RA, Ataxia-telangiectasia. Dermatol Clin 1995; 13:1–6.

22. German J, Bloom's syndrome. Dermatol Clin 1995; 13:7–18.

23. Lambert WC, Kuo HR, Lambert MW, Xeroderma pigmentosum. Dermatol Clin 1995; 13:169–209.

24. Ellis NA, Groden J, Ye TZ, et al, The Bloom's syndrome gene product is homologous to RecQ helicases. Cell 1995; 83:655–66.

25. Savitsky K, Bar-Shira A, Gilad S, et al, A single ataxia telangiectasia gene with a product similar to PI-3 kinase. Science 1995; 268:1749–53.

26. Bohr VA, Phillips DH, Hanawalt PC, Heterogeneous DNA damage and repair in the mammalian genome. Cancer Res 1987; 47:6426–36.

27. Hanawalt PC, Transcription-coupled repair and human disease. Science 1994; 266:1957–8.

28. Spitz MR, Wu X, Wang Y, et al, Modulation of nucleotide excision repair capacity by XPD polymorphisms in lung cancer patients. Cancer Res 2001; 61:1354–7.

29. David-Beabes GL, London SJ, Genetic polymorphism of XRCC1 and lung cancer risk among African-Americans and Caucasians. Lung Cancer 2001; 34:333–9.

30. Zhou W, Liu G, Miller DP, et al, Gene–environment interaction for the ERCC2 polymorphisms and cumulative cigarette smoking exposure in lung cancer. Cancer Res 2002; 62:1377–81.

31. Zhou W, Liu G, Miller DP, et al, Polymorphisms in the DNA repair genes XRCC1 and ERCC2, smoking, and lung cancer risk. Cancer Epidemiol Biomarkers Prev 2003; 12:359–65.

32. Liang G, Xing D, Miao X, et al, Sequence variations in the DNA repair gene XPD and risk of lung cancer in a Chinese population. Int J Cancer 2003; 105:669–73.

33. Ito H, Matsuo K, Hamajima N, et al, Gene–environment interactions between the smoking habit and polymorphisms in the DNA repair genes, APE1 Asp148Glu and XRCC1 Arg399Gln, in Japanese lung cancer risk. Carcinogenesis, 2004 (Epub ahead of print).

34. Tokuhata GK, Lillienfeld AM. Familial aggregation of lung cancer in humans. J Natl Cancer Inst 1963; 30:289–312.

35. Ooi WL, Elston RC, Chen VW, Bailey-Wilson

JE, Rothschild H, Increased familial risk for lung cancer. J Natl Cancer Inst 1986; 76:217–22.

36. Sellers TA, Ooi WL, Elston RC, et al, Increased familial risk for non-lung cancer among relatives of lung cancer patients. Am J Epidemiol 1987; 126:237–46.

37. Sellers TA, Elston RC, Stewart C, Rothschild H, Familial risk of cancer among randomly selected cancer probands. Genet Epidemiol 1988; 5: 381–91.

38. Shaw GL, Falk RT, Pickle LW, Mason TJ, Buffler PA, Lung cancer risk associated with cancer in relatives. J Clin Epidemiol 1991; 44:429–37.

39. Knudson AG Jr, Mutation and cancer: statistical study of retinoblastoma. Proc Natl Acad Sci USA 1971; 68:820–3.

40. Sellers TA, Bailey-Wilson JE, Elston RC, et al, Evidence for mendelian inheritance in the pathogenesis of lung cancer. J Natl Cancer Inst 1990; 82:1272–9.

41. Schwartz AG, Yang P, Swanson GM, Familial risk of lung cancer among nonsmokers and their relatives. Am J Epidemiol 1996; 144:554–62.

42. Mayne ST, Buenconsejo J, Janerich DT, Familial cancer history and lung cancer risk in United States nonsmoking men and women. Cancer Epidemiol Biomarkers Prev 1999; 8:1065–9.

43. Wiencke JK, Kelsey KT, Varkonyi A, et al, Correlation of DNA adducts in blood mononuclear cells with tobacco carcinogen-induced damage in human lung. Cancer Res 1995; 55:4910–14.

44. Wogan GN, Gorelick NJ, Chemical and biochemical dosimetry of exposure to genotoxic chemicals. Environ Health Perspect 1985; 62:5–18.

45. Christiani DC, Occupational lung cancer. In Banks DE, Parker JE (eds) Occupational Lung Diseases. London, Chapman and Hall, 1998.

46. Selikoff IJ, Hammond EC, Seidman H, Mortality experience of insulation workers in the United States and Canada, 1943–1976. Ann NY Acad Sci 1979; 330:91–116.

47. Field RW, A review of residential radon case-control epidemiologic studies performed in the United States. Rev Environ Health 2001; 16(3):151–67.

48. The Alpha Tocopheral Beta Carotene Study Group (ATBCSG), The effect of vitamin E and beta carotene on the incidence of lung cancer and other cancers in male smokers. The Alpha-Tocopherol, Beta Carotene Cancer Prevention Study Group. N Engl J Med 1994; 330: 1029–35.

49. Paisley JA, Beta-carotene and lung cancer: a review of randomized clinical trials. Can J Diet Pract Res 1999; 60:160–5.

50. Breslow RA, Graubard BI, Sinha R, Subar AF, Diet and lung cancer mortality: a 1987 National Health Interview Survey cohort study. Cancer Causes Control 2000; 11:419–31.

51. Ruano-Ravina A, Figueiras A, Barros-Dios JM, Diet and lung cancer: a new approach. Eur J Cancer Prev 2000; 9:395–400.

52. Williams MD, Sandler AB, The epidemiology of lung cancer. Cancer Treat Res 2001; 105:31–52.

53. De Stefani E, Brennan P, Boffetta P, et al, Diet and adenocarcinoma of the lung: a case-control study in Uruguay. Lung Cancer 2002; 35: 43–51.

54. Holick CN, Michaud DS, Stolzenberg-Solomon R, et al, Dietary carotenoids, serum beta-carotene, and retinol and risk of lung cancer in the alpha-tocopherol, beta-carotene cohort study. Am J Epidemiol 2002; 156:536–47.

55. Watanabe M, Polymorphic CYP genes and disease predisposition – what have the studies shown so far? Toxicol Lett 1998; 102–3: 167–71.

56. Bartsch H, Nair U, Risch A, et al, Genetic polymorphism of CYP genes, alone or in combination, as a risk modifier of tobacco-related cancers. Cancer Epidemiol Biomarkers Prev 2000; 9:3–28.

57. Reszka E, Wasowicz W, Significance of genetic polymorphisms in glutathione S-transferase multigene family and lung cancer risk. Int J Occup Med Environ Health 2001; 14:99–113.

58. Gelboin HV, Benzo[α]pyrene metabolism, activation and carcinogenesis: role and regulation of mixed-function oxidases and related enzymes. Physiol Rev 1980; 60:1107–66.

59. Badawi AF, Hirvonen A, Bell DA, Lang NP, Kadlubar FF, Role of aromatic amine acetyltransferases, *NAT1* and *NAT2*, in carcinogen-DNA adduct formation in human urinary bladder. Cancer Res 1995; 55:5230–7.
60. Hein DW, Doll MA, Rustan TD, Ferguson RJ, Metabolic activation of N-hydroxyarylamines and N-hydroxyarylamides by 16 recombinant human NAT2 allozymes: effects of 7 specific *NAT2* nucleic acid substitutions. Cancer Res 1995; 55:3531–6.
61. Raunio H, Husgafvel-Pursiainen K, Anttila S, et al, Diagnosis of polymorphisms in carcinogen-activating and inactivating enzymes and cancer susceptibility – a review. Gene 1995; 159: 113–21.
62. Hengstler JG, Arand M, Herrero ME, Oesch F, Polymorphisms of N-acetyltransferases, glutathione S-transferases, microsomal epoxide hydrolase and sulfotransferases: influence on cancer susceptibility. Recent Results Cancer Res 1998; 154:47–85.
63. Hirvonen A, Polymorphic NATs and cancer predisposition. IARC Sci Publ 1999; 148: 251–70.
64. Xu LL, Wain JC, Miller DP, et al, The NAD(P)H:quinone oxidoreductase 1 gene polymorphism and lung cancer: differential susceptibility based on smoking behavior. Cancer Epidemiol Biomarkers Prev 2001; 10:303–9.
65. Zhou W, Liu G, Thurston SW, et al, Genetic polymorphisms in N-acetyltransferase-2 and microsomal epoxide hydrolase, cumulative cigarette smoking, and lung cancer. Cancer Epidemiol Biomarkers Prev 2002; 11:15–21.
66. Lee WJ, Brennan P, Boffetta P, et al, Microsomal epoxide hydrolase polymorphisms and lung cancer risk: a quantitative review. Biomarkers 2002; 7:230–41.
67. Benhamou S, Lee WJ, Alexandrie AK, et al, Meta- and pooled analyses of the effects of glutathione S-transferase M1 polymorphisms and smoking on lung cancer risk. Carcinogenesis 2002; 23:1343–50.
68. Williams JA, Single nucleotide polymorphisms, metabolic activation and environmental carcinogenesis: why molecular epidemiologists should think about enzyme expression. Carcinogenesis 2001; 22:209–14.
69. Kiyohara C, Otsu A, Shirakawa T, Fukuda S, Hopkin J, Genetic polymorphisms and lung cancer susceptibility: a review. Lung Cancer 2002; 37:241–56.
70. Miller DP, Neuberg D, de Vivo I, et al, Smoking and the risk of lung cancer: susceptibility with GSTP1 polymorphisms. Epidemiology 2003; 14:545–51.
71. Benford DJ, Bridges JW, Xenobiotic metabolism in lung. In Bridges JW, Chasseaud LF (eds) Progress in Drug Metabolism. London, Taylor and Francis, 1986, pp 53–94.
72. Marshall CJ, Vousden KH, Phillips DH, Activation of c-Ha-ras-1 proto-oncogene by in vitro modification with a chemical carcinogen, benzo(a)pyrene diol-epoxide. Nature 1984; 310:586–9.
73. Vousden KH, Bos JL, Marshall CJ, Phillips DH, Mutations activating human c-Ha-ras1 proto-oncogene (HRAS1) induced by chemical carcinogens and depurination. Proc Natl Acad Sci USA 1986; 83:1222–6.
74. Liu G, Miller DP, Zhou W, et al, Differential association of the codon 72 p53 and GSTM1 polymorphisms on histological subtype of non-small cell lung carcinoma. Cancer Res 2001; 61:8718–22.
75. Miller DP, Liu G, De Vivo I, et al, Combinations of the variant genotypes of GSTP1, GSTM1, and p53 are associated with an increased lung cancer risk. Cancer Res 2002; 62:2819–23.
76. Feyler A, Voho A, Bouchardy C, et al, Point: myeloperoxidase −463G→a polymorphism and lung cancer risk. Cancer Epidemiol Biomarkers Prev 2002; 11:1550–4.
77. Xu LL, Liu G, Miller DP, et al, Counterpoint: the myeloperoxidase −463G→A polymorphism does not decrease lung cancer susceptibility in Caucasians. Cancer Epidemiol Biomarkers Prev 2002; 11:1555–9.
78. Wu X, Zhao H, Amos CI, et al, p53 Genotypes

and haplotypes associated with lung cancer susceptibility and ethnicity. J Natl Cancer Inst 2002; 94:681–90.

79. Matakidou A, Eisen T, Houlston RS, TP53 polymorphisms and lung cancer risk: a systematic review and meta-analysis. Mutagenesis 2003; 18:377–85.

80. National Research Council, Biological markers in environmental health research. Environmental Health Perspectives 1987; 77:333–9.

3 Tobacco, lung cancer and tobacco control

David M Burns

Contents Introduction • Epidemiology of tobacco and lung cancer • Smoking behavior • Tobacco control • Summary

INTRODUCTION

Native Americans who greeted Columbus on his arrival in the New World introduced his crew to the use of tobacco, and tobacco use rapidly spread throughout Europe and much of the rest of the world. However, for most of its history tobacco was burned in pipes or cigars and applied to the mucosa in oral or nasal forms.[1] The use of tobacco as cigarettes was largely a development of the 20th century (Figure 3.1). The shift toward tobacco use as cigarettes was associated with the introduction of mass marketing techniques by Camel cigarettes in 1913 and the rapid adoption of these techniques by other cigarette manufacturers.[2]

Cigarettes also use a different blend of tobacco leaf which generates a more acidic smoke than that of pipes and cigars.[3] Nicotine can be easily absorbed across the oral mucosa from the alkaline smoke of pipes and cigars, but the more acidic smoke of a cigarette must be inhaled into the larger absorptive surface of the lungs in order to absorb amounts of nicotine sufficient to satisfy the smoker's addiction. It is this inhalation into the lung, with its concomitant deposition and absorption of the toxic and carcinogenic compounds in the smoke, which

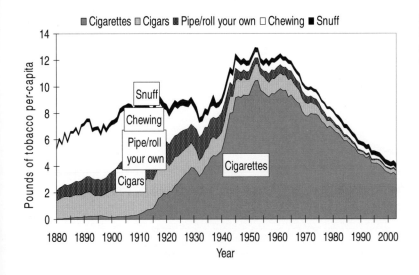

Figure 3.1
Per-capita consumption of different forms of tobacco in the US 1880–2003.

resulted in the epidemic of tobacco-related diseases in the last century.

EPIDEMIOLOGY OF TOBACCO AND LUNG CANCER

Cigarette smoking is the predominant cause of lung cancer, with 80–90% of lung cancers that occur in the US attributable to tobacco use.[4,5] Approximately 15% of continuing smokers, and 25% of heavy smokers, will develop lung cancer over their lifetime.[6] Lung cancer is currently the largest cause of cancer death in the United States and in many developed countries;[5,7]

however, a review of lung cancer published early in the last century concluded that it was one of the rarest of human cancers.[8] During the 1920s Dr Alton Oschner, a leading US thoracic surgeon and founder of the Oschner Clinic in New Orleans, described being called out of his medical school dormitory in the 1920s to witness an autopsy on a lung cancer patient and being told that it was such a rare disease that he might never see another case of it in the rest of his professional life. During his first year as a surgeon he saw four cases of lung cancer and concluded that there must be an epidemic of that disease (Oschner A, personal communication, 1980). Figure 3.2 presents this epidemic

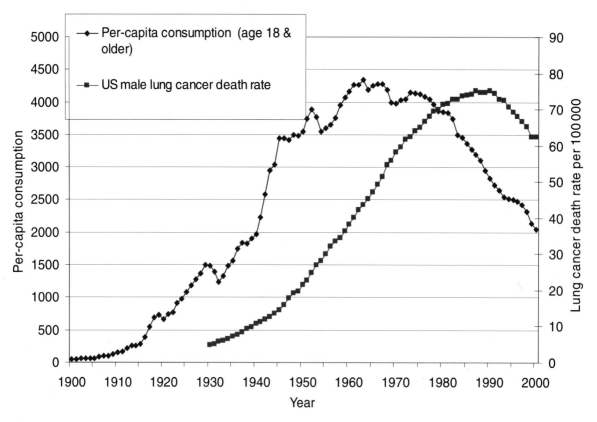

Figure 3.2
Comparison of per-capita consumption and US male lung cancer death rates.

of lung cancer for US males and demonstrates that it tracked closely, with approximately a 20-year lag, the rise in per-capita cigarette consumption in the US.

Quantification of lung cancer risks due to smoking

The role of cigarette smoking in causing lung cancer for a population can be quantified in at least two ways. Relative risk is the ratio of the rate of disease in smokers compared to that in never smokers. Excess risk is the death rate that remains when the death rate in never smokers is subtracted from that of smokers and reflects the absolute amount of disease that results from smoking.

A relative risk of ten for a population of smokers suggests that the smokers in that population have ten times the risk of developing lung cancer compared to the non-smokers. Because relative risks are a ratio of disease frequency in two populations, they are powerfully influenced by the rates of disease in the comparison population. When rates are low in the comparison population, as they are for lung cancer among never smokers particularly at younger ages, modest levels of absolute risk can produce very high relative risks. These high relative risks indicate that the disease in question (lung cancer) occurs almost exclusively in the population of smokers and correspondingly that smoking is the dominant cause of disease in the population. If there are multiple causes of a disease in the population, as is true for heart disease, the relative risk found for smokers will be substantially lower even for the same absolute amount of disease caused by smoking. As a result, relative risk is a useful measure of the proportion of the disease occurring in a population due to the exposure being examined, but it is not a measure of the magnitude of the risk in absolute terms, and therefore it does not quantify well the risk an individual smoker has of dying of lung cancer at any point of time.

Calculation of excess death rates (the death rate in smokers minus the death rate in never smokers) presents a more accurate description of the increased risk produced by smoking for an individual smoker and better quantifies the disease burden produced by smoking in the population[9] since it provides a measure of the absolute rate of disease produced by smoking rather than simply a ratio.

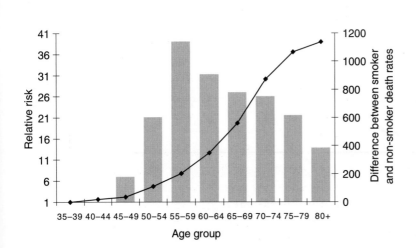

Figure 3.3
White male age-specific lung cancer relative risks (solid bars) and differences in lung cancer mortality rates between smokers and non-smokers (solid line with filled diamonds). Relative risk is the ratio of age-specific death rates between current smokers and never smokers. The difference in lung cancer mortality is the age-specific rate for never smokers subtracted from the same age-specific rate for current smokers.

Figure 3.3 presents the relative risks and excess risks among cigarette smokers compared to never smokers for male deaths due to lung cancer at different age derived from the American Cancer Society Cancer Prevention Study II.[9] Lung cancer relative risks peak at a ratio of 39.0 for ages 55–59 and then decline with increasing age. This relative risk presentation might suggest to the reader that the risk of smoking declines with age, and the decline in relative risk with age has been used to suggest that the benefits of cessation for older smokers are smaller and less worthy of intervention. This distortion of the relationship between smoking behavior and lung cancer risk with increasing age is evident when excess death rates are examined. Excess death rates for smokers by age group are presented as the solid line in Figure 3.3, and this line presents a very different picture of the disease burden produced by smoking at different ages. The high relative risks at younger ages can be seen to be partly due to the low rate among never smokers at those ages, and the absolute increase in death rate produced by smoking increases steadily with

increasing age. Clearly, in contrast to the impression created by examining relative risks, examination of excess mortality rates demonstrates that smoking is a substantial problem for older smokers and that the magnitude of the disease burden produced by smoking increases rather than deceases with age. In contrast to peaking at age 55–59, the absolute excess risk of dying of lung cancer at age 50–59 is only one quarter of that at the oldest ages.

The increase in risk due to cigarette smoking is not uniform across age groups for the major diseases caused by smoking. The age of onset of substantial excess risk is different for the different major tobacco-induced diseases. Figure 3.4 shows age-specific relative risks for smokers for coronary heart disease (CHD), lung cancer, and chronic obstructive pulmonary disease (COPD) for the American Cancer Society CPS II.[9] CHD is the tobacco-related disease which is evident earliest in life. Under the age of 45, CHD is the dominant cause of increased mortality due to cigarette smoking. Lung cancer rates increase steeply after age 50 and excess death from COPD is largely confined to the seventh and

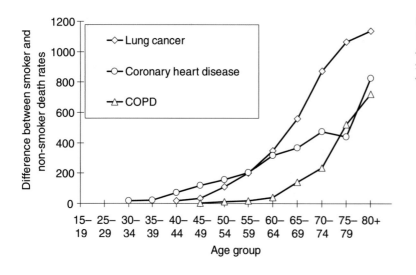

Figure 3.4
Difference between smokers and non-smokers in cause specific mortality rates for white males by age.

eighth decades of life. In late life, excess death from COPD, CHD and lung cancer are roughly similar. Thus, the contribution of cigarette smoking to the disease burden is a function of the age range of the population examined as well as the smoking behaviors of the population.

Exposure response relationships of cigarette smoking and lung cancer

The risk of developing lung cancer increases with increasing intensity of smoking, with increasing duration of smoking and with the age of the smoker.[10,11]

There is a roughly proportional increase in the lung cancer relative risks with increasing number of cigarettes smoked per day for current cigarette smokers.[11-14] The relative risks also increase progressively with increasing duration of smoking as seen in Figure 3.5 for the American Cancer Society Cancer Prevention Study I data.[14] By the time a smoker has been smoking for 55–60 years, a duration reached at age 70–75 years for the average smoker who begins smoking at age 15, the risk is 17 times higher than that for never smokers.

Duration of smoking is the most powerful predictor of lung cancer risk.[10,15] However, once the duration of smoking is fixed, chronological age and age of initiation become co-linear, that is when one specifies the age of a current smoker of a given duration one also specifies the age at which that smoker started smoking. This co-linearity makes it difficult to define the independent contributions of age of initiation and chronological age for lung cancer risk. Starting to smoke at an earlier age clearly increases the risk of smoking at any given age due to the effect on increased duration; however, once duration is specified, the risk of smoking for a given duration is greater if that duration occurs later in life than if it occurs earlier in life. It remains unclear whether this effect is due to the relatively lower number of cigarettes smoked per day as the smoking behavior is initiated, the smaller number of cells at risk within a developing lung,[16] an increased vulnerability to carcinogenesis with advancing age,[10] or some other factor.

With cessation of cigarette smoking, both the absolute and relative risks of developing lung cancer decline compared to continuing smokers, but the decline is slow, requiring about 10 years for the excess disease risk to decline by more than one half.[17] The risk of developing lung cancer among former cigarette

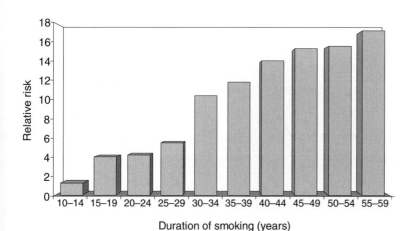

Figure 3.5
Relative risk of lung cancer with increasing duration of smoking.

smokers never returns to that of never smokers, however, and there is a twofold increased lung cancer risk even among long-term former smokers.[18] While the risk of developing lung cancer following cessation declines in comparison to a smoker's other choice (continuing to smoke), the actual death rate from lung cancer does not decline following cessation.[19] Figure 3.6 presents these relationships. The risk for a continuing smoker of 40+ cigarettes per day in the figure continues to increase with advancing age and duration of smoking. If that smoker quits at age 50, lung cancer risk (both relative risk and excess risk) is lower than that for the continuing smoker within a few years of quitting; however the actual lung cancer death rate for those smokers remains relatively constant following cessation and does not decline with advancing duration of cessation and age. This leaves the former smoker with a continuing excess risk of developing lung cancer due to smoking, and the age-specific lung cancer death rate does not decline to that of the never smoker.

The ability to alter lung cancer rates through tobacco control programs that promote cessation has recently become evident in California where the rate of decline in male lung cancer rates has exceeded that of the rest of the US and where female lung cancer rates are declining in contrast to their continued increase in the rest of the country.[20] These changes are attributable to changes in smoking behavior in California over the past decades and a substantial part of the excess decline in smoking behavior can be attributed to the tobacco control efforts in California funded by a portion of the Proposition 99 increase in cigarette taxes.

Pipes and cigars

Smoking pipes and cigars results in oral and laryngeal cancer risks that are similar to those of cigarette smokers, but the risks of developing lung cancer are much lower for pipe and cigar smokers.[3] This difference is likely a result of differences in exposure to these structures secondary to a difference in the extent of inhalation with use of these different forms of tobacco. The more alkaline smoke generated by burning pipe and cigar tobacco allows nicotine to be easily absorbed across the oral mucosa, and smokers who have only used these products tend not to

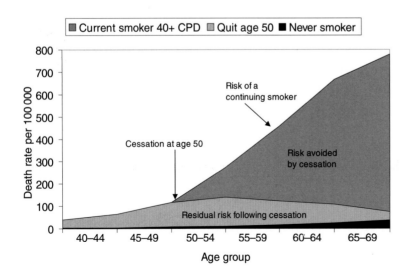

Figure 3.6
Lung cancer mortality rates for smokers of 40+ CPD, never smokers and smokers who quit at age 50.

inhale smoke into the lung. The more acidic smoke from cigarette tobacco protonates the nicotine making oral absorption more difficult. Cigarette smoke must then be inhaled into the larger absorptive surface of the lung to facilitate the absorption of nicotine. Unfortunately cigarette smokers who switch to smoking cigars are likely to continue inhaling, negating any potential benefit of switching.[3]

Low-tar cigarettes

The type of cigarette smoked has transformed over the last half century largely due to the introduction and marketing of filtered and low-tar cigarettes. There has been a 60% fall in the sales weighted average tar values for US cigarettes over the last 50 years and a transition from less than 5% of cigarettes being filtered to the current level of over 97%.[21] This transition was supported by statements from public health agencies based on the expectation that lower yield cigarettes might reduce the disease risks caused by smoking by reducing exposure to cigarette tar. Epidemiological studies appeared to support a reduction in lung cancer, but not other tobacco-related disease risks among smokers who chose to use filtered cigarettes or cigarettes with lower machine-measured tar and nicotine values. However, smokers compensate for any reduction in nicotine delivery by increasing the intensity of smoking or the number of cigarettes smoked, and compensation prevents low-yield cigarette designs from altering the amount of tar actually delivered to smokers. The epidemiological studies were unable to adequately control for these compensatory smoking behaviors and for differences between the smokers who chose to use low-yield cigarettes. They therefore identified a difference in risk due to the difference between the populations of smokers who used the different products rather than due to a difference in cigarette smoked.

There is now a scientific consensus that all of the changes in cigarettes over the last 50 years have not resulted in a meaningful benefit to public health and that smokers should not expect a reduction in disease risks from cigarettes with lower machine-measured tar and nicotine yields.

Cigarettes are designed with an elasticity of yield so they can be made to yield whatever dose of nicotine the smoker desires simply by changing the way the cigarette is smoked. This elasticity of delivery is enhanced by placing holes in the filters in locations where they can be blocked by the fingers or lips of the smoker. These design changes resulted in cigarettes that could be marketed as lower yield but which delivered a full dose of nicotine, and risk, to smokers. Machine-measured tar and nicotine yields using the FTC method do not estimate exposure of smokers to tar or nicotine from a given cigarette, and comparisons of machine-measured yields between brands are likely to mislead the smoker about the exposure they will receive when they switch brands. Current medical recommendations for smokers interested in reducing their risks are to quit smoking completely, and medical and public health authorities do not recommend switching to lower-yield brands as a means of reducing risk.

SMOKING BEHAVIOR

The natural history of cigarette smoking in developed countries reveals a consistent pattern across gender and ethnic groups. This natural history is presented in Figure 3.7. Young teens and pre-teens experiment with cigarette smoking often by sneaking cigarettes from parents or older siblings or by being provided cigarettes by their peers. They then may become

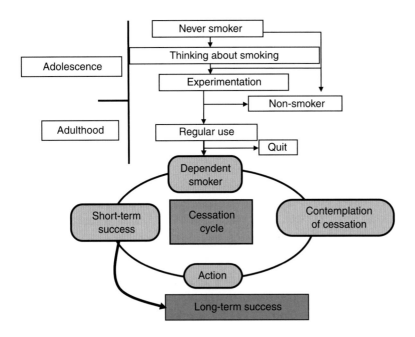

Figure 3.7
Smoking initiation and cessation.

episodic smokers largely for the psychological and sociologic utility of smoking which allows them to interact with their peer group and to superimpose on their own inadequate self image the 'super-adequate' image promoted by tobacco advertising.

Lower economic status and having a parent or older sibling who smoke are important predictors of adolescent smoking.[22] Educational aspirations and school performance have also long been established as strong correlates of cigarette smoking,[23,24] and adolescents who report three or more friends who smoke have a smoking prevalence approximately ten times that of adolescents who report no friends who smoke. However, tobacco advertising and promotional activities are also important in the smoking initiation process, and it is likely that they play a causal role. Tobacco advertisements may be particularly attractive to adolescents who identify with the image offered by the images in the ads. These are the youth who are likely to retain tobacco promotional items,

while those whose identity needs are met in other ways would likely lose, discard or forget about them. Owning the items offers the opportunity to 'try on the image of a smoker',[25] and doing so is likely part of a longer-term process of accepting the image and eventually the smoking behavior that goes with it.

As adolescents find a greater utility of smoking for adjusting their perception of their own internal and external sense of wellbeing, they smoke more frequently. With a greater frequency of smoking, the adolescent transitions from an episodic smoker largely seeking the image enhancement of smoking to a dependent smoker addicted to nicotine and having great difficulty going for extended periods without smoking.

Initiation of smoking is largely complete by young adulthood, and after age 30, the predominant smoking behavioral change is cessation. This life experience is presented in Figure 3.8 which presents the ever smoking and current smoking prevalence of US white males born

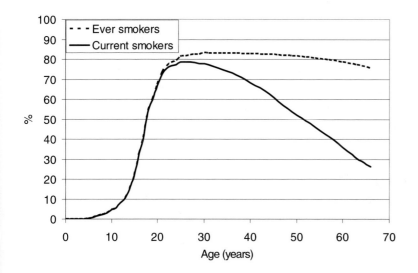

Figure 3.8
Prevalence of current and ever smoking by age among US white males born 1920–24.

between 1920 and 1924 as they age. The two curves superimpose early in adolescence and cessation begins to create a difference between the ever and current smoking prevalence lines in late adolescence and early adulthood. Initiation is complete by age 25–30, but cessation continues to reduce current smoking prevalence for the rest of adulthood. The ever smoking prevalence declines at older ages due to the higher mortality of smokers compared to never smokers which leads to the surviving population having a higher fraction of never smokers as the smokers more rapidly die off.

Cessation of smoking during adulthood is a dynamic process involving a large fraction of the smoking population. In any given year one third to one half of current smokers make a serious attempt to quit smoking, but only 2–5% of them are successful in achieving long-term abstinence. Cessation is therefore best viewed as a cycle where large numbers of smokers are interested in quitting and are attempting to stop smoking, with a few being successful on each trip around the cycle. This concept is presented in Figure 3.7 and it divides the population of smokers into those not thinking about quitting,

those contemplating cessation, those taking action and those recent quitters who are at high risk of relapse. This concept envisions smokers moving, or being moved by tobacco control intervention, from one stage to another with the goal of continuing to cycle them through the process of cessation until they achieve long-term abstinence. Understanding the dynamic nature of the cessation process facilitates appropriate intervention by health care practitioners and tobacco control programs. The goal is to create motion within a population of smokers through persistent and inescapable messages to quit with provision of support for their cessation efforts.

Trends in initiation over time in the US
Adolescent smoking prevalence peaked in the US during the 1940s for males and during the early 1970s for females.[22] Among males there has been a substantial decline in smoking prevalence from that peak; however, among female adolescents, the decline has been less dramatic. Smoking initiation rates among males and females are now similar for both genders. The fall in adolescent initiation over time has been

greatest among older adolescents and young adults, with initiation rates among 12–14-year-old adolescents changing much less.[22] Both genders also demonstrated an increase in prevalence during the mid 1990s before once again rapidly declining at the end of the 1990s and the start of the current century.[26] This increase in initiation demonstrates that gains in preventing smoking initiation are not permanent. The increased adolescent initiation observed in the mid 1990s is felt to be the result of shifts in cigarette marketing strategies particularly sponsorships of events and promotional items (hats, tee-shirts, etc.).

There were small differences in smoking prevalence rates among whites, Hispanics, and African-American 12th grade adolescents in 1976.[26] However, during a period of general decline in use (1977–81) smoking prevalence among African-American and Hispanic 12th grade students declined more than among whites. Thereafter, cigarette smoking prevalence among Hispanic adolescents remained stable, but at lower levels than whites. Smoking prevalence among African-American students continued to decline steadily from 1981–92, opening a very large differential with white smoking rates, and a sizeable differential with Hispanic rates.

Stages of the tobacco epidemic around the world

Current lung cancer mortality is the result of smoking initiation rates two to seven decades ago and cessation rates five or more years ago. As a result, differences in current smoking prevalence in different countries may not match differences in lung cancer rates; and this pattern has been described as falling into four stages of the tobacco epidemic.[27] The pattern of smoking behavior described above is common in most of the developed countries of the Americas and

northern Europe, and lung cancer rates are falling for males and the increase in rates for females is leveling off in these countries. In the former Eastern Bloc and Soviet countries, smoking prevalence remains high for males with less cessation, and females are either continuing heavy smokers or increasing in prevalence. Lung cancer rates are continuing to rise among both males and females in these countries.

Earlier stages in the tobacco epidemic are reflected by patterns of use in Asia, Latin America and some countries in southern Europe. Smoking is high among males and until recently was low among females. Aggressive marketing of cigarettes to women has led to a relatively recent rapid rise in female smoking prevalence. The net result of this pattern is a high rate of lung cancer in males with a much lower rate of lung cancer among women in comparison to males and in comparison to what one would expect if current female smoking prevalence rates had existed over the past several decades. In these areas an epidemic of lung cancer among women will begin to be evident in the next decades.

The earliest stage in the tobacco epidemic is represented by countries in sub-Saharan Africa where tobacco use was uncommon among both males and females until recently. There rates of lung cancer and other tobacco-related diseases are low due to both the low prevalence of smoking in the past and the low life expectancy of the population. As cigarettes are marketed to these countries and smoking prevalence increases, they will begin down the path of the tobacco-related disease epidemic observed over the last century in the developed world. It is hoped that the recent adoption and entry into force of the international Framework Convention on Tobacco Control may enable these countries, and others around the world, to avoid the tragic experiences of the developed world with tobacco use and its subsequent disease burden.

TOBACCO CONTROL

Tobacco control efforts are predominantly focused on prevention of initiation and promotion of cessation and abstinence on the part of those who have initiated. Other areas, such as harm reduction through introduction or substitution of less hazardous products, are sometimes included as tobacco control strategies but they are beyond the scope of this chapter.

For both prevention and cessation the problem can be viewed from the perspective of the individual as the target of the intervention or with the target being the environment in which the behavior occurs. The goal can be to give an individual the information, tools and personal resources to resist the omnipresent influences to start smoking, continue smoking or relapse back to smoking; or the goal can be to reduce the omnipresent

nature or power of those environmental influences to drive the smoking behavior of the individual. Both of these goals are complementary, and most current tobacco control programs combine both approaches because there is substantial evidence that they reinforce each other in reducing initiation and promoting cessation.[28]

Preventing initiation

The obvious conclusion that the best way to avoid the disease consequences of smoking is to never start smoking, and the near universal agreement that children should not smoke, has made prevention of cigarette smoking a popular and somewhat painless political choice for the focus of tobacco control efforts. Unfortunately, dealing with preventing initiation without simultaneously dealing with adult smoking is often self defeating because much of the cigarette marketing, and of adolescent motivation for starting to smoke, is to model adult behavior.

Figure 3.9 presents the stages of adolescent initiation described in Figure 3.7 with the forces

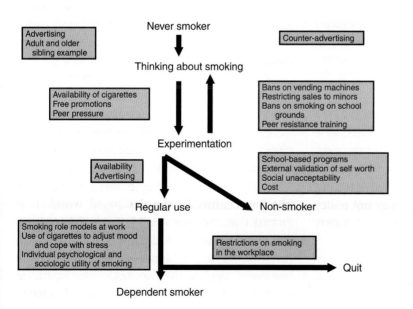

Figure 3.9
Preventing initiation.

and interventions that either promote or help prevent initiation placed in the figure based on the stage where they are most likely to influence smoking initiation. Transitions between the different stages of initiation are driven by different influences and are therefore susceptible to different interventions. At ages 10–14, adolescents transition from the belief that they will never smoke, a near universal response of pre-teens, to a status of thinking about smoking. Issues of autonomy, adolescent rebellion and a desire to mimic adult behavior drive this thinking. Tobacco advertising, with its themes of smokers being secure, confident, sexually and physically attractive, exciting, and dominant over their environment, plays on these issues; and the advertising is most effective on adolescents who have the least objective validation of their self worth and are therefore most in need of superimposing the imagery from the advertising on their own inadequate self image.

Bans on advertisements, restriction of advertising themes or locations and elimination of the distribution of advertising promotional items are interventions intended to interrupt the powerful effect of tobacco advertising and marketing approaches on adolescents. In addition, counter-marketing efforts through paid media campaigns have had some success in preventing younger adolescents from moving toward initiating smoking.[29]

Transition from thinking about smoking to experimentation and episodic use is influenced by the availability of cigarettes, both from peers and family and by purchase, and by association with other adolescents who smoke or who are thought to smoke. There is some evidence that giving away tobacco promotional items as a marketing approach changed the normative expectation of adolescents toward believing that most of their age group peers smoked, and this change in norms played an important role in the increase in adolescent smoking prevalence noticed in the US during the mid 1990s.[22] Restricting adolescent purchase of cigarettes through bans on vending machines and merchant-targeted programs to enforce laws banning underage purchasing of cigarettes are widely supported interventions, and they are effective themes for community mobilization in support of tobacco control efforts. These efforts can alter the frequency with which adolescents are able to purchase cigarettes and will reduce the number of merchants who sell cigarettes to adolescents; however, there is little evidence that they are able to reduce the actual experimentation or occasional use of cigarettes by adolescents.[22] The reason for this apparent discrepancy may be the observation that most younger adolescents get their cigarettes from others rather than by purchasing them and the reality that it only takes a few merchants willing to sell to adolescents in a community to supply the experimentation needs of young smokers. Peer resistance training programs delivered independently or as part of a comprehensive school health curriculum are effective at delaying the uptake of smoking by adolescents, but studies with longer term follow-up of these interventions usually do not demonstrate a difference in the prevalence of smoking during early adulthood.[28]

The transition between experimentation and regular smoking is an important one because many adolescents who experiment do not go on to become regular smokers, suggesting that this transition may be one where interventions could be effective. A key to understanding this transition is recognizing the utility of cigarette smoking for the adolescent smoker. This utility is critically important since the adolescent is still at a stage where addiction is not the powerful determinant of smoking behavior that it becomes later in the smoker's life. Smoking must have a profound value for the adolescent who is beginning to smoke otherwise the initial symptoms of cough and nausea that accompany initial smoking would be more effective barriers to initiation. The symbolic value and image-based adjustment of internal mood create this utility. By smoking, the adolescent is able to signal their adulthood and independence of the constraints of childhood, declare their inclusion in peer groups, and mistakenly feel that they are acting similarly to the majority of their age group peers. Adolescence is characterized by feelings of insecurity and inadequacy about the self and its role in the world. Adolescents do not consciously believe that cigarette smoking makes them like the images in the advertisements, however they are able to transiently superimpose the image from smoking in advertisements and movies on their own inadequate self image, and that superimposition makes them feel better, providing a meaningful utility for the adolescent smoker. Tobacco control programs attempt to disrupt this utility through restrictions on advertising and media counter-marketing that de-normalizes smoking behavior, demonstrates the deceptive and predatory marketing practices of the tobacco companies, and uses 'edgy' themes and styles. It is often the advertisements that are least appealing or even offensive to adults that are the most effective with adolescents.

Cost is arguably the most powerful tobacco control tool. Increases in the cost of cigarettes have repetitively been demonstrated to produce a decline in adult consumption, and the effect on adolescent smoking is even more powerful. Successful tobacco control programs in California and Massachusetts, among other states, have been funded through increases in tobacco taxes that were earmarked for tobacco control programs.

Cost is probably a powerful determinant in preventing both regular use and the transition to dependent use through creating a higher economic barrier to frequent use. Other barriers to regular use are likely to act in the same way. For example, restrictions on smoking in the workplace reduce the frequency of smoking and may act as a barrier to transition from occasional use to dependence. Similarly, restrictions on smoking in other locations and social norms against public smoking may decrease the utility of smoking and reduce frequency of use. As a result, efforts to promote restrictions on smoking and to change social norms about exposing others to smoke are major parts of tobacco control programs interested in either prevention or cessation.

There are few interventions that have been proven to be effective in aiding the dependent adolescent smoker to quit. Pharmacological and counseling interventions proven to be effective with adults have much less efficacy with adolescents. Recent efforts to develop customized, internet based interventions offer some promise, but approaches to adolescent cessation remain an urgent problem awaiting new methods.

Prevention of initiation is an achievable goal and tobacco control efforts in California, Florida, Massachusetts and the national campaign conducted by the American Legacy Foundation are examples of comprehensive, well-designed programs that can alter adolescent initiation. However, these programs are more effective if they are supplemented with programs that also focus on adult smoking behavior, rather than trying to treat adolescent smoking as an isolated problem of childhood.

Promoting cessation

Individual approaches

Many approaches to cessation treat smoking as an individual issue and focus on providing the smoker with the counseling and pharmacological assistance necessary to achieve sustained abstinence. This view of cessation is based on a clinical model where the goal is to strengthen the smoker so that he or she can break their addiction and resist pressures to relapse. Current scientific understanding of how to assist smokers in their cessation attempts recognizes that there is no single approach that works best for all smokers, and therefore cessation assistance should include a menu of different approaches offered through different channels in a continuously available mode over a prolonged time period.[28] Nicotine replacement and other pharmacotherapy, telephone counseling, physician advice, and clinic-based cessation programs are all proven methods of increasing cessation success.[30] Smokers can also be reached by consultations during acute hospitalizations for both tobacco-related diagnoses (i.e., a non-fatal heart attack) and non-tobacco-related conditions (i.e., a broken limb or childbirth). Smokers need to be able to select from a menu of these services and have those services readily available at the time that they are motivated to quit.

Those cessation approaches that are most effective (i.e. a 6–8-week cessation clinic approach) are also the most time intensive; and only a small fraction of smokers are ready to access them at any given point in time. An effective program must include both programs with a range of intensities and a promotional campaign that makes smokers aware of the program and supports a cessation attempt. That program needs to be consistently provided over a prolonged interval since many smokers will have to make multiple attempts before they are ultimately successful. Cessation assistance also needs to be integrated into existing health care delivery systems, public health programs, community organizations and insurance structures.

Chapter 4 deals in detail with these individual approaches and they will not be discussed further here except to note that they are essential components of any comprehensive tobacco control program.

Cessation in the context of screening for lung cancer

A number of studies are currently underway to demonstrate the effectiveness of using CT to screen for lung cancer. One traditional concern about screening for lung cancer has been that smokers may see screening as an alternative to smoking cessation and participation in a screening program may inhibit successful cessation. No existing set of observations supports this concern, and two independent screening programs have demonstrated that high rates of cessation occur among those patients who are screened when they are simultaneously provided with cessation advice and assistance.[31,32] Screening programs represent an opportunity to reach populations of smokers when they are receptive to smoking cessation interventions and screening programs should be viewed as an adjunct, rather than an alternative, to cessation.

Population approaches

Since the 1970s tobacco control strategies have shifted away from a focus on the individual smoker and toward changing the environment within which the smoker smokes.[33] These efforts include changing community norms, increasing the cost of cigarettes, restricting where smoking is allowed and providing societal-based persistent and inescapable messages to quit coupled with support for cessation. The best practices for these strategies, and estimates of program costs for each state, have been published by the US Centers for Disease Control and Prevention.[34] Programs in California and Massachusetts using these approaches have been associated with reductions in various measures of smoking behavior.[35,36]

Differences in cessation that exist between California, Massachusetts and the remaining states support an overall effect of a comprehensive tobacco control program, but it is not possible to completely separate out the individual effects of specific components because the components are not delivered in isolation and their effects may be created by synergistic interactions between program elements. However, it is possible to describe which program elements are effective. The effectiveness of the program components and their relation to the various stages of change in the process of cessation are presented in Figure 3.10.

Changes in the cost of cigarettes are associated with reductions in measures of total and per-capita consumption of cigarettes, with most studies showing a 4% decline in consumption for each 10% increase in price. More limited data are available for cessation, but when differences across states in cost of cigarettes are compared to differences in state-specific rates of cessation, there is a significant association between higher cost and higher rates of cessation.[29]

There has been a dramatic increase in the fraction of the working population protected by

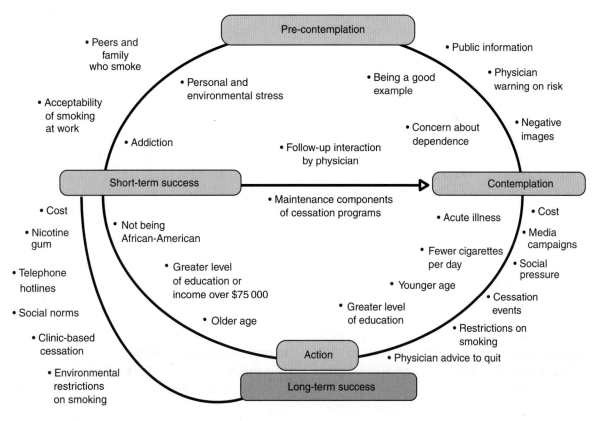

Figure 3.10
The process of cessation.

total bans on smoking in the workplace in the US, increasing from 3% in 1986 to 70% in 1999.[37] Multiple workplace observations have demonstrated that instituting a change in workplace smoking restrictions is accompanied by an increase in cessation attempts and a reduction in number of cigarettes smoked per day.[29] Once restrictions on smoking in the workplace have been successfully implemented, they continue to have an effect. Working in a workplace where smoking is banned is associated with a reduction in the number of cigarettes smoked per day and an increase in the success rate of smokers who are attempting to quit.

The health care system has long been recognized as a logical and potentially productive means of reaching smokers with a cessation message and promoting their successful cessation. Approximately 70% of smokers see a physician each year creating the potential to reach large numbers of smokers with a cessation message. The fraction of patients who report having been advised in the last year by their physician to quit smoking remains too low, but it has been increasing over time and now exceeds 50% of smokers.

One approach to improving the results with physician advice or with pharmacological interventions is to increase the fraction of smokers who receive advice or use cessation assistance. However, the principal limitation for these two interventions is not simply that they are utilized by too few individuals, but rather that the promise of these interventions established in clinical trials is not fulfilled in their real world application. An answer to improving the effectiveness of these interventions may be to try to supplement these interventions and improve their effectiveness by linking them with other existing components of a comprehensive tobacco control program. For example, linking physician advice with telephone hotline coun-

seling, providing information on how to effectively utilize over-the-counter medications at community cessation events, and encouraging health care systems to view cessation as a population-based intervention delivered across all interactions with the system rather than initiated exclusively by physicians.

Comprehensive tobacco control programs commonly use both mass media and self-help materials. These channels share the ability to reach large numbers of individuals at relatively low cost. However, they also share the misconception that they are autonomous interventions where the goals are achieved by delivering the self-help materials to the smoker or having the smoker exposed to the media message. Both of these tobacco control channels simply are methods by which other tobacco control interventions can be facilitated, reinforced, publicized and by which agendas can be set; but in isolation, without integration into a more comprehensive approach to cessation, they have little effect. California and Massachusetts have effectively used media in conjunction with community-based programs and public policy interventions.

Public information about the risks of smoking, negative images about being a smoker and physician warnings about the risk of smoking can all convert a smoker who is not interested in quitting into one who is considering a cessation attempt, and the desire to set a good example for children and concern about being dependent on smoking are reasons smokers give for wanting to quit. An acute illness can often trigger cessation activity. Smokers at younger ages, with higher levels of education and income, and who smoke fewer cigarettes per day are more likely to try to quit.

A variety of environmental influences and interventions have substantial impact on successful cessation. Changes in cost and environmental restrictions on smoking in the workplace have an effect on long-term success. Nicotine replacement therapy and other pharmacological interventions are associated with improved cessation success. Telephone counseling and clinic-based cessation are also effective interventions

Community approaches and interaction across channels

Changing the environment in which the smoker lives and smokes to provide persistent and inescapable messages to quit coupled with support for cessation has been a goal of most comprehensive tobacco control programs,[33] but accomplishing this goal is often a challenge. Community activation approaches, such as the NCI COMMIT trial,[38,39] have yielded modest results and have not impacted heavy smokers. The limited impact may be due to an underestimate of the time required for activation and the decision to intervene at the level of small communities rather than at the state level where more powerful policy options such as tax increases are possible.

Telephone counseling services are provided in California and other states, and there are considerable data supporting their effectiveness.[30,34] Their utility is dependent on the resources provided in terms of the number of smokers that can be reached, but it is even more critically dependent on their links to other community organizations for referrals and to media and community-based promotions for self referral of smokers.

Community and local programmatic activity are the foundation on which comprehensive tobacco control programs are built, but because they are so broad-based in their implementation it is difficult to independently quantify them as interventions, and correspondingly difficult to demonstrate their association with individual or population-based cessation activity and success. However, the fact that we have limited tools to accurately measure interventions at the community level should not be confused with a limited effect for these community-level programs.

If the model of smoking behavior change presented in Figure 3.10 is used as a framework, smokers cycle through stages where they are disinterested in cessation, contemplate quitting, make a quit attempt and are either successful or relapse to smoking. The relapse to smoking may be followed by a period of disinterest in cessation or the smoker may think about making an additional cessation attempt. In this figure, cessation influences are located based on the stage of this process that they are likely to influence, with internal personal characteristics presented inside the circle and external environmental influences presented outside the circle.

Individual components of a comprehensive tobacco control program may affect the process of cessation at different stages. Public information campaigns may get smokers to think about the need to quit, physician advice may trigger a cessation attempt and working in a smoke-free environment may facilitate cessation once the cessation attempt is made. An additional advantage of this formulation is that it facilitates identification of potential synergistic interactions among different program components. For example, physician advice seems to have its largest impact on a smoker making a quit attempt, but is less effective in achieving long-term abstinence; so as an isolated cessation intervention it has little impact on smoking prevalence. But if smokers who are attempting to quit based on physician advice can be linked to interventions which have their effect predominantly on improving long-term success (e.g. telephone counseling, clinic-based cessation assistance or pharmacological treatment), the net effect on long-term cessation is likely to be substantially greater that the sum of the effects of these interventions offered independently.

Media have been used to set the agenda for changing the restrictions on where smoking is allowed, to trigger contemplation of cessation and cessation attempts, to promote referral to telephone counseling cessation services, and as one component of a multilevel campaign to denormalize tobacco use. The role played by the media campaign in cessation is usually to move smokers from the stage of pre-contemplation to contemplation or to trigger a quit attempt. The media is supported in promoting a quit attempt by changing community norms about smoking and other persistent and inescapable messages to quit in the smoker's environment. Cessation success is then facilitated by referral to cessation assistance and other environmental factors including restrictions on smoking in the workplace.

SUMMARY

Cigarette smoking is the largest preventable cause of disease in the US and in most other developed countries. The risk of lung cancer increases with increasing intensity and duration of smoking and with increasing age. Disease risks diminish relative to the continuing smoker once smoking ceases. Approximately one half of current ever smokers have become former smokers, and this cessation has coincided with a 40-year effort to educate and inform smokers about the risks of smoking. Restrictions on where people can smoke, increasing the cost of cigarettes, providing physician advice to quit coupled with cessation

assistance, pharmacological assistance, and telephone hotlines can have substantial effects on cessation. However, many of these interventions are being implemented in the general population in ways that are less effective than they were expected to be based on clinical trials. Increasing the effectiveness of these interventions, and linking multiple interventions to provide synergy, offer great opportunities to improve rates of population-based cessation.

ACKNOWLEDGMENT

Supported in part by a grant from the Flight Attendant Medical Research Institute.

REFERENCES

1. Burns D, Lee L, Shen Z, et al, Cigarette smoking behavior in the United States. In Burns D, Garfinkel L, Samet J (eds) Changes in Cigarette-Related Disease Risks and Their Implication for Prevention and Control. Smoking and Tobacco Control Monograph No. 8. USDHHS, National Institutes of Health, National Cancer Institute, NIH Pub. No. 97-4213, pp. 13–112, 1997.
2. Kluger RL, Ashes to ashes. New York, Alfred A Knopf Publishers, 1996.
3. National Cancer Institute, In: Burns D, Cummings KM, Hoffman D (eds) Cigars: Health Effects and Trends. Smoking and Tobacco Control Monograph No. 9, USDHHS, National Institutes of Health, National Cancer Institute, NIH Pub. No. 98-4302, 1998.
4. US Department of Health and Human Services, Women and Smoking: A Report of the Surgeon General. USDHHS, Public Health Service, Centers for Disease Control and Prevention, National Center for Chronic Disease Prevention

and Health Promotion, Office on Smoking and Health, 2001.

5. US Department of Health and Human Services, The Health Consequences of Tobacco Use: A Report of the Surgeon General. USDHHS, Public Health Service, Centers for Disease Control and Prevention, National Center for Chronic Disease Prevention and Health Promotion, Office on Smoking and Health, 2004.

6. Peto R, Darby S, Deo H, Silcocks P, Whitley E, Doll R, Smoking, smoking cessation, and lung cancer in the UK since 1950: Combination of national statistics with two case-control studies. BMJ 2000; 321(7257):323–9.

7. US Department of Health and Human Services, The health consequences of smoking: Cancer. A report of the surgeon general. US DHHS, Public Health Service, Office of the Assistant Secretary for Health, Office on Smoking and Health, DHHS Pub. No. 82-50179, 1982.

8. Adler I, Primary Malignant Growths of the Lungs and Bronchus. New York, Longmans, Green and Co. Publishers, 1912.

9. Thun M, Myers D, Day-Lally C, et al, Age and the exposure-response relationships between cigarette smoking and premature death in cancer prevention study II. Changes in cigarette-related disease risks and their implications for prevention and control. Smoking and Tobacco Control Monograph 8. USDHHS, National Institutes of Health, National Cancer Institute, NIH Pub. No. 97-4213, pp. 383–476, 1997.

10. Flanders WD, Lally CA, Zhu BP, Henley SJ, Thun MJ, Lung cancer mortality in relation to age, duration of smoking, and daily cigarette consumption: Results from Cancer Prevention Study II. Cancer Res 2003; 63(19):6556–62.

11. Knoke JD, Shanks TG, Vaughn JW, Thun MJ, Burns DM, Lung cancer mortality is related to age in addition to duration and intensity of cigarette smoking: An analysis of CPS-I data. Cancer Epidemiol Biomarkers 2004; Prev 13(6): 949–57.

12. Doll R, Peto R, Boreham J, Sutherland I, Mortality in relation to smoking: 50 years' observations on male British doctors. BMJ 2004; 328(7455): 1519.

13. Doll R, Peto R, Wheatley K, Gray R, Sutherland I, Mortality in relation to smoking: 40 years' observations on male British doctors. BMJ 1994; 309(6959):901–11.

14. Burns D, Shanks T, Choi W, et al, The American Cancer Society Cancer prevention study #1, 12-year follow-up on one million men and women. In Burns D, Garfinkel L, Samet J (eds) Changes in Cigarette-Related Disease Risks and Their Implication for Prevention and Control. Smoking and Tobacco Control Monograph No. 8. USDHHS, National Institutes of Health, National Cancer Institute, NIH Pub. No. 97-4213, pp. 113–304, 1997.

15. Doll R, Peto R, Cigarette smoking and bronchial carcinoma: Dose and time relationships among regular smokers and lifelong non-smokers. J Epidem Comm Health 1978; 32:303–13.

16. Moolgavkar SH, Venzon DJ, Two-event models for carcinogenesis: Incidence curves for childhood and adult tumors. Mathematical Biosci 1979; 47:55–77.

17. US Department of Health and Human Services, The health benefits of smoking cessation. A report of the surgeon general. USDHHS, Public Health Service, Centers for Disease Control, Center for Chronic Disease Prevention and Health Promotion, Office on Smoking and Health, DHHS Pub. No. (CDC) 90-8416, 1990.

18. National Cancer Institute, Changes in cigarette-related disease risks and their implication for prevention and control. In: Burns D, Garfinkel L, Samet J (eds) Changes in Cigarette-Related Disease Risks and Their Implication for Prevention and Control. Smoking and Tobacco Control Monograph No. 8. USDHHS, National Institutes of Health, National Cancer Institute, NIH Pub. No. 97-4213, 1997.

19. Halpern MT, Gillespie BW, Warner KE, Patterns of absolute risk of lung cancer mortality in former smokers. J Natl Cancer Inst 1993; 85(6): 457–64.

20. Cowling DW, Kwong SL, Schlag R, et al, Declines in lung cancer rates – California 1988–1997. MMWR 2000; 49:1066–9.

21. National Cancer Institute, Risks associated with smoking cigarettes with low machine-measured yields of tar and nicotine. Smoking and Tobacco Control Monograph No. 13. USDHHS, National Institutes of Health, National Cancer Institute, NIH Pub. No. 02-5047, 2001.

22. National Cancer Institute, Changing Adolescent Smoking Prevalence: Where It Is and Why, Smoking and Tobacco Control Monograph No. 14. Burns D (ed.) USDHHS, NIH, NCI, NIH Pub. No. 02-5086, 2001b.

23. Bachman JG, O'Malley PM, Johnston J, Youth in Transition. Vol. 6. Adolescence to Adulthood: Change and Stability in the Lives of Young Men. Ann Arbor, MI, Institute for Social Research, 1978.

24. Johnston LD, Drugs and American youth. Ann Arbor, MI, Institute for Social Research, 1973.

25. Feighery E, Borzekowski DLG, Schooler C, Flora J, Seeing, wanting, owning: The relationship between receptivity to tobacco marketing and smoking susceptibility in young people. Tob Contr 1998; 7:123–8.

26. Johnston LD, O'Malley PM, Bachman JG, Schulenberg JE, Monitoring the future national survey results on drug use, 1975–2003. Volume I: Secondary school students. National Institutes of Health, National Cancer Institute, NIH Publication No. 04-5507. National Institute on Drug Abuse 545, 2004.

27. Lopez AD, Collishaw NE, Piha T, A descriptive model of the cigarette epidemic in developed countries. Tob Contr 1994; 3:242–7.

28. US Department of Health and Human Services, Reducing Tobacco Use: A Report of the Surgeon General. Atlanta, Georgia, US Department of Health and Human Services, Public Health Service, Centers for Disease Control and Prevention, National Center for Chronic Disease Prevention and Health Promotion, Office on Smoking and Health, 2000.

29. Bauer UE, Johnson TM, Hopkins RS, Brooks RG, Changes in youth cigarette use and intentions following implementation of a tobacco control program: findings from the Florida Youth Tobacco Survey, 1998–2000. JAMA 2000; 284(6):723–8.

30. US Public Health Service, Treating Tobacco Use and Dependence. Clinical Practice Guideline, Public Health Service, DHHS, 2000.

31. Ostroff JS, Buckshee N, Mancuso CA, Yankelevitz DF, Henschke CI, Smoking cessation following CT screening for early detection of lung cancer. Prev Med 2001; 33(6):613–21.

32. Cox LS, Clark MM, Jett JR, et al, Change in smoking status after spiral chest computed tomography scan screening. Cancer 2003; 98(11):2495–501.

33. National Cancer Institute, Strategies to Control Tobacco Use In the United States: a blueprint for public health action in the 1990s, Smoking and Tobacco Control Monograph No. 1, USDHHS NIH NCI, 1991.

34. Centers for Disease Control and Prevention, Best Practices for Comprehensive Tobacco Control Programs – August 1999. Atlanta, GA, US Department of Health and Human Services, Centers for Disease Control and Prevention, National Center for Chronic Disease Prevention and Health Promotion, Office on Smoking and Health, August 1999.

35. Biener I, Roman AM, 1996 Massachusetts Adult Tobacco Survey: Tobacco Use and Attitudes after Three Years of the Massachusetts Tobacco Control Program. Technical Report and Tables. Boston: Center for Survey Research, University of Massachusetts, 1997.

36. Pierce JP, Gilpin EA, Emery SL, et al, Tobacco Control in California: Who's Winning the War? La Jolla, CA, University of California, San Diego, 1998.

37. Shopland DR, Gerlach KK, Burns DM, Hartman AM, Gibson JT, State-specific trends in smoke-free workplace policy coverage. The Current Population Survey Tobacco Use Supplement, 1993 to 1999. J Occup Environ Med 2001; 43:680–6.

38. COMMIT Research Group, Community Intervention Trial for Smoking Cessation (COMMIT): I. Cohort results from a four-year community intervention. Am J Public Health 1995; 85:183–92.

39. COMMIT Research Group, Community Intervention Trial for Smoking Cessation (COMMIT): II. Changes in adult cigarette smoking prevalence. Am J Public Health 1995; 85:183–200.

4 Clinical approaches to smoking cessation

Patricia L Mabry, Erik M Augustson, Glen D Morgan, Scott J Leischow

Contents Introduction • Etiology • The role of the oncologist • Clinical interventions • Non-pharmacological approaches • Pharmacological approaches • Bupropion hydrochloride (Zyban) • Nicotine replacement therapies (NRTs) • Summary

INTRODUCTION

Prevalence

Smoking patterns and the demographics of smokers vary substantially across countries.[1] However, despite its known risks and significant efforts in North America and many European countries to reduce tobacco use, smoking remains the number one cause of morbidity and mortality in developed countries.[2] In addition, while tobacco use is on the decline in many developed countries, it is on the increase in other parts of the world as less developed countries are becoming more frequent targets of the tobacco companies. The WHO estimates that worldwide 1.3 billion individuals smoke or use other tobacco products,[1] and it is predicted that by 2020 the global burden will exceed nine million deaths annually[3] with seven million of these occurring in economically developing countries.[4] Even without an increase in the number of smokers in less developed countries, the current impact of cigarettes is extensive, accounting for an estimated 4.83 million deaths per year worldwide.[5] In the United States alone, recent estimates blame approximately 440 000 annual deaths on tobacco,[6] while a staggering 800 000 tobacco-attributable deaths per year are estimated in Europe[7,8] and 800 000 more in China.[9]

Tobacco use and cancer

In addition to being a leading risk factor for cardiac and pulmonary disease, smoking is responsible for nearly one-third of all cancers.[10] The clearest example of a smoking-related cancer is lung cancer, with nearly 90% of lung cancers in the United States being caused by smoking.[11] No other cluster of risk factors, including biological and genetic factors, environmental factors, and health behaviors other than smoking, has as strong an association with lung cancer. Lung cancer is currently the number one cause of cancer deaths for both men and women in the United States, Canada and the United Kingdom.[12–14] It is expected that this pattern will be replicated in a wide range of other countries as the global prevalence of smoking increases.[1]

The importance of cessation

Although prevention of smoking initiation is important, smoking cessation is crucial to any efforts to reduce the morbidity and mortality of smoking, as illustrated in Figure 4.1.[15] It has been well demonstrated that stopping smoking significantly reduces the risk of subsequent smoking-related disease. The earlier one stops smoking, the greater the reduction in health risk, but stopping at any age can be beneficial.[6]

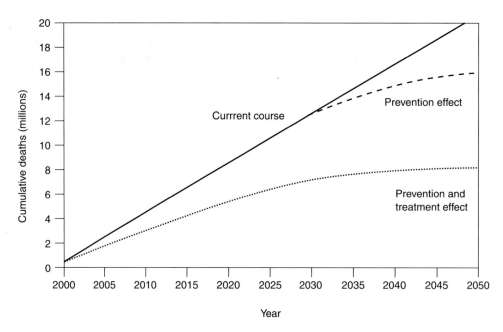

Figure 4.1
Projections of smoking-related mortality based on present trends (current course), compared with projections of effective prevention (prevention effect) and effects of combined prevention and treatment (prevention and treatment effect).
Source: reproduced with permission from Henningfield and Slade, 1998[15].

Some estimates indicate that stopping smoking before middle age decreases the tobacco-attributable risk of lung cancer by 90%,[16] with significant reductions in risk being demonstrated even if one stops smoking well into middle age.

The benefits of quitting are seen even after a diagnosis of cancer. Many smokers and their physicians are under the mistaken belief that quitting smoking at this point is too late. A substantial body of evidence has established a link between continued smoking and a number of negative outcomes in cancer patients, including poorer survival rates, less-effective responses to treatment and higher incidence of secondary tumors.[17] This has been demonstrated to be true for a number of cancers including those clearly related to smoking such as lung and head/neck cancers,[18–22] as well as those not believed to be etiologically associated with smoking such as prostate cancer.[23–27] Moreover, the benefits of quitting smoking may be more pronounced for cancer patients; it has been suggested that continued smoking has detrimental effects on anti-tumor therapy and that quitting smoking is as important as the type of chemotherapy used.[28]

Despite the clear negative outcomes associated with continued smoking, a significant proportion of cancer patients continue to smoke following their diagnosis. Recent studies have reported rates of continued smoking to be 17–45%.[29–35] The true rates of smoking may be underestimated, as many of these studies have relied solely on self-report and have not performed biochemical verification of smoking status.

Of note, stopping smoking may affect the pharmacokinetics of certain medications, and patients with current or a history of depressive disorders may experience an increase in related symptoms. This should be considered when advising medicated patients to quit and such patients should be closely monitored. However, the benefits of quitting far outweigh the known risks and there are no patient populations for which smoking cessation is contraindicated.

ETIOLOGY

It is now widely recognized that a central reason for continuing to smoke in spite of the risk of dire health consequences is physiological dependence to nicotine.[36] Unfortunately, nicotine is one of the most difficult addictive behaviors to break, rivaling cocaine and heroin.[37] Nicotine's addiction potential is largely due to the pharmacokinetic actions that arise when the route of nicotine administration is inhalation, as it is with cigarette smoking. The huge surface area of the alveolar capillary interface permits high nicotine absorption, while high rates of pulmonary capillary blood flow mean rapid onset of drug action. Thus, nicotine enters the brain more rapidly (7–10 seconds after taking a puff[38]) following inhalation of cigarette smoke and in a larger quantity (bolus) than following any other common route of administration, and even faster than by IV administration.[39,40] Rapid onset of drug action, cyclic variations in levels of a drug within the body requiring repeated dosing at regular intervals, and the resulting reinforcing effects are important determinants of addiction potential.[41] Typical patterns of tobacco use behavior match this profile and explain, to a great extent, tobacco use and dependence, even in the face of severe health consequences. This phenomenon is illustrated in Figure 4.2, which shows the hypothetical pharmacokinetic profile of blood nicotine that would be observed in a typical smoker over a 24-hour period.

The most typical feature of nicotine dependence is a distinct withdrawal syndrome following cessation, which includes irritability, frustration, anger, anxiety, difficulty concentrating, restlessness, decreased heart rate and increased appetite.[42] Also within the

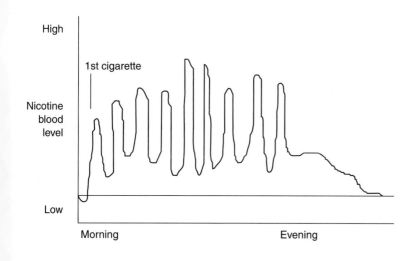

Figure 4.2
Nicotine levels during smoking
Source: reproduced with permission from Tsoh et al., 1997[105].

characterization of dependence are cravings, compulsive use, tolerance and a dose-dependent physiologic response.[43]

Although nicotine dependence is a key factor, a wide range of social, environmental, psychological and physiological factors (see Figure 4.3) can play a large role in the initiation and maintenance of smoking, and in determining how likely it is that someone will attempt to quit and their ability to successfully stay quit.[43–46] For example, psychological determinants of smoking such as personality factors, susceptibility to stress, perceived self efficacy and risk, and depression and other psychiatric co-morbidities have been associated with smoking onset and persistence as well as relapse.[43–45,47] In addition, behavioral and molecular genetics studies have demonstrated that there is a heritable component to the acquisition and persistence of smoking behavior.[48,49] These individual factors do not operate independently, but rather interact with each other.[50] The relative importance of various factors may wax and wane across the smoker's lifetime.[45]

THE ROLE OF THE ONCOLOGIST

Oncologists and their staff can and should play a key role in promoting successful cessation in their patients. First, by nature of their clinical practice, these health care providers are highly likely to encounter smokers in need of assistance with smoking cessation. Second, a diagnosis of cancer presents a unique opportunity to intervene with smokers. These have been referred to as "teachable moments" or times when individuals are highly motivated due to circumstances such as an illness to attempt to change a health behavior.[51] Feelings of personal vulnerability are high, increasing motivation to quit, especially among those with smoking-

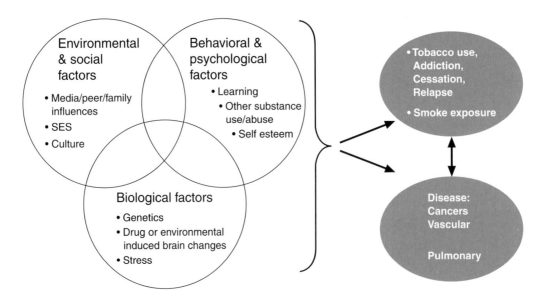

Figure 4.3
Behavioral model of nicotine addiction and tobacco-related disease. Source: reproduced with permission from Morgan et al., 2003.[110]

related diagnoses, such as cancer.[52] In fact, the highest rates of cessation among cancer patients are among head and neck cancer patients.[53]

Intervening with patients during active treatment or hospitalization may be especially effective for several reasons. First, patients are essentially a "captive audience". Moreover, opportunities to smoke in hospital settings are greatly reduced if not eliminated. Perhaps most importantly, smokers are removed from smoking cues present in their home environment, allowing them to experience physiological withdrawal prior to and separate from encounters with the psychosocial factors in their natural environment that maintain their addiction. Abstinence rates as high as 70% have been reported in post-myocardial infarction patients receiving cessation intervention.[54] This compares to the more typical abstinence rates of less than 20% in most smoking treatment contexts. Treatment components that have been proven efficacious for hospitalized and cancer patients are the same as those that have been shown to work with smokers in general[55] and are discussed in detail subsequently.

Generally speaking, oncologists and other medical personnel are highly respected by their patients and are seen as credible, experienced authorities whose advice should be heeded. A number of studies have demonstrated that physicians can in fact have a significant impact on smoking cessation success, even with brief interventions such as merely strongly advising the patient to quit.[56] However, cancer patients who continue to smoke in spite of their diagnosis may be "hard core".[57] Thus, intensive initial interventions that are followed by relapse prevention are advocated, as they are associated with greater long-term abstinence rates.[58]

Given the busy nature of the typical medical practice, most physicians will only have time for brief cessation interventions. Even brief advice from a physician can have substantial impact on both subsequent quit attempts by the patient and long-term success.[59] Table 4.1 contains the US government's '5 As' strategy for helping smokers to quit. The particular method of assistance offered is to some degree dependent on situational factors, such the patient's

Table 4.1 The '5 As' for provider intervention in smoking cessation[59]	
Ask about tobacco use	Identify and document tobacco use status for every patient at every visit
Advise to quit	In a clear, strong, and personalized manner, urge every tobacco user to quit
Assess willingness to make a quit attempt	During the visit, determine whether the tobacco user is willing to make a quit attempt this time
Assist in quit attempt	For the patient willing to make a quit attempt, use counseling and pharmacotherapy to help him or her quit
Arrange follow up	Schedule follow-up contact, preferably within the first week after the quit date

preference and the clinician's prior experience and training.

With any approach, a key is thought to be the patient's readiness to change. These stages are summarized in Table 4.2.[60] Patients who are not yet ready or willing to set a quit date should be offered motivational materials or information tailored to their own health history and personal health risk. For example, a patient with diabetes mellitus or asthma should be counseled regarding the impact smoking has on their present condition as well as the future course of their disease. Similarly, a patient with a strong family history of cancer or heart disease should be made aware that while they cannot change their heritable risk for these diseases, they can reduce their overall risk by quitting smoking.

For patients in the preparation and action stages, formal assistance with cessation should be offered. Patients in the maintenance stage should be reinforced for their continued abstinence and relapse prevention strategies should be employed if they appear at heightened risk of relapse. For example, patients who have quit

successfully should be congratulated and encouraged to stay on track. It can be valuable to discuss potential relapse situations and how to handle them.

CLINICAL INTERVENTIONS

The health benefits of quitting smoking are widely publicized and nearly all smokers in countries with well-developed tobacco control programs are aware of them. Unfortunately, knowledge of health risks has proven insufficient as a strategy in itself to eradicate smoking. To be sure, public health campaigns have been instrumental in cutting prevalence rates from their high in the US in 1965 of 42.4%, to the 23.3% prevalence in 2000,[61,62] and similar successes have been seen. However, quitting smoking is a difficult task for the majority of smokers and most require repeated attempts before successfully maintaining abstinence. National surveys in the US indicate that 70% of adult smokers say that they would like to quit

Table 4.2 Stages of change*	
1. Pre-contemplation	The smoker is not considering cessation and may not acknowledge that smoking is a problem behavior
2. Contemplation	The smoker has not yet made the decision to quit but is thinking about cessation and processes information about the health effects of smoking and ways to quit
3. Preparation/ready for action	The smoker has developed a plan and strategies to help them stop smoking
4. Action	The smoker has been smoke-free for up to 6 months
5. Maintenance	Long-term abstinence from smoking is being established, as the ex-smoker has not smoked in over 6 months

*Relapse can occur during action or maintenance, in which case the smoker may recycle back to any of the previous stages.[60]

smoking, yet only about 6.0% stay abstinent for at least 1 month[63] and only approximately 5.0% of those who quit are able to maintain their abstinence for 3–12 months.[64]

A wide variety of treatments for tobacco dependence have been developed and investigated, and several national and global organizations have issued guidelines or recommendations for treating tobacco dependence.[59,65,66] These clinical practice guidelines are all founded on empirical evidence derived from expert reviews of scientific publications and come to highly similar conclusions, which are summarized in Table 4.3.

Non-pharmacological and pharmacological approaches are reviewed below.

NON-PHARMACOLOGICAL APPROACHES

Behavioral treatments for tobacco dependence range from brief 3-minute advice to quit to multiple sessions of individual or group therapy. These behavioral treatments can be administered by health care professionals and trained non-professionals alike and can be used as stand-alone treatments or in combination with medication. As noted above, it may be more appropriate, given time constraints, for physicians to focus on briefer interventions. More intensive approaches have been developed which require substantial time and professional training. Meta-analyses have revealed that there is a strong dose–response relationship between treatment intensity (frequency and duration of contact) and success at quitting smoking.[59] Moreover, a variety of treatment delivery formats are effective, including face-to-face individual and group counseling, and phone-based counseling. When behavioral treatments are combined, the likelihood that a particular quit attempt will succeed increases. For all treatments, more frequent contact is recommended in the early quit period when risk of relapse is highest.[67,68]

While non-specific counseling can be effective, there are differences in the efficacy of counseling and behavioral treatment approaches. Counseling which focuses on social support and

---

Table 4.3 Clinical practice guidelines for health care providers

- Monitor smoking status of patients
- Offer cessation advice to all smokers
- Assist smokers who are ready to quit:
  - Unless contraindicated, offer approved pharmacotherapy (nicotine replacement and bupropion hydrochloride are considered first-line treatments)
  - Behavioral counseling and social support are important adjuncts to pharmacology
  - There is a strong dose–response relationship between frequency and duration of counseling and outcome (more is better)
- Motivate smokers who are not ready to quit
- Telephone counseling is effective
- Tobacco dependence is a chronic condition with high risk for relapse. Thus, effective treatment often requires repeated intervention

problem solving techniques such as how to manage craving and effectively preparing for a quit date are effective. Other components, which are commonly integrated into comprehensive smoking cessation treatments with unclear effectiveness, include relaxation training, breathing exercises, stress management, cigarette fading and weight management.

There are also a number of more complicated but promising approaches. Although not yet fully explored, there is some support for scheduled reduced smoking in which the smoker is prompted to smoke only at specific times of the day based on set time intervals between cigarettes. These intervals are increased, and the number of cigarettes is decreased, each day, over a period of weeks until smoking is eliminated.[69] Note that this method differs in an important way from cigarette fading, in that the schedule, not the smoker, controls the specific cigarettes to eliminate. Another approach that has proven useful in the substance abuse field that is receiving increasing attention with regard to smoking cessation is contingency management in which the smoker is offered incentives (e.g. cash, vouchers for prizes, lottery tickets) for providing biochemical evidence of quitting smoking. Evidence also supports the use of aversive approaches such as rapid smoking techniques, but these strategies are not well tolerated by patients and as such are not commonly used.

An additional behavioral treatment resource is the use of telephone quitlines in which smokers can call for counseling services. Quitlines are becoming more widely available and in some countries are available through national or regional initiatives. Research has supported the effectiveness of quitlines as a cessation delivery method[70–74] and recent treatment guidelines encourage the promotion of quitlines to enhance the number of individuals who use these services.[75] They are advantageous because they have a wide reach, offer immediate assistance, and provide some degree of anonymity which smokers cannot achieve in the clinician's office.

Acupuncture and hypnosis are among other non-pharmacological methods that have been touted as tools for smoking cessation. However, the scientific evidence supporting them is limited and expert reviews have concluded that there is insufficient evidence at this time to endorse either of these methods.[59]

PHARMACOLOGICAL APPROACHES

Nicotine's short half-life (approximately 2 hours[76,77]) precipitates the onset of withdrawal symptoms if the smoker does not get multiple doses of nicotine throughout the day. This contributes to the difficulty smokers have in breaking their dependence by causing them to experience the discomfort of withdrawal and the reward of smoking to avoid withdrawal several times a day. Heavily dependent smokers may even wake up in the middle of the night to smoke in order to attenuate withdrawal symptoms.

Pharmacological treatments for cessation are typically targeted at reducing symptoms of nicotine withdrawal. In addition, as many smokers use the effects of tobacco to manage mood and affect, some pharmacological treatments are thought to work by performing this same function. Reducing the reinforcing effects of smoking is another way that medications may help smokers quit.

Tobacco dependence treatment medications can be classified as those that contain nicotine and those that do not. Those that contain nicotine are commonly referred to as "nicotine replacement therapies" (NRTs), and include patch, gum, nasal spray, inhalator and lozenge. By far the most widely used non-nicotine medication is bupropion hydrochloride (Zyban®), and it, along with the nicotine replacements, is considered to be a "first-line" pharmacological intervention.[59] In general, no differences in efficacy have been found between products, with bupropion and all NRTs showing 1.5–2-fold increases in quit rates over placebo (see Table 4.4).

Nortriptyline (a tricyclic antidepressant medication) and clonidine (an antihypertensive) also do not contain nicotine and have been demonstrated to be efficacious as treatments for tobacco dependence. However, because they both have significant side-effect profiles, they are considered second-line treatments and are rarely used in practice.[59]

Currently the only widely available pharmaceuticals for smoking cessation are nicotine replacement therapies and bupropion. As such, they are the only ones to be reviewed in any detail in this chapter. Additional products are under development and becoming available that are worth brief mention. These include a nicotine vaccine, a nicotine receptor blocker (varenicline tartrate, Pfizer) and a selective cannabinoid CB_1 receptor antagonist (SR141716, rimonabant, Sanofi Synthelabo). Mecamylamine, an acetylcholine receptor antagonist and nicotine antagonist has been studied as an adjunct to the nicotine patch.[78,79] In addition, several new tobacco products have been advertised as reduced harm products or are suggested for use in situations where smoking is either prohibited or undesirable. These include: tobacco lozenges (marketed as Ariva in the US), reduced nitrosamine cigarettes (e.g., Eclipse), and uncured smokeless tobacco (e.g. Snus available in some Scandinavian countries). The reader is cautioned that these products are not pharmacological tools and have not yet been fully evaluated so they cannot be considered to be "safe".

BUPROPION HYDROCHLORIDE (ZYBAN)

Bupropion hydrochloride was originally used as a non-traditional antidepressant (also marketed under the tradename, Wellbutrin). Moreover, bupropion is well tolerated, has few and mild side effects,[80] and the dosing is more straightforward than for many of the NRT products. Bupropion is now available in the sustained release formula; dosing begins with 150 mg once per day for three days followed by twice daily (300 mg/day) for 12 weeks. Patients are typically instructed to quit smoking 7–10 days after starting the medication in order to have the drug reach therapeutic levels in the body. This level of dosing has been found to be efficacious, safe and well tolerated.[80,81] The most common side effects are insomnia and dry mouth. Bupropion may be the best pharmacotherapy for depressed patients and for cancer

Table 4.4 Meta-analyses: efficacy of FDA-approved smoking cessation medications		
Pharmacology	**n***	**Estimated odds ratio (95% CI)****
Bupropion SR	2	2.1 (1.5, 3.0)
Nicotine gum	13	1.5 (1.3, 1.8)
Nicotine inhaler	4	2.5 (1.7, 3.6)
Nicotine nasal	3	2.7 (1.8, 4.1)
Nicotine patch	27	1.9 (1.7, 2.2)
Two NRTs	3	1.9 (1.3, 2.6)

*n = number of studies included in each meta-analysis.
**Odds ratios when compared with placebo.
(Adapted from Tables 25–29 and 32 in [59]).

patients who are experiencing psychological distress in connection with their cancer. Bupropion is contraindicated for persons at increased risk for seizure including patients with a history of head injury, prior seizure, eating disorder, benzodiazapine withdrawal or immoderate alcohol use.[59]

NICOTINE REPLACEMENT THERAPIES (NRTs)

Approximately 80% of those who choose to quit smoking with pharmacological assistance choose some form of nicotine replacement.[82] Nicotine replacement therapies (NRTs) offer a way to replace the physiologically addictive substance in tobacco (i.e., nicotine) while removing the habitual behavior (e.g. smoking) that ordinarily supports the addiction. The rationale of this approach is that the tobacco user can learn to cope with the psychological and behavioral aspects of quitting separately, before he/she must go through physiological withdrawal. Nicotine replacement comes in a variety of forms, which share some commonalities, yet each form has unique properties.

While nicotine is responsible for physiological addiction to tobacco, it is not believed to be a carcinogen in itself[83–85] (however, for alternative perspective see: Rubin;[86] West et al[87]). Rather, the nitrosamines, particularly in cured tobacco, have been identified as the primary carcinogens in tobacco.[84,85] Nicotine replacement therapies have been shown to be safe and to have minimal abuse liability, even over the long term,[88] in those who continue to smoke[89] and in stable cardiovascular patients.[90] Moreover, while surgery patients are routinely counseled to cease smoking because smoking impairs wound healing, NRT does not, and can be safely used by such patients.[91] There is some debate about whether pregnant smokers should be offered NRT. While the benefits of quitting smoking may outweigh the risks associated with NRT, some believe that non-pharmacological options should be exhausted before resorting to any pharmacotherapy during pregnancy.

Nicotine replacements are available in a variety of forms and understanding each product will help the clinician to make use of the different products depending on the particular patient. As noted above, the efficacy of various NRT delivery systems within well-controlled clinical trials is largely equivalent. However, important differences do exist among the products which are worthy of consideration. For example, the products vary in how rapidly they deliver nicotine and maximum dose available. For comparison purposes, Figure 4.4 illustrates actual venous blood levels of nicotine resulting from a single administration of various nicotine replacement products as well as cigarettes and oral snuff. Note that none of the nicotine replacement therapies yields the bolus of nicotine seen with smoking. For a comprehensive review of pharmacokinetics in nicotine addition and nicotine replacement therapy, the reader is encouraged to read LeHouzac.[92]

Identifying the appropriate dose of an NRT product is more difficult than often believed as matching to approximately the same dose as received when smoking is extremely challenging. The amount of nicotine entering the body when smoking depends on a number of factors including the brand of cigarette being smoked, the percentage free-base nicotine (which is more readily absorbed)[93] and additives that may enhance nicotine absorption.[36] Furthermore, the amount of nicotine absorbed per cigarette also depends on the characteristics of the smoker. Smokers differ in smoking "topography", which refers to such variables as puff frequency and volume, whether or not vent holes

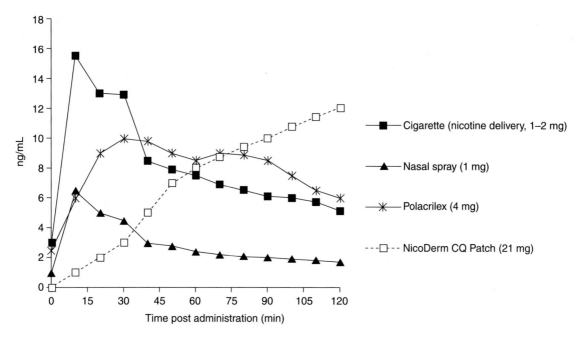

Figure 4.4
Plasma nicotine concentrations by nicotine delivery system. Venous plasma concentrations in nanograms of nicotine per millimeter of blood as a function of time for various nicotine delivery systems. Adapted with permission from: Fant R et al., 1999[106]. Data on the cigarette and nicotine gum are from those published by[107]; data on nicotine spray are from[52]; data on transdermal nicotine are from[108]. For more information, see[109].

(intentionally or not) are covered, and how much of the cigarette is smoked.[36] Finally, individual differences in nicotine metabolism vary according to gender, race and other heritable traits[94,95] and are so large that there is no way to predict the resultant blood nicotine levels from a given dose of nicotine.[96]

In practice, overdose is rarely observed to be a problem, rather underdosing is far more likely. One suggested method for "individualization of dosage" is for the patient to use at least the minimum recommended dose and adjust upward (within manufacturer's guidelines) to address any persisting withdrawal symptoms (e.g., see manufacturer's instructions for Nicotrol® nicotine nasal spray). For acutely dosed NRTs (i.e. gum, inhaler, nasal spray and

sublingual tablet), patients should be encouraged to use the product on a fixed schedule, such as every hour, so that blood levels of nicotine do not drop precipitously, increasing risk for relapse.

Some evidence suggests that women have less success at quitting with nicotine replacement therapy than men[97,98] although this latter finding has been debated.[95] These findings have been interpreted as possibly indicating that women smoke for different reasons than men (e.g., to reduce negative affect and to control body weight) and may require higher doses of nicotine replacement therapy to reach optimal treatment conditions compared to men.[95] It may also be that men are more responsive to the nicotine delivery aspect of smoking than women are, and thus they may be more likely to benefit from nicotine replacement.

Nicotine transdermal patch

Known simply as "the patch" (Nicotrol® Patch, Glaxo Smith Kline, USA), this product is available over-the-counter in the US. It stands apart from the other NRTs, in that the one-per-day dosing provides continuous, but relatively low, levels of nicotine. The once-per-day dosing is a feature that may account for the patch's popularity among patients and is certainly a significant advantage over the other NRTs in terms of compliance. The most common side effect of the patch is the potential in some patients for local skin irritation and rash, and patients who are allergic to adhesive tape or with other dermatological concerns should not use this product.

Depending on the brand, the patch is designed for 24-hour or 16-hour use. Patients who report vivid dreams as a side effect generally do better on the 16-hour patch. Dosing ranges from 7–21 mg per patch, and patches are designed for use in a stepped fashion, with the patient using stronger patches first, switching to weaker patches over the recommended 8 weeks of treatment as the dependency on cigarettes and nicotine wanes. Patients should be cautioned not to cut or reuse patches as exposure to air reduces product efficacy. Smoking while wearing the patch is contraindicated and in direct contrast to the presumed goal of quitting. However, occasional smoking during treatment with the patch is fairly common, is not believed to be dangerous, and is probably not grounds for discontinuing patch therapy unless the smoker has ceased making a concerted effort to quit, is demonstrating signs of nicotine overdose, or is smoking more than a few cigarettes per day.[89] Patch wearers should be encouraged to report any smoking lapses so that they

may be addressed with counseling and so that appropriate adjustments to pharmacotherapy can be made.

Nicotine gum

Nicotine gum is a popular NRT available over-the-counter in the US in 2- and 4-mg dosages. The manufacturer instructs the smoker to select dosage strength based on the number of cigarettes he/she smokes per day (i.e., ≥25 cigarettes per day indicates 4 mg). While this method of dosing is intuitive and easy, as noted previously, the number of cigarettes per day is not an accurate indicator of nicotine intake and as such should only be used as a preliminary dosing guide from which a patient can increase until the desired effect is reached.

There is preliminary evidence that gum is best used on a schedule[99] and the manufacturer advises chewing one piece every 1–2 hours for the first 6 weeks. Many people fail to use the gum as directed even for a short period of time. It is commonplace for gum users to report using less than half of the amount prescribed on the box. The underdosing problem is rooted in many things, including the fact that there are undesirable side effects (jaw soreness and fatigue, stomach upset and hiccups, mouth sores). Nicotine gum is not likely to be the best choice for patients with temporomandibular joint disease, dentures or other dental work. Many patients dislike the taste of the gum; mint and orange flavors are now available. Moreover, dosing is not precise (manufacturer instructions are to use 10–20 pieces per day).

One common problem is that many persons trying to quit may fail to heed instructions regarding the proper use of the product. The gum should be used with the chew/park method of using the gum which entails chewing the gum only briefly until a tingling sensation or peppery taste is detected in the mouth at which time the person "parks" the gum between their gum and cheek. The nicotine from the gum is absorbed through the oral mucosa. However, it is not well absorbed in the gut. Therefore, if chewing is too vigorous, nicotine will be pressed out of the gum into the saliva where it will be transported to the gut where absorption is poor. Because nicotine is best absorbed in a basic environment (pH < 7.4), patients using nicotine gum should be cautioned about drinking acidic beverages within 30 minutes of using gum. Given that the vast majority of beverages are acidic (e.g., coffee, most soft drinks, juices), and that dosing is at regular intervals throughout the day, this inconvenience should be strongly considered when selecting a pharmaceutical aid for cessation.

Nicotine nasal spray

Of the currently available nicotine replacement therapies, nicotine nasal spray is the one that most closely approximates the pharmacokinetic profile of cigarettes (e.g., the nicotine enters circulation and the brain more rapidly than any of the other nicotine replacement therapy delivery modes and faster than IV administration).[38,100] Because of this, the dependency profile for this product is somewhat higher than for other forms of NRT, but still well within an acceptable range.[59] Unfortunately, another distinguishing characteristic of nicotine nasal spray is that the side effects are rather aversive. Burning in the nasal passage, sneezing, coughing, sore throat, watering eyes and runny nose are commonly reported and most people report at least one of these symptoms of at least moderate intensity. These symptoms are most intense for only a few minutes following spray use and do abate significantly with repeated administrations. However, the aversive nature of the product almost certainly contributes to the widespread problem of underdosing.

Patients and clinicians will undoubtedly experience some difficulty in determining the best initial dose of spray to use. Each puff of spray delivers 1 mg of nicotine in a saline solution, of which 0.5 mg is absorbed. Manufacturer's instructions indicate that the range for appropriate dosing is 8–40 doses per day (one dose = two sprays, one in each nostril), not to exceed five doses in any 1-hour period.

Nicotine inhaler

The nicotine oral inhaler or inhalator (Nicotrol®, Glaxo Smith Kline), is available only by prescription in the US and is on the British Formulary. The oral inhaler consists of a cartridge containing a sponge impregnated with nicotine and a plastic reusable mouthpiece. When placed inside the mouthpiece the seal on the cartridge is broken allowing the nicotine to be inhaled as a vapor through the mouthpiece. Contrary to what might be expected, nicotine from the oral inhaler is not absorbed through the lungs, but rather, is absorbed in the buccal mucosa. Thus, the side-effect profile is substantially similar to that of nicotine gum; in particular side effects are mouth sores, hiccups. The unique feature of the nicotine inhaler is that it is most similar to the act of smoking itself. While some patients may favor this likeness, for others the conspicuous nature of the product is a definite drawback.

Nicotine lozenge

The Commit® nicotine lozenge (Glaxo Smith Kline) was approved by the Food and Drug Administration for over-the-counter sale in the US in 2002. Studies have found that the 2- and 4-mg lozenges yield 8–10% higher maximal plasma nicotine concentrations and 25–27% higher nicotine AUC values (area under the concentration–time curve) compared with 2- and 4-mg nicotine gum.[101] Choi and colleagues conclude that the difference stems from the fact that some residual nicotine is retained in the gum whereas the entire lozenge is consumed.[101] This difference may have implications in practice; at least one study has demonstrated that the lozenge has succeeded where other NRTs failed.[102]

Nicotine tablet

The nicotine sublingual tablet (Nicorette Microtab®; Pharmacia & Upjohn Consumer Healthcare, Lund, Sweden) has been demonstrated to be a safe and effective aid to smoking cessation, doubling quit rates over placebo at 6 and 12 months.[103] It is available in 2 mg strength with an average 1 mg of nicotine absorbed. Although not yet approved by the FDA for use in the US, the sublingual tablet and nicotine lozenge are on the British National Formulary.

Other NRT products

There are a number of new products under development and it is anticipated that the array of potential NRT cessation tools will expand significantly in the coming years. Examples of new nicotine replacement products include a "rapid-release" nicotine gum (JSR, LLC, Maryland, USA, and Biovail Corporation, Mississauga, Ontario, Canada), a biphasic nicotine pill that delivers both acute and slow-release nicotine (School of Pharmacy, The Robert Gordon University, Schoolhill, Aberdeen, UK), and a straw that delivers a bolus of nicotine with the first sip of a drink (Recovery Pharmaceuticals, Inc., Wayland, MA).

Other issues pertinent to nicotine replacement therapy

All forms of NRT, particularly the acute forms, which are dosed multiple times per day, suffer from the problem of underdosing. For a variety of reasons, patients fail to take the recommended doses for the minimum period of time. For some, the side effects are too aversive, others may underdose out of a desire to reduce their out-of-pocket expenses, or perhaps because they do not understand the importance of keeping blood nicotine levels stable. Patient education about the importance of adequate dosing may be the best tool for ensuring compliance.

The ideal duration of NRT is not clear; the manufacturer's instructions for most NRT products indicate that the products are to be used for a 7–12-week period. However, research suggests that risks from continued long-term use of the products are likely minimal and extending pharmacological treatment to a year or more may be appropriate for many smokers, considering the high rate of relapse back to smoking and the chronic nature of tobacco dependence.[88]

Combining the nicotine patch with an acute form of nicotine replacement, such as nicotine gum, has received some empirical support as a strategy,[104] and may be especially useful for difficult-to-treat patients who have not succeeded with one or more previous attempts with a single medication.

SUMMARY

- Substantial benefits can be gained by quitting even after a diagnosis of cancer.
- Physicians and other health care professionals can play a key role in helping patients initiate and maintain cessation.
- Many smokers, even those experiencing significant health effects related to smoking, find quitting difficult and may require multiple attempts at quitting before succeeding. However, a variety of

effective behavioral and pharmacological treatments are available.

- Physicians should be actively involved in helping their patients attempt to quit and in discussing various treatment options which may be appropriate, considering which approaches seem to best match their patient's needs.

REFERENCES

1. Shafey ODS, Guindon G, Tobacco Control Country Profiles 2003. Atlanta, GA: American Cancer Society, Inc., World Health Organization, International Union Against Cancer, 2003.
2. Peto R, Lopez AD, Boreham J, Thun M, Heath C Jr. Mortality from tobacco in developed countries: indirect estimation from national vital statistics. Lancet 1992; 339:1268–78.
3. Peto R, Lopez AD, Future Worldwide Health Effects of Current Smoking Patterns. In: Koop CE, Pearson CE, Schwartz MR (eds) Critical Issues in Global Health. San Francisco, Jossey-Bass, 2001.
4. Mackay J, Eriksen M, The Tobacco Atlas. Geneva, World Health Organization, 2002.
5. Ezzati M, Lopez AD, Estimates of global mortality attributable to smoking in 2000. Lancet 2003; 362:847–52.
6. Centers for Disease Control and Prevention, Annual Smoking – Attributable Mortality, Years of Potential Life Lost, and Economic Costs – United States 1995–1999. Morbidity & Mortality Weekly Report 2002; 51:300–3.
7. Jamison DT, Creese A, Prentice T, et al, The World Health Report. Geneva, World Health Organization, 1999.
8. Murray CJ, Lopez AD, Assessing the burden of disease that can be attributed to specific risk factors. In: Ad Hoc Committee on Health Research Relating to Future Intervention Options (ed.) Investing in Health Research and Development. Geneva, World Health Organization, 1996.
9. Liu BQ, Peto R, Chen ZM, et al, Emerging tobacco hazards in China: 1. Retrospective proportional mortality study of one million deaths. BMJ 1998; 317:1411–22.
10. Doll R, Peto R, The causes of cancer: quantitative estimates of avoidable risks of cancer in the United States today. J Nat Cancer Inst 1981; 66:1191–308.
11. Centers for Disease Control. Reducing the Health Consequences of Smoking: 25 Years of Progress – A Report of the Surgeon General. Rockville: US Department of Health and Human Services, 1989.
12. American Cancer Society, Cancer Facts and Figures 2003. Atlanta, 2003.
13. National Cancer Institute of Canada, Canadian Cancer Statistics 2003. Toronto, Canada, 2003.
14. Quinn MBP, Brock A, Kirby L, Jones J, Cancer trends in England and Wales 1950–1999. National Statistics 2001, Studies on Medical and Populations Subjects no. 66.
15. Henningfield JE, Slade J, Tobacco-dependence medications: public health and regulatory issues. Food Drug Law J 1998; 53 (suppl):75–114.
16. Peto R, Darby S, Deo H, et al, Smoking, smoking cessation, and lung cancer in the UK since 1950: combination of national statistics with two case-control studies. BMJ 2000; 321:323–9.
17. Gritz R, Lazev A, Vidrine D, Smoking cessation in cancer patients: never too late to quit. In: Given C, Given B, Champion V, Kozachik S, DeVoss D (eds) Evidence-Based Cancer Care and Prevention: Behavioral Interventions. New York, Springer Publishing Company, 2003.
18. Browman GP, Wong G, Hodson I, et al, Influence of cigarette smoking on the efficacy of radiation therapy in head and neck cancer. N Engl J Med 1993; 328:159–63.
19. Goodman MT, Kolonel LN, Wilkens LR, Yoshizawa CN, Le Marchand L, Smoking

history and survival among lung cancer patients. Cancer Causes Control 1990; 1: 155–63.

20. Day GL, Blot WJ, Shore RE, et al, Second cancers following oral and pharyngeal cancers: role of tobacco and alcohol. J Natl Cancer Inst 1994; 86:131–7.

21. Tucker MA, Murray N, Shaw EG, et al, Second primary cancers related to smoking and treatment of small-cell lung cancer. Lung Cancer Working Cadre. J Natl Cancer Inst 1997; 89:1782–8.

22. Kawahara M, Ushijima S, Kamimori T, et al, Second primary tumours in more than 2-year disease-free survivors of small-cell lung cancer in Japan: the role of smoking cessation. Br J Cancer 1998; 78:409–12.

23. Coughlin SS, Neaton JD, Sengupta A, Cigarette smoking as a predictor of death from prostate cancer in 348,874 men screened for the Multiple Risk Factor Intervention Trial. Am J Epidemiol 1996; 143:1002–6.

24. Hsing AW, McLaughlin JK, Schuman LM, et al, Diet, tobacco use, and fatal prostate cancer: results from the Lutheran Brotherhood Cohort Study. Cancer Res 1990; 50:6836–40.

25. Hsing AW, McLaughlin JK, Hrubec Z, Blot WJ, Fraumeni JF Jr, Tobacco use and prostate cancer: 26-year follow-up of US veterans. Am J Epidemiol 1991; 133:437–41.

26. Rodriguez C, Tatham LM, Thun MJ, Calle EE, Heath CW Jr, Smoking and fatal prostate cancer in a large cohort of adult men. Am J Epidemiol 1997; 145:466–75.

27. Yu GP, Ostroff JS, Zhang ZF, Tang J, Schantz SP, Smoking history and cancer patient survival: a hospital cancer registry study. Cancer Detect Prev 1997; 21:497–509.

28. Dresler CM, Is it more important to quit smoking than which chemotherapy is used? Lung Cancer 2003; 39:119–24.

29. Sanderson Cox L, Sloan JA, Patten CA, et al, Smoking behavior of 226 patients with diagnosis of stage IIIA/IIIB non-small cell lung cancer. Psychooncology 2002; 11:472–8.

30. Dresler CM, Bailey M, Roper CR, Patterson GA, Cooper JD, Smoking cessation and lung cancer resection. Chest 1996; 110:1199–202.

31. Gritz ER, Schacherer C, Koehly L, Nielsen IR, Abemayor E, Smoking withdrawal and relapse in head and neck cancer patients. Head Neck 1999; 21:420–7.

32. Hasuo S, Koyama Y, Kinoshita N, et al, [Smoking behavior and cognition for smoking cessation after diagnosis of head and neck cancer or stomach cancer]. Nippon Koshu Eisei Zasshi 1998; 45:732–9.

33. Ostroff J, Garland J, Moadel A, et al, Cigarette smoking patterns in patients after treatment of bladder cancer. J Cancer Educ 2000; 15: 86–90.

34. Ostroff JS, Jacobsen PB, Moadel AB, et al, Prevalence and predictors of continued tobacco use after treatment of patients with head and neck cancer. Cancer 1995; 75:569–76.

35. Vander Ark W, DiNardo LJ, Oliver DS, Factors affecting smoking cessation in patients with head and neck cancer. Laryngoscope 1997; 107:888–92.

36. US Dept of Health and Human Services, The Health Consequences of Smoking: Nicotine Addiction. A Report of the Surgeon General. Atlanta, GA: National Institutes of Health, Centers for Disease Control, US Dept of Health and Human Services, 1988.

37. Royal College of Physicians, Nicotine Addiction in Britain: A Report of the Tobacco Advisory Group of the Royal College of Physicians, 2000.

38. Schneider NG, Lunell E, Olmstead RE, Fagerstrom KO, Clinical pharmacokinetics of nasal nicotine delivery. A review and comparison to other nicotine systems. Clin Pharmacokinet 1996; 31:65–80.

39. Russell MA, Feyerabend C, Cigarette smoking: a dependence on high-nicotine boli. Drug Metab Rev 1978; 8:29–57.

40. Benowitz NL, The human pharmacology of nicotine. Res Advances Alcohol Drug Prob 1986; 9:1–51.

41. Henningfield JE, Keenan RM, Nicotine delivery

kinetics and abuse liability. J Consult Clin Psychol 1993; 61:743–50.

42. Hughes J, Higgens S, Hatsukami DK, Effects of abstinence from tobacco. In: Kozlowski L, Annis H, Cappell H, Glaser F (eds) Recent Advances in Alcohol and Drug Problems. New York: Plenum, 1990, pp. 317–98.

43. Shadel WG, Shiffman S, Niaura R, Nichter M, Abrams DB, Current models of nicotine dependence: what is known and what is needed to advance understanding of tobacco etiology among youth. Drug Alcohol Depend 2000; 59 (Suppl 1):S9–22.

44. Bergen A, Caparaso N, Cigarette smoking. J Nat Cancer Inst 1999; 91:1365–75.

45. Haire-Joshu D, Morgan G, Fisher EB Jr, Determinants of cigarette smoking. Clin Chest Med 1991; 12:711–25.

46. Jarvis MJ, A profile of tobacco smoking. Addiction 1994; 89:1371–6.

47. Romer D, Jamieson P, The role of perceived risk in starting and stopping smoking. In: Slovic P (ed.) Smoking: Risk, Perception and Policy. Thousand Oaks, CA: Sage Publications and the American Academy of Political and Social Science, 2001, pp. 64–80.

48. True WR, Heath AC, Scherrer JF, et al, Genetic and environmental contributions to smoking. Addiction 1997; 92:1277–87.

49. Munafo M, Johnstone E, Murphy M, Walton R, New directions in the genetic mechanisms underlying nicotine addiction. Addict Biol 2001; 6:109–17.

50. Mayhew KP, Flay BR, Mott JA, Stages in the development of adolescent smoking. Drug Alcohol Depend 2000; 59 (Suppl 1):S61–81.

51. McBride CM, Emmons KM, Lipkus IM, Understanding the potential of teachable moments: the case of smoking cessation. Health Educ Res 2003; 18:156–70.

52. Halpern MT, Schmier JK, Ward KD, Klesges RC, Smoking cessation in hospitalized patients. Respir Care 2000; 45:330–6.

53. Christensen AJ, Moran PJ, Ehlers SL, et al, Smoking and drinking behavior in patients with head and neck cancer: effects of behavioral self-blame and perceived control. J Behav Med 1999; 22:407–18.

54. Frid D, Ockene IS, Ockene JK, et al, Severity of angiographically proven coronary artery disease predicts smoking cessation. Am J Prev Med 1991; 7:131–5.

55. Schnoll RA, Miller SM, Smoking – cessation initiatives for cancer patients. Primary Care and Cancer 2000; 20:10–15.

56. Silagy C, Stead LF, Physician advice for smoking cessation. Cochrane Database Syst Rev 2001:CD000165.

57. Schnoll RA, Zhang B, Rue M, et al, Brief physician-initiated quit-smoking strategies for clinical oncology settings: a trial coordinated by the Eastern Cooperative Oncology Group. J Clin Oncol 2003; 21:355–65.

58. France EK, Glasgow RE, Marcus AC, Smoking cessation interventions among hospitalized patients: what have we learned? Prev Med 2001; 32:376–88.

59. Fiore MC, Bailey WC, Cohen SJ, Treating Tobacco Use and Dependence. Clinical Practice Guideline. Rockville, MD, US Department of Health and Human Services, 2000.

60. Prochaska JO, DiClemente CC, Norcross JC, In search of how people change. Applications to addictive behaviors. Am Psychol 1992; 47:1102–14.

61. Centers for Disease Control and Prevention, Surveillance for Selected Tobacco-Use Behaviors – United States, 1900–1994. Morbidity & Mortality Weekly Report 1994; 43:SS–3.

62. Centers for Disease Control and Prevention, Cigarette smoking among adults – United States, 2001. Morbidity & Mortality Weekly Report 2003; 52:953–6.

63. Centers for Disease Control and Prevention, Cigarette smoking among adults – United States 1991. Morbidity & Mortality Weekly Report 1993; 42:230–3.

64. Zhu S, Melcer T, Sun J, Rosbrook B, Pierce JP, Smoking cessation with and without

assistance: a population-based analysis. Am J Prev Med 2000; 18:305–11.

65. West R, McNeill A, Raw M, Smoking cessation guidelines for health professionals: an update. Health Education Authority. Thorax 2000; 55:987–99.

66. World Health Organization, WHO Evidence-Based Recommendation on the Treatment of Tobacco Dependence. Copenhagen, Denmark, 2001.

67. Hughes JR, Keely J, Naud S, Shape of the relapse curve and long-term abstinence among untreated smokers. Addiction 2004; 99: 29–38.

68. Zhu S, Pierce JP, A new scheduling method for time-limited counseling. Professional Psychology: Research and Practice 1995; 26:624–5.

69. Cinciripini PM, Wetter DW, McClure JB, Scheduled reduced smoking: effects on smoking abstinence and potential mechanisms of action. Addictive Behaviors 1997; 22:759–67.

70. Wakefield M, Borland R, Saved by the bell: the role of telephone helpline services in the context of mass-media anti-smoking campaigns. Tob Control 2000; 9:117–19.

71. Ossip-Klein DJ, Giovino GA, Megahed N, et al, Effects of a smoker's hotline: results of a 10-county self-help trial. J Consult Clin Psychol 1991; 59:325–32.

72. Zhu SH, Anderson CM, Johnson CE, Tedeschi G, Roeseler A, A centralized telephone service for tobacco cessation: the California experience. Tob Control 2000; 9:II48–55.

73. Zhu SH, Stretch V, Balabanis M, et al, Telephone counseling for smoking cessation: effects of single-session and multiple-session interventions. J Consult Clin Psychol 1996; 64:202–11.

74. Zhu SH, Tedeschi G, Anderson CM, et al, Telephone counseling as adjuvant treatment for nicotine replacement therapy in a 'real-world' setting. Prev Med 2000; 31:357–63.

75. Fiore MC, Croyle RT, Curry SJ, et al, Preventing 3 million premature deaths and helping 5 million smokers quit: a national action plan for tobacco cessation. Am J Public Health 2004; 94:205–10.

76. Benowitz NL, Jacob P 3rd, Jones RT, Rosenberg J, Interindividual variability in the metabolism and cardiovascular effects of nicotine in man. J Pharmacol Exp Ther 1982; 221:368–72.

77. Feyerabend C, Ings RM, Russel MA, Nicotine pharmacokinetics and its application to intake from smoking. Br J Clin Pharmacol 1985; 19:239–47.

78. Rose JE, Behm FM, Westman EC, et al, Mecamylamine combined with nicotine skin patch facilitates smoking cessation beyond nicotine patch treatment alone. Clin Pharmacol Ther 1994; 56:86–99.

79. Rose JE, Behm FM, Westman EC, Nicotine-mecamylamine treatment for smoking cessation: the role of pre-cessation therapy. Exp Clin Psychopharmacol 1998; 6:331–43.

80. Johnston JA, Fiedler-Kelly J, Glover ED, et al, Relationship between drug exposure and the efficacy and safety of bupropion sustained release for smoking cessation. Nicotine Tob Res 2001; 3:131–40.

81. Hurt RD, Sachs DP, Glover ED, et al, A comparison of sustained-release bupropion and placebo for smoking cessation. N Engl J Med 1997; 337:1195–202.

82. Burton SL, Gitchell JG, Shiffman S, Use of FDA-approved pharmacologic treatments for tobacco dependence – United States, 1984–1998. Morbidity & Mortality Weekly Report 2000; 49:665–8.

83. Hecht SS, Tobacco carcinogens, their biomarkers and tobacco-induced cancer. Nat Rev Cancer 2003; 3:733–44.

84. Hecht SS, Cigarette smoking and lung cancer: chemical mechanisms and approaches to prevention. Lancet Oncol 2002; 3:461–9.

85. Hecht SS, Tobacco smoke carcinogens and lung cancer. J Natl Cancer Inst 1999; 91:1194–210.

86. Rubin H, Synergistic mechanisms in carcinogenesis by polycyclic aromatic hydrocarbons and by tobacco smoke: a bio-historical per-

spective with updates. Carcinogenesis 2001; 22:1903–30.

87. West KA, Brognard J, Clark AS, et al, Rapid Akt activation by nicotine and a tobacco carcinogen modulates the phenotype of normal human airway epithelial cells. J Clin Invest 2003; 111:81–90.

88. Sims TH, Fiore MC, Pharmacotherapy for treating tobacco dependence: what is the ideal duration of therapy? CNS Drugs 2002; 16: 653–62.

89. Hasford J, Fagerstrom KO, Haustein KO, A naturalistic cohort study on effectiveness, safety and usage pattern of an over-the-counter nicotine patch. Cohort study on smoking cessation. Eur J Clin Pharmacol 2003; 59:443–7.

90. Benowitz NL, Gourlay SG, Cardiovascular toxicity of nicotine: implications for nicotine replacement therapy. J Am Coll Cardiol 1997; 29:1422–31.

91. Sorensen LT, Karlsmark T, Gottrup F, Abstinence from smoking reduces incisional wound infection: a randomized controlled trial. Ann Surg 2003; 238:1–5.

92. Le Houezec J, Role of nicotine pharmacokinetics in nicotine addiction and nicotine replacement therapy: a review. Int J Tuberc Lung Dis 2003; 7:811–19.

93. Pankow JF, Tavakoli AD, Luo W, Isabelle LM, Percent free base nicotine in the tobacco smoke particulate matter of selected commercial and reference cigarettes. Chem Res Toxicol 2003; 16:1014–18.

94. Benowitz NL, Perez-Stable E, Herrera B, Jacob P, African American–Caucasian differences in nicotine and cotinine metabolism. Clin Pharmacol Ther 1995; 57:159.

95. Benowitz NL, Hatsukami DK, Gender differences in the pharmacology of nicotine addiction. Addiction Biology 1998; 3:383–404.

96. Benowitz NL, Zevin S, Jacob P 3rd, Sources of variability in nicotine and cotinine levels with use of nicotine nasal spray, transdermal nicotine, and cigarette smoking. Br J Clin Pharmacol 1997; 43:259–67.

97. Perkins K, Sex differences in nicotine vs. non-nicotine reinforcement as determinants of tobacco smoking. Exp Clin Psychopharmacol 1996; 4:166–77.

98. Wetter DW, Fiore MC, Young TB, et al, Gender differences in response to nicotine replacement therapy: objective and subjective indexes of tobacco withdrawal. Exp Clin Psychopharmacol 1999; 7:135–44.

99. Killen JD, Fortmann SP, Newman B, Varady A, Evaluation of a treatment approach combining nicotine gum with self-guided behavioral treatments for smoking relapse prevention. J Consult Clin Psychol 1990; 58:85–92.

100. Gourlay SG, Benowitz NL, Arteriovenous differences in plasma concentration of nicotine and catecholamines and related cardiovascular effects after smoking, nicotine nasal spray, and intravenous nicotine. Clin Pharmacol Ther 1997; 62:453–63.

101. Choi JH, Dresler CM, Norton MR, Strahs KR, Pharmacokinetics of a nicotine polacrilex lozenge. Nicotine Tob Res 2003; 5:635–44.

102. Shiffman S, Dresler CM, Rohay JM, Successful treatment with a nicotine lozenge of smokers with prior failure in pharmacological therapy. Addiction 2004; 99:83–92.

103. Glover ED, Glover PN, Franzon M, et al, A comparison of a nicotine sublingual tablet and placebo for smoking cessation. Nicotine Tob Res 2002; 4:441–50.

104. Sweeney CT, Fant RV, Fagerstrom KO, McGovern JF, Henningfield JE, Combination nicotine replacement therapy for smoking cessation: rationale, efficacy and tolerability. CNS Drugs 2001; 15:453–67.

105. Tsoh JY, Skaar KL, McClure JB, et al, Smoking cessation 2: components of effective intervention. Behav Med 1997; 23:15–27.

106. Fant RV, Owen LL, Hemingfield JE, Nicotine replacement therapy. Primary Care: Clinics in Office Practice 1999; 26(3):633–52.

107. Benowitz NL, Porchet H, Sheiner L, Jacob P 3rd, Nicotine absorption and cardiovascular effects with smokeless tobacco use: comparison

with cigarettes and nicotine gum. Clin Pharmacol Ther 1988; 44:23–8.

108. Benowitz NL, Nicotine replacement therapy. What has been accomplished – can we do better? Drugs 1993; 45:157–70.

109. Henningfield JE, Fant RV, Shiffman S, et al, Tobacco dependence: scientific and public health basis of treatment. Econ Neurosci 2000; 2:42–6.

110. Morgan GD, Kobus K, Gerlach KK, et al, Nicotine Tob Res. 2003; 5 Suppl 1:S11–9. http://www.tandf.co.uk.

5 Pathology of lung preneoplasia

William D Travis, Elisabeth Brambilla

Contents   Introduction • Preinvasive bronchial squamous lesions • Microinvasive squamous cell carcinoma • Molecular pathology of preinvasive bronchial lesions • Atypical adenomatous hyperplasia • Molecular, immunohistochemical and morphometric studies of AAH • Diffuse idiopathic pulmonary neuroendocrine cell hyperplasia • Conclusion

INTRODUCTION

Lung cancer is currently the most common cause of cancer incidence and mortality worldwide.[1] In 2004 it is estimated that lung cancer will account for over 173 000 new cases in the United States and over 160 000 cancer deaths.[2] While lung cancer incidence has been decreasing in males since the early 1980s, it appears to be near its peak and starting to decline in women.[2] Despite all of the efforts at treatment of lung cancer, the 5-year survival has remained between 10–15% over the past few decades.[3,4] For this reason, there is great interest in early detection of lung cancer utilizing a variety of approaches including fluorescence bronchoscopy and screening of high-risk patients by spiral or helical CT.[5,6] Along with the interest in early diagnosis of lung cancer there has been considerable evolution in the concepts of preinvasive lesions for lung carcinoma in the past few decades as well as in lung cancer classification.[7,8] This is reflected by the absence of preinvasive lesions in the 1967 WHO classification, the addition of squamous dysplasia/carcinoma 'in situ' in the 1981 classification and the addition of atypical adenomatous hyperplasia and diffuse idiopathic neuroendocrine cell hyperplasia in the 1999 and 2004 WHO classifications (Table 5.1). While minor changes were made in

Table 5.1 History of classification of preinvasive lesions by the WHO

1967 WHO classification[84]	1981 WHO classification[85]	1999 WHO/IASLC classification[7]	2004 WHO classification[7,8]
No category of preinvasive lesions	Squamous dysplasia/ carcinoma in situ	Squamous dysplasia/ carcinoma in situ	Squamous dysplasia/ carcinoma in situ
		Atypical adenomatous hyperplasia	Atypical adenomatous hyperplasia
		Diffuse idiopathic pulmonary neuroendocrine cell hyperplasia	Diffuse idiopathic pulmonary neuroendocrine cell hyperplasia

WHO = World Health Organization; IASLC = International Association for the Study of Lung Cancer.

classification of several invasive tumors in the 2004 WHO classification compared to the 1999 WHO classification, there were no changes made with regard to preinvasive lesions.

PREINVASIVE BRONCHIAL SQUAMOUS LESIONS

Bronchial carcinogenesis is conceptualized as a multistep and multicentric process involving transformation of the normal bronchial mucosa through a continuous spectrum of lesions, including basal cell hyperplasia, squamous metaplasia, dysplasia and carcinoma in situ (Table 5.2).[8–16] In addition to these epithelial changes, alterations of the extracellular matrix, particularly destruction of the epithelial basement membrane, are critical events in the development of invasion and in the eventual occurrence of metastases.[17,18]

In the new 2004 WHO classification squamous dysplasia and CIS are grouped together under the term preinvasive bronchial squamous

lesions.[8] These lesions are considered only to be potential precursors to squamous cell carcinoma. Lesions such as goblet cell hyperplasia, basal cell (reserve cell) hyperplasia and squamous metaplasia are not thought to be preinvasive lesions.

Squamous metaplasia and dysplasia

Squamous metaplasia occurs when squamous cells replace the pseudostratified and ciliated respiratory epithelium.[7,8] Squamous differentiation is evident either by keratinization or intercellular bridges. The squamous cells show maturation from the basal layer to a layer of surface keratinized cells.

Squamous dysplasia may be graded as mild, moderate (Figure 5.1) or severe depending on the spectrum of morphologically atypical changes and the thickness of epithelium involved. In dysplasia, the changes do not reach the full thickness involvement that characterizes carcinoma in situ.[7,8] The 2004 WHO criteria for the grades of dysplasia and for carcinoma in situ are summarized in Table 5.2. However, there is

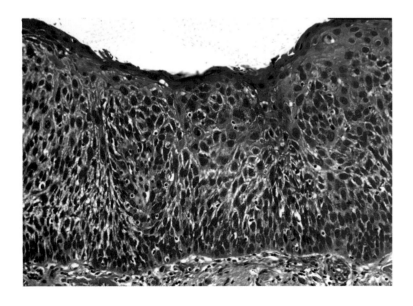

Figure 5.1
Moderate dysplasia. The squamous epithelium shows maturation and keratinization at the surface. However, up to the middle third of the epithelium shows nuclear crowding and hyperchromasia with numerous prominent nucleoli. Mitoses are lacking.

Table 5.2 Microscopic features of squamous dysplasia and carcinoma in situ				
Abnormality	**Thickness**	**Cell size**	**Maturation/orientation**	**Nuclei**
Mild dysplasia	Mildly increased	Mildly increased Mild anisocytosis, Pleomorphism	Continuous progression of maturation from base to luminal surface Basilar zone expanded with cellular crowding in lower third Distinct intermediate (prickle cell) zone present Superficial flattening of epithelial cells	Mild variation of N/C ratio Finely granular chromatin Minimal angulation Nucleoli inconspicuous or absent Nuclei vertically oriented in lower third Mitoses absent or very rare
Moderate dysplasia	Moderately increased	Mild increase in cell size; cells often small May have moderate anisocytosis, pleomorphism	Partial progression of maturation from base to luminal surface Basilar zone expanded with cellular crowding in lower two thirds of epithelium Intermediate zone confined to upper third of epithelium Superficial flattening of epithelial cells	Moderate variation of N/C ratio Finely granular chromatin Angulations, grooves and lobulations present Nucleoli inconspicuous or absent Nuclei vertically oriented in lower two thirds Mitotic figures present in lower third

continued

Table 5.2 continued				
Abnormality	Thickness	Cell size	Maturation/orientation	Nuclei
Severe dysplasia	Markedly increased	Markedly increased May have marked anisocytosis, pleomorphism	Little progression of maturation from base to luminal surface Basilar zone expanded with cellular crowding well into upper third Intermediate zone greatly attenuated Superficial flattening of epithelial cells	N/C ratio often high and variable Chromatin coarse and uneven Nuclear angulations and folding prominent Nucleoli frequently present and conspicuous Nuclei vertically oriented in lower two thirds Mitotic figures present in lower two thirds
Carcinoma in situ	May or may not be increased	May be markedly increased May have marked anisocytosis, pleomorphism	No progression of maturation from base to luminal surface; epithelium could be inverted with little change in appearance Basilar zone expanded with cellular crowding throughout epithelium Intermediate zone absent Surface flattening confined to the most superficial cells	N/C ratio often high and variable Chromatin coarse and uneven Nuclear angulations and folding prominent Nucleoli may be present or inconspicuous No consistent orientation of nuclei in relation to epithelial surface Mitotic figures present through full thickness

From references [7,8].

a spectrum of morphology within each of the grades of dysplasia/CIS which rarely gather all of the criteria listed in lesions from the various categories.

Rarely micropapillary change can occur in squamous metaplastic or dysplastic epithelium.[19] The term angiogenic squamous dysplasia (ASD) has been proposed for this lesion.[20] It is characterized by papillary projections above the mucosal surface with a fibrovascular core within the papillae. Grading of dysplasia and the distinction from either squamous metaplasia or carcinoma in situ can be difficult due to disorientation of the mucosa associated with micropapillary change.[21,22]

Carcinoma in situ

In carcinoma in situ (CIS) squamous cells with malignant cytologic features replace the entire thickness of the bronchial epithelium.[7,8] Invasive growth or penetration past the level of the subepithelial basement membrane is lacking (Figure 5.2). The tumor cells may have marked cytologic changes with variation in size and shape and an increase in the nuclear to cytoplasmic ratio. Nuclear enlargement and hyperchromasia are common with prominent nucleoli and nuclear angulation. Mitoses occur throughout the thickness of the epithelium, including near the mucosal surface. The stratification and orientation seen in normal mucosa is lost and maturation is lacking. These changes may alter the appearance of the mucosa so it would appear the same if it were inverted, despite some flattening of the superficial cells. CIS may spread into submucosal glands but if the basement membrane is intact or if the tumor cells do not spread beyond the border of the glands, this does not represent invasive growth (Figure 5.2). The basement membrane may be difficult to evaluate in CIS since it is often markedly thinned and breaks may be present. Occasion-

ally CIS may undermine adjacent mucosa so cytologically malignant cells are present within benign respiratory epithelial cells. Submucosal chronic inflammation is often present in association with CIS.

There are several clinical implications to the presence of CIS. If an in situ component is present within or adjacent to a tumor this finding supports that it arose primarily within the lung.[23] If a carcinoma is completely in situ,

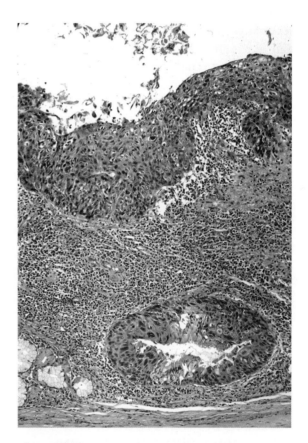

Figure 5.2
Carcinoma in situ with submucosal gland involvement. The mucosal surface is diffusely involved by CIS. There is full-thickness involvement by cytologically malignant-appearing squamous cells. There is extension into the underlying submucosal gland, but this does not qualify as invasive carcinoma.

clinically it is not capable of metastasizing.[23] The finding of CIS also raises concern for potential multicentricity, future recurrence and for concurrent or subsequent invasive carcinoma.[23] Therefore, chemoprevention and close clinical follow-up are considerations for patients diagnosed with severe dysplasia and/or CIS, in the absence of invasive carcinoma.

Atypical squamous metaplasia associated with bronchial inflammation or fibrosis as well as radiation- and/or chemotherapy-induced atypia are often in the differential diagnosis for squamous dysplasia and CIS. If there is acute and/or chronic inflammation of the airways or a history of previous biopsy or treatment, the threshold for diagnosis of malignancy must be increased.

MICROINVASIVE SQUAMOUS CELL CARCINOMA

Invasion requires the passage of tumor cells through the basement membrane into the underlying submucosa and is identified by the presence of carcinoma cells, singly or in clumps, invading the underlying stroma. This can be very difficult in small bronchoscopic specimens. In cases where invasion is suspected but not certain, deeper sections may be helpful to resolve the matter. These microinvasive tumors are T1 squamous cell carcinoma.

MOLECULAR PATHOLOGY OF PREINVASIVE BRONCHIAL LESIONS

Molecular studies have demonstrated that lung carcinogenesis is a multistep process with accumulation of genetic changes in the epithelial cells and alterations in the extracellular matrix.

Early genetic changes in squamous cell lung carcinogenesis include loss of heterozygosity (LOH) at chromosome regions 3p (including 3p12, 3p14.2 (FHIT gene),[24,25] 3p14.1–21.3, 3p21, 3p22–24, 3p25)[26] and 9p21.[27] Wistuba et al showed that these changes can be found even in histologically normal bronchial mucosa of former cigarette smokers.[28] In later stages, LOH of other chromosome regions including 17p13 (P53 gene), 13q (RB gene), and 5q (APC-MCC region) and K-ras mutations can be found.[27,29] Brambilla et al demonstrated alteration in the p53 transcription pathway (Bcl2, Bax, waf-1) and the RB pathway (rb, p16, cyclin D1) in preinvasive squamous bronchial lesions.[11,30] With immunohistochemistry for p53, an increasing percentage of staining can be found with progression through dysplasia, CIS and invasive carcinoma.[13,26,31] With laser capture microdissection one can analyze specific areas of abnormal mucosa.

Correlation with increasing grades of dysplasia or CIS can be found with other genetic alterations ncluding telomerase,[32] aneuploidy and proliferating cell nuclear antigen (PCNA).[33]

Only few immunohistochemical and/or molecular biology studies have been made of the extracellular matrix, matrix metalloproteinases (MMPs) or tissue inhibitors of metalloproteinases (TIMPs) in preinvasive bronchial lesions.[34–36] An increasing degree of matrix rearrangement of the basement membrane was shown in one study with increasing severity of epithelial changes in squamous preinvasive bronchial lesions.[34] Bolon et al found using immunohistochemical staining of frozen sections, that stromelysin-1 (MMP-3) was inconsistently expressed in 31% of preinvasive lesions, while stromelysin-3 (MMP-11) and urokinase type plasminogen activator were frequently expressed in such lesions.[35] Galateau et al demonstrated a series of changes in MMP and

TIMP expression in the epithelial cells in bronchial preinvasive lesions.[37] In this study it was shown that MMP-1, MMP-2, MMP-9, and to a lesser extent MMP-3, play important roles in the remodeling of the basement membrane and extracellular matrix associated with progression of bronchial squamous preinvasive lesions. By confocal microscopy a progressive decrease was shown in colocalization of TIMP-1 and type IV collagen beginning with dysplasia, suggesting a TIMP-1 has a protective effect on basement membranes in early preinvasive lesions that is lost in progression to carcinoma in situ and invasive carcinoma.[37]

ATYPICAL ADENOMATOUS HYPERPLASIA

Atypical adenomatous hyperplasia (AAH) was added to the list of preinvasive lesions for lung cancer in the 1999 WHO classification[7] and it is retained in the 2004 WHO classification.[8] It is a bronchioloalveolar proliferation regarded to be a precursor to adenocarcinoma (Figures 5.3 and 5.4).[8,38] AAH resembles, but falls short of, criteria for the diagnosis of bronchioloalveolar carcinoma, non-mucinous type.[7,8,31,40] AAH is most often encountered as an incidental histologic finding in lung specimens removed for other reasons, commonly a lung carcinoma.

The finding of AAH mostly in lung adenocarcinoma specimens and cases of multiple AAH and multiple adenocarcinomas supports the concept that they are precursor lesions to adenocarcinoma. Depending on the extent of the search and the criteria used for the diagnosis the incidence of AAH varies from 5.7–21.4%.[41–43] Weng et al examined lobectomy and pneumonectomy specimens of 165 primary and 45 metastatic tumor cases processing an average of 51 blocks per specimen[41] and found AAH in 16.4% of lung cancer resection specimens. It was present in 20% of males and 9.1%

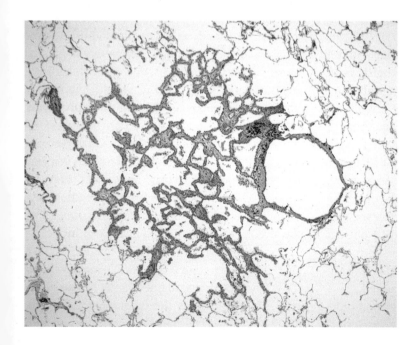

Figure 5.3
Atypical adenomatous hyperplasia. An ill-defined bronchioloalveolar proliferation is situated in a peribronchiolar location.

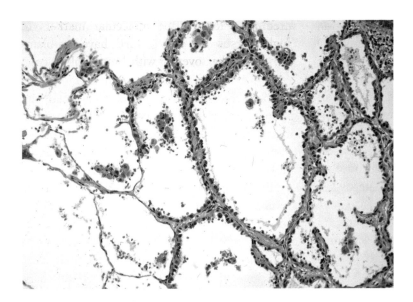

Figure 5.4
Atypical adenomatous hyperplasia. The bronchioloalveolar proliferation shows atypical pneumocytes proliferating along the alveolar walls. The alveolar architecture is preserved. The edge of the lesion shows the transition to normal alveolar epithelium.

of females.[41] However, in lung specimens resected for metastases and not lung cancer, they found AAH in 4.4% of cases with 4.8% in males and 4% in females.[41]

AAH frequently presents as multiple lesions. Multiple AAH were found in 6.7% of lung cancer resection specimens and 2% of lung specimens resected for metastases.[41]

The size of AAH is generally less than 5 mm in diameter, although the lesions can measure up to 10 mm.[40,41] AAH appears histologically as a small nodular lesion, in which the alveoli and respiratory bronchioles are lined by monotonous, slightly atypical cuboidal to low columnar pneumocytes (Figures 5.3 and 5.4). There is dense nuclear chromatin, nucleoli are inconspicuous and cytoplasm is scant. The alveolar septa may be slightly thickened. Mild lymphocytic infiltration and lymphoid aggregates may be present. The degree of atypia varies from mild to moderate. When it is severe, the possibility of bronchioloalveolar carcinoma must be considered.

AAH must be separated from the non-mucinous subtype of bronchioloalveolar carcinoma, type II pneumocyte hyperplasia with interstitial inflammation and/or fibrosis,[44–47] micronodular pneumocyte hyperplasia,[48] respiratory bronchiolitis,[49] peribronchiolar fibrosis with peribronchiolar metaplasia,[50] and papillary adenoma.[51,52] Separation of AAH from BAC can be very difficult and subjective.[7,8,39,53] Adenocarcinoma is favored if there is marked cell crowding and/or overlapping of nuclei, cytologic atypia with nuclear hyperchromasia and/or prominent nucleoli, large cell size, and loss of alveolar architecture with prominent papillary or invasive growth. When AAH becomes larger than 0.5 cm one must be more concerned about BAC, but a small percentage of AAH lesions are larger and a small percentage of bronchioloalveolar carcinomas may be smaller. Other features favoring adenocarcinoma include extensive papillary growth with loss of the alveolar architecture and invasive growth.

It is difficult enough to make the diagnosis of AAH and to separate it from BAC. Some authors have attempted to define 'high- versus low-grade AAH'.[54] This is not recommended by the 1999 or 2004 WHO panels.[7,8]

The concept of AAH and the new definition of bronchioloalveolar carcinoma by the WHO classification as an adenocarcinoma with lepidic growth and lacking invasion makes it tempting to propose the latter as an adenocarcinoma 'in situ'.[7,8] However, this has some conceptual problems in that bronchioloalveolar carcinomas are often multicentric, especially the mucinous subtype, and they can invade extensively along the surface of the alveolar walls causing lobar consolidation ultimately causing respiratory death. No other 'in situ' carcinoma is known to be potentially fatal. The WHO panel in both 1999 and 2004 considered this possible terminology and chose not to adopt it.[7,8] Another problem with the concept of AAH, is the uncertain clinical implication of the diagnosis in a patient without a lung carcinoma. Since virtually the entire literature on AAH has been reported in surgically resected specimens for lung cancer or metastases, little is known about the potential for progression to carcinoma.[55]

MOLECULAR, IMMUNOHISTOCHEMICAL AND MORPHOMETRIC STUDIES OF AAH

Many different special techniques have been used to study AAH including molecular,[33,56–61] cell proliferation, immunohistochemical,[62,63] DNA quantification,[60] ultrastructural,[64] and morphometric[65,66] methods.

The concept that AAH represents a preneoplastic and even possibly a neoplastic lesion is based on demonstration of multiple molecular abnormalities. p53 alterations by immunohistochemistry have been reported in 8–58% of cases.[56,57,59,67,68] Interestingly, some have reported a greater percentage of cases staining with 'higher-grade atypia'.[57,67] However, grading of AAH is very difficult and studies of AAH

attempting to describe molecular markers in 'high- versus low-grade AAH' have problems with cases that overlap with bronchioloalveolar carcinoma. LOH of chromosome 3p, 9p and 17p in 18%, 13% and 6% was found by Kitaguchi et al respectively in the AAH lesions, while the corresponding carcinomatous lesions showed LOH of 67%, 50% and 17% respectively.[56] Kurasono showed that cyclin D1 is highly expressed in AAH but it is lost in adenocarcinomas.[58] AAH has been shown to have K-ras codon 12 mutations in 17–50% of cases suggesting it is an early lesion in development of adenocarcinoma.[69–71]

DIFFUSE IDIOPATHIC PULMONARY NEUROENDOCRINE CELL HYPERPLASIA

Diffuse idiopathic pulmonary neuroendocrine cell hyperplasia (DIPNECH) is characterized by widespread proliferation of neuroendocrine cells in the peripheral airways.[7,8] This ranges from neuroendocrine cell hyperplasia to multiple tumorlets. This condition is very rare with less than 30 cases reported.[7,72–74] DIPNECH may present with airway obstruction due to the frequent association with bronchiolar fibrosis. Such patients often appear to have an interstitial lung disease. DIPNECH is thought to represent a precursor lesion for carcinoid tumors since a subset of these patients has one or more carcinoid tumors.[7,8]

Aguayo et al described DIPNECH in 1992 and proposed that the neuroendocrine cell proliferation was the primary lesion and that substances such as bombesin produced by the neuroendocrine cells were causes of the airway fibrosis.[74] Neuroendocrine cell hyperplasia, tumorlets and carcinoid tumors represent a continuum of neuroendocrine cell proliferation. Tumorlets represent micronodular proliferations of neuroendocrine cells that usually infiltrate beyond the bronchial/bronchiolar wall. The cut off in size between tumorlets and carcinoid tumors is arbitrarily set at 0.5 cm so carcinoid tumor is diagnosed for neuroendocrine proliferations measuring greater than 0.5 cm in diameter.[7]

DIPNECH typically presents in the fifth or sixth decades of life and there appears to be a female predominance.[74–77] Patients present with slowly progressive dry cough and dyspnea, often over many years. Pulmonary function tests show an obstructive or mixed obstructive/restrictive pattern of impairment with reduced diffusing capacity.

Chest radiographs may be normal, but computerized tomographic scanning (particularly with an expiration study) demonstrates a mosaic pattern of air trapping, sometimes with nodules and thickened bronchial and bronchiolar walls.[72,76] Multiple nodules that correspond to tumorlets or carcinoid tumors may be present.[74,76]

Patients with DIPNECH typically have a favorable clinical course. Rare patients have required lung transplantation due to severe obstructive airway disease. The carcinoid tumors that occur in DIPNECH so far have all been typical carcinoids.

Histologically, lung biopsies from patients with DIPNECH show a neuroendocrine cell hyperplasia that can consist of increased numbers of scattered single cells, small nodules (neuroendocrine bodies) or linear proliferations of neuroendocrine cells within the bronchiolar epithelium (Figures 5.5 and 5.6). Micronodular masses represent tumorlets and if they are 0.5 cm in size or greater they are called carcinoid tumors. The neuroendocrine proliferations and tumorlets may cause airway narrowing and/or obliteration. No distinguishing molecular features are recognized, but the loss of heterozygosity found in carcinoid tumors at the 11q13 region that closely approximates to the MEN1 tumor suppressor gene is rare in tumorlets.[78] Cohen et al demonstrated high expression of neutral endopeptidase in DIPNECH.[79]

There are no clinical and/or radiologic features that would allow for the diagnosis of

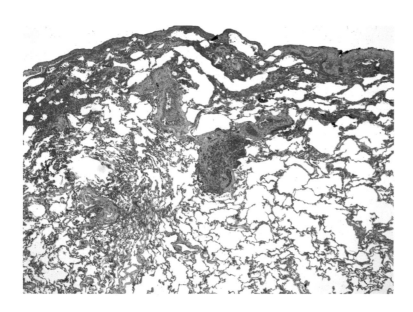

Figure 5.5
Diffuse idiopathic neuroendocrine cell hyperplasia. The bronchial lumen is obliterated by a nodular proliferation of neuroendocrine cells.

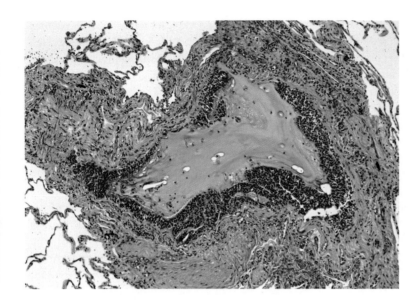

Figure 5.6
Diffuse idiopathic neuroendocrine cell hyperplasia. The bronchiolar mucosa is partly replaced by a proliferation of neuroendocrine cells.

DIPNECH without surgical lung biopsy. The presenting clinical findings of cough, dyspnea, mixed obstructive/restrictive pulmonary impairment and a nodular pattern of pulmonary infiltration could be seen in many diffuse parenchymal lung disorders. The finding of a mosaic pattern of air trapping on expiration CT could be seen in small airway disorders due to a wide variety of causes.

The pathologic differential diagnosis includes NE cell hyperplasia and/or tumorlets that can occur as a secondary lesion in a wide variety of inflammatory and fibrotic lung conditions such as bronchiectasis and chronic lung abscess.[80–83] DIPNECH must also be distinguished from the NE cell hyperplasia that can be seen in the normal lung adjacent to up to 75% of peripheral carcinoid tumors.[77]

CONCLUSION

In summary, it is important to understand the pathology of preinvasive lesions for lung cancer.

With increasing focus on early detection of lung cancer, screening trials and chemoprevention, patients with this group of lesions represent an attractive cohort for chemoprevention research. Given the paucity of clinical correlative information about the natural history of some of the early lesions, this is an important area for clinicians to work with clinical and molecular pathologists to conduct additional research to further elucidate this critical but poorly understood area.

REFERENCES

1. Parkin DM, Pisani P, Ferlay J, Global cancer statistics. CA-A Cancer J Clin 1999; 49:33–64.
2. Jemal A, Tiwari RC, Murray T, et al, Cancer statistics, 2004. CA Cancer J Clin 2004; 54:8–29.
3. Jemal A, Clegg LX, Ward E, et al, Annual report to the nation on the status of cancer, 1975–2001, with a special feature regarding survival. Cancer 2004; 101:3–27.
4. Travis WD, Travis LB, Devesa SS, Lung cancer [published erratum appears in Cancer 1995 Jun 15; 75(12):2979]. Cancer 1995; 75:191–202.

5. Bepler G, Goodridge CD, Djulbegovic B, Clark RA, Tockman M, A systematic review and lessons learned from early lung cancer detection trials using low-dose computed tomography of the chest. Cancer Control 2003; 10:306–14.

6. Bach PB, Kelley MJ, Tate RC, McCrory DC, Screening for lung cancer: a review of the current literature. Chest 2003; 123:72S–82S.

7. Travis WD, Colby TV, Corrin B, Shimosato Y, Brambilla E, in collaboration with LH Sobin and pathologists from 14 countries, Histological Typing of Lung and Pleural Tumors. Berlin, Springer, 1999.

8. Travis WD, Brambilla E, Müller-Hermelink HK, Harris CC, Pathology and Genetics: Tumours of the Lung, Pleura, Thymus and Heart. Lyon, IARC, 2004.

9. Auerbach O, Gere B, Forman JB, et al, Changes in the bronchial epithelium in relation to smoking and cancer of the lung. N Engl J Med 1957; 256:97–104.

10. Becci PJ, McDowell EM, Trump BF, The respiratory epithelium. IV. Histogenesis of epidermoid metaplasia and carcinoma in situ in the hamster. J Natl Cancer Inst 1978; 61:577–86.

11. Brambilla E, Gazzeri S, Lantuejoul S, et al, p53 mutant immunophenotype and deregulation of p53 transcription pathway (Bcl2, Bax, and Waf1) in precursor bronchial lesions of lung cancer. Clin Cancer Res 1998; 4:1609–18.

12. Colby TV, Koss MN, Travis WD, Tumors of the Lower Respiratory Tract; Armed Forces Institute of Pathology Fascicle, Third Series. Washington, DC, Armed Forces Institute of Pathology, 1995.

13. Bennett WP, Colby TV, Travis WD, et al, p53 protein accumulates frequently in early bronchial neoplasia. Cancer Res 1993; 53: 4817–22.

14. Carter D, Pathology of early squamous cell carcinoma of the lung. Pathol Ann 1978; 13 (Pt 1): 131–47.

15. McDowell EM, McLaughlin JS, Merenyl DK, et al, The respiratory epithelium. V. Histogenesis of lung carcinomas in the human. J Natl Cancer Inst 1978; 61:587–606.

16. Woolner LB, Lung. In: Henson DE, Albores-Saavedra J (eds) Pathology of Incipient Neoplasia. Philadelphia, W.B. Saunders Company, 1993, 191–221.

17. Flug M, Kopf-Maier P, The basement membrane and its involvement in carcinoma cell invasion. Acta Anat (Basel) 1995; 152:69–84.

18. Bosman FT, The borderline:basement membranes and the transition from premalignant to malignant neoplasia. Microsc Res Tech 1994; 28:216–25.

19. Müller KM, Muller G, The ultrastructure of preneoplastic changes in the bronchial mucosa. Curr Top Pathol 1983; 73:233–63.

20. Keith RL, Miller YE, Gemmill RM, et al, Angiogenic squamous dysplasia in bronchi of individuals at high risk for lung cancer. Clin Cancer Res 2000; 6:1616–25.

21. Kerr KM, Pulmonary preinvasive neoplasia. J Clin Pathol 2001; 54:257–71.

22. Travis WD, Pathology of pulmonary incipient neoplasia. In: Albores-Saavedra J, Henson DE (eds) Pathology of Incipient Neoplasia. Philadelphia, W.B. Saunders Co., 2000.

23. Woolner LB, Fontana RS, Cortese DA, et al, Roentgenographically occult lung cancer: pathologic findings and frequency of multicentricity during a 10-year period. Mayo Clin Proc 1984; 59:453–66.

24. Fong KM, Biesterveld EJ, Virmani A, et al, FHIT and FRA3B 3p14.2 allele loss are common in lung cancer and preneoplastic bronchial lesions and are associated with cancer-related FHIT cDNA splicing aberrations. Cancer Res 1997; 57:2256–67.

25. Sozzi G, Pastorino U, Moiraghi L, et al, Loss of FHIT function in lung cancer and preinvasive bronchial lesions. Cancer Res 1998; 58:5032–7.

26. Sundaresan V, Ganly P, Hasleton P, et al, p53 and chromosome 3 abnormalities, characteristic of malignant lung tumours, are detectable in preinvasive lesions of the bronchus. Oncogene 1992; 7:1989–97.

27. Wistuba II, Behrens C, Milchgrub S, et al, Sequential molecular abnormalities are involved

in the multistage development of squamous cell lung carcinoma [in process citation]. Oncogene 1999; 18:643–50.

28. Wistuba II, Lam S, Behrens C, et al, Molecular damage in the bronchial epithelium of current and former smokers. J Natl Cancer Inst 1997; 89:1366–73.

29. Chung GT, Sundaresan V, Hasleton P, et al, Sequential molecular genetic changes in lung cancer development. Oncogene 1995; 11: 2591–8.

30. Brambilla E, Gazzeri S, Moro D, et al, Alterations of Rb pathway (Rb-p16INK4-cyclin D1) in pre-invasive bronchial lesions. Clin Cancer Res 1999; 5:243–50.

31. Sozzi G, Miozzo M, Donghi R, et al, Deletions of 17p and p53 mutations in preneoplastic lesions of the lung. Cancer Res 1992; 52:6079–82.

32. Yashima K, Litzky LA, Kaiser L, et al, Telomerase expression in respiratory epithelium during the multistage pathogenesis of lung carcinomas. Cancer Res 1997; 57:2373–7.

33. Smith AL, Hung J, Walker L, et al, Extensive areas of aneuploidy are present in the respiratory epithelium of lung cancer patients. Br J Cancer 1996; 73:203–9.

34. Fisseler-Eckhoff A, Prebeg M, Voss B, Muller KM, Extracellular matrix in preneoplastic lesions and early cancer of the lung. Pathol Res Pract 1990; 186:95–101.

35. Bolon I, Brambilla E, Vandenbunder B, et al, Changes in the expression of matrix proteases and of the transcription factor c-Ets-1 during progression of precancerous bronchial lesions. Lab Invest 1996; 75:1–13.

36. Imai T, Saito Y, Nagamoto N, et al, Electron microscopic observations in in situ and micro-invasive bronchogenic squamous cell carcinoma. J Pathol 1988; 156:241–9.

37. Galateau-Salle FB, Luna RE, Horiba K, et al, Matrix metalloproteinases (MMPs) and tissue inhibitors of metalloproteinases (TIMPs) in bronchial squamous preneoplastic lesions. Mod Pathol 1998; 11:175A(abstract)

38. Noguchi M, Shimosato Y, The development and progression of adenocarcinoma of the lung. Cancer Treat Res 1995; 72:131–42.

39. Kitamura H, Kameda Y, Ito T, Hayashi H, Atypical adenomatous hyperplasia of the lung. Implications for the pathogenesis of peripheral lung adenocarcinoma [in process citation]. Am J Clin Pathol 1999; 111:610–22.

40. Miller RR, Bronchioloalveolar cell adenomas. Am J Surg Pathol 1990; 14:904–12.

41. Weng SY, Tsuchiya E, Kasuga T, Sugano H, Incidence of atypical bronchioloalveolar cell hyperplasia of the lung: relation to histological subtypes of lung cancer. Virchows Arch A Pathol Anat Histopathol 1992; 420:463–71.

42. Carey FA, Wallace WA, Fergusson RJ, Kerr KM, Lamb D, Alveolar atypical hyperplasia in association with primary pulmonary adenocarcinoma: a clinicopathological study of 10 cases. Thorax 1992; 47:1041–3.

43. Nakanishi K, Alveolar epithelial hyperplasia and adenocarcinoma of the lung. Arch Pathol Lab Med 1990; 114:363–8.

44. Meyer EC, Liebow AA, Relationship of interstitial pneumonia, honeycombing, and atypical epithelial proliferation to cancer of the lung. Cancer 1965; 18:322–51.

45. Raeburn C, Spencer H, A study of the origin and development of lung cancer. Thorax 1953; 8, 1–10.

46. Spencer H, Raeburn C, Pulmonary (bronchiolar) adenomatosis. J Pathol Bacteriol 1956; 71:145–54.

47. Fraire AE, Greenberg SD, Carcinoma and diffuse interstitial fibrosis of lung. Cancer 1973; 31: 1078–86.

48. Muir TE, Leslie KO, Popper H, et al, Micronodular pneumocyte hyperplasia. Am J Surg Pathol 1998; 22:465–72.

49. Myers JL, Veal CF Jr, Shin MS, Katzenstein AL, Respiratory bronchiolitis causing interstitial lung disease. A clinicopathologic study of six cases. Am Rev Respir Dis 1987; 135:880–4.

50. Colby TV, Bronchiolitis. Pathologic considerations. Am J Clin Pathol 1998; 109:101–9.

51. Sanchez-Jimenez J, Ballester-Martinez A, Lodo-

Besse J, et al, Papillary adenoma of type 2 pneumocytes. Pediatr Pulmonol 1994; 17:396–400.

52. Mori M, Chiba R, Tezuka F, et al, Papillary adenoma of type II pneumocytes might have malignant potential. Virchows Arch 1996; 428:195–200.

53. Ritter JH, Pulmonary atypical adenomatous hyperplasia. A histologic lesion in search of usable criteria and clinical significance. Am J Clin Pathol 1999; 111:587–9.

54. Nakanishi K, Kawai T, Kumaki F, et al, Survivin expression in atypical adenomatous hyperplasia of the lung. Am J Clin Pathol 2003; 120:712–19.

55. Suzuki K, Nagai K, Yoshida J, et al, The prognosis of resected lung carcinoma associated with atypical adenomatous hyperplasia: a comparison of the prognosis of well-differentiated adenocarcinoma associated with atypical adenomatous hyperplasia and intrapulmonary metastasis. Cancer 1997; 79:1521–6.

56. Kitaguchi S, Takeshima Y, Nishisaka T, Inai K, Proliferative activity, p53 expression and loss of heterozygosity on 3p, 9p and 17p in atypical adenomatous hyperplasia of the lung. Hiroshima J Med Sci 1998; 47:17–25.

57. Kitamura H, Kameda Y, Nakamura N, et al, Proliferative potential and p53 overexpression in precursor and early stage lesions of bronchioloalveolar lung carcinoma. Am J Pathol 1995; 146:876–87.

58. Kurasono Y, Ito T, Kameda Y, Nakamura N, Kitamura H, Expression of cyclin D1, retinoblastoma gene protein, and p16 MTS1 protein in atypical adenomatous hyperplasia and adenocarcinoma of the lung. An immunohistochemical analysis. Virchows Arch 1998; 432:207–15.

59. Pueblitz S, Hieger LR, Expression of p53 and CEA in atypical adenomatous hyperplasia of the lung [letter; comment]. Am J Surg Pathol 1997; 21:867–8.

60. Nakayama H, Noguchi M, Tsuchiya R, Kodama T, Shimosato Y, Clonal growth of atypical adenomatous hyperplasia of the lung: cytofluorometric analysis of nuclear DNA content. Mod Pathol 1990; 3:314–20.

61. Niho S, Yokose T, Suzuki K, et al, Monoclonality of atypical adenomatous hyperplasia of the lung. Am J Pathol 1999; 154:249–54.

62. Rao SK, Fraire AE, Alveolar cell hyperplasia in association with adenocarcinoma of lung. Mod Pathol 1995; 8:165–9.

63. Mori M, Tezuka F, Chiba R, et al, Atypical adenomatous hyperplasia and adenocarcinoma of the human lung. Their heterology in form and analogy in immunohistochemical characteristics. Cancer 1996; 77:665–74.

64. Mori M, Kaji M, Tezuka F, Takahashi T, Comparative ultrastructural study of atypical adenomatous hyperplasia and adenocarcinoma of the human lung. Ultrastruct Pathol 1998; 22:459–66.

65. Kodama T, Biyajima S, Watanabe S, Shimosato Y, Morphometric study of adenocarcinomas and hyperplastic epithelial lesions in the peripheral lung. Am J Clin Pathol 1986; 85:146–51.

66. Mori M, Chiba R, Takahashi T, Atypical adenomatous hyperplasia of the lung and its differentiation from adenocarcinoma. Characterization of atypical cells by morphometry and multivariate cluster analysis. Cancer 1993; 72:2331–40.

67. Kerr KM, Carey FA, King G, Lamb D, Atypical alveolar hyperplasia: relationship with pulmonary adenocarcinoma, p53, and c-erbB-2 expression. J Pathol 1994; 174:249–56.

68. Slebos RJ, Baas IO, Clement MJ, et al, p53 alterations in atypical alveolar hyperplasia of the human lung. Hum Pathol 1998; 29:801–8.

69. Ohshima S, Shimizu Y, Takahama M, Detection of c-Ki-ras gene mutation in paraffin sections of adenocarcinoma and atypical bronchioloalveolar cell hyperplasia of human lung. Virchows Arch 1994; 424:129–34.

70. Sugio K, Kishimoto Y, Virmani AK, Hung JY, Gazdar AF, K-ras mutations are a relatively late event in the pathogenesis of lung carcinomas. Cancer Res 1994; 54:5811–15.

71. Westra WH, Baas IO, Hruban RH, et al, K-ras oncogene activation in atypical alveolar hyperplasias of the human lung. Cancer Res 1996; 56:2224–8.

72. Brown MJ, English J, Muller NL, Bronchiolitis obliterans due to neuroendocrine hyperplasia: high-resolution CT – pathologic correlation. AJR. Am J Roentgenol 1997; 168:1561–2.

73. Sheerin N, Harrison NK, Sheppard MN, et al, Obliterative bronchiolitis caused by multiple tumourlets and microcarcinoids successfully treated by single lung transplantation. Thorax 1995; 50:207–9.

74. Aguayo SM, Miller YE, Waldron JA Jr, et al, Brief report: idiopathic diffuse hyperplasia of pulmonary neuroendocrine cells and airways disease. N Engl J Med 1992; 327:1285–8.

75. Miller MA, Mark GJ, Kanarek D, Multiple peripheral pulmonary carcinoids and tumorlets of carcinoid type, with restrictive and obstructive lung disease. Am J Med 1978; 65:373–8.

76. Lee JS, Brown KK, Cool C, Lynch DA, Diffuse pulmonary neuroendocrine cell hyperplasia: radiologic and clinical features. J Comput Assist Tomogr 2002; 26:180–4.

77. Miller RR, Muller NL, Neuroendocrine cell hyperplasia and obliterative bronchiolitis in patients with peripheral carcinoid tumors. Am J Surg Pathol 1995; 19:653–8.

78. Finkelstein SD, Hasegawa T, Colby T, Yousem SA, 11q13 allelic imbalance discriminates pulmonary carcinoids from tumorlets. A microdissection-based genotyping approach useful in clinical practice. Am J Pathol 1999; 155: 633–40.

79. Cohen AJ, King TE Jr, Gilman LB, Magill-Solc C, Miller YE, High expression of neutral endopeptidase in idiopathic diffuse hyperplasia of pulmonary neuroendocrine cells. Am J Respir Crit Care Med 1998; 158:1593–9.

80. Gosney JR, Pulmonary neuroendocrine cell system in pediatric and adult lung disease. Microsc Res Tech 1997; 37:107–13.

81. Bonikos DS, Archibald R, Bensch KG, On the origin of the so-called tumorlets of the lung. Hum Pathol 1976; 7:461–9.

82. Churg A, Warnock ML, Pulmonary tumorlet. A form of peripheral carcinoid. Cancer 1976; 37: 1469–77.

83. Ranchod M, The histogenesis and development of pulmonary tumorlets. Cancer 1977; 39:1135–45.

84. World Health Organization, Histological typing of lung tumours. Geneva, World Health Organization, 1967.

85. World Health Organization, Histological typing of lung tumors. Geneva, World Health Organization, 1981.

6 Lung carcinogenesis: biology

Gabriella Sozzi, Francesca Andriani, Luca Roz,
Tommaso A Dragani, Giacomo Manenti,
Manuela Gariboldi, Elisabeth Brambilla

Contents   Introduction • Alterations in positive growth signal: proto-oncogenes • Alterations in apoptotic pathways • Alterations of negative growth signals: tumor suppressor genes • Genotypic and somatic markers

INTRODUCTION

Lung cancer is the leading cause of cancer-related deaths and is projected to reach epidemic levels in the world during the 21st century. Identification of individuals at the earliest stages of lung cancer in which curative resection is feasible could greatly reduce mortality. In this respect, the elucidation of genetic and biological changes characterizing the malignant transformation of cells and the development of sensitive techniques able to detect molecular signatures of tumorigenesis in tissues and also in body fluids could actually contribute to improve early detection, risk assessment and disease monitoring which ultimately might result in reduction of lung cancer-related mortality.

It is now well established that lung carcinogenesis is a stepwise process whereby multiple and sequential genetic changes must occur in the bronchial epithelial cell to achieve transformation into cancerous cell. Of crucial interest was the demonstration that genetic abnormalities were already present in normal appearing bronchial cells not only from lung cancer patients but also from disease-free chronic, current or former, smokers as a result of the genotoxic effect of tobacco smoking.[1–3]

In addition while in lung cancer, as for the majority of sporadic cancers, evidence of genes conferring strong susceptibility to the onset of the disease has not been conclusively proved so far, genetic polymorphisms might likely have a larger quantitative effect on the risk of lung cancer.[4]

It is quite apparent that in lung cancer conventional histopathology including the classification system and technologies have their limits in providing additional novel markers to improve the management of lung cancer patients. For this reason numerous molecular aberrations have been explored as potential new diagnostic markers and markers for molecular sub-staging. The completion of the human genome sequencing program is recently impacting in the development of new global approaches and high-throughput technologies for profiling the genetic basis of cancer. In particular, high-throughput approaches such as array-CGH for genomic profiling, cDNA microarrays for expression profiling and tissue arrays for DNA, RNA and protein status analyses are highly promising tools for refinement of histopathological classification and clinical outcome.[5–7] In addition, integration of microarray technologies such as large-scale profiling of the genome, transcriptome and proteome might lead to the identification of novel targets and also to prioritization of targets. This chapter is not meant to be exhaustive but will attempt to summarize the current understanding on the role of selected molecular changes at the clinical level, especially with respect to their use as diagnostic and prognostic/predictive markers as well as early detection biomarkers.

We will focus particularly on alterations in positive and negative growth-control signals and apoptosis and on the molecular mechanisms of these alterations that include genetic changes like amplification, LOH and point mutations as well as down-regulation of gene expression through epigenetic silencing. We will highlight the possible role of these alterations for predicting prognosis or for their use as therapeutical targets and we will discuss the present knowledge on the identification of somatic and constitutional lesions in peripheral blood and how they could advance early detection and risk assessment of lung cancer disease.

ALTERATIONS IN POSITIVE GROWTH SIGNAL: PROTO-ONCOGENES

Table 6.1 summarizes the frequency in NSCLC and SCLC histotypes of the major molecular alterations described below in the text.

Receptor tyrosine kinases

Autocrine and paracrine growth stimulation loops are produced as a consequence of the expression of growth factors and their receptors by both lung cancer and adjacent stromal cells. Receptor tyrosine kinases and particularly the *ERBB* family receptors constitute major components in positive signaling cascade and are overexpressed in lung cancer cells. Upon binding with their respective ligands *ERBB* receptors homo-heterodimerize thereby initiating intracellular signal transduction cascades through various pathways, including *RAS*-mediated pathways such as *MAP* kinases.

Table 6.1 Frequency of molecular changes in lung cancer		
Alteration	**Small-cell lung cancer**	**Non-small cell lung cancer**
Receptor tyrosine kinases	c-kit 70%	EGFR overexpression: 90% (SCC); 50% (ADC)
		HER2/neu: 30% (ADC)
	MET point mutations (rare)	MET overexpression: 25%
RAS point mutations	–	10–30% (ADC)
MYC family amplification	65% high level	50% low level
p53 inactivation	75–100%	50%
Rb inactivation	90%	15–30%
p16^{INK4A} inactivation	0–10%	30–40%
FHIT inactivation	80%	50–70%
3p, 9p, 13q, 17p allelic loss	90%	70%
Bcl2 overexpression	75–90%	30%

SCC = squamous cell carcinoma; ADC = adenocarcinoma; EGFR = epidermal growth factor receptor; Rb = retinoblastoma gene; FHIT = Fragile histidine triad.

The tyrosine kinase receptors involved in lung cancer are the epidermal growth factor receptor (*EGFR*), *HER2/neu*, *c-KIT* and *c-MET*. These members are expressed independently of one another in the various subtypes of NSCLC and in SCLC.

EGFR regulates proliferation and differentiation of epithelial cells, and together with its ligands epidermal growth factor (EGF) and transforming growth factor-alpha (TGF-α), is overexpressed in NSCLCs, especially in squamous cell carcinoma (SCC), but rarely in SCLC. By immunohistochemistry (IHC) high expression of *EGFR* has been reported in >90% of SCC and in about 50% of adenocarcinoma (ADC)[8] as well as in preneoplasia, with an apparent stepwise increase in its expression from uninvolved bronchial mucosa to epithelial hyperplasia to cancer, particularly in subjects who had developed lung cancer compared with those who had not, suggesting its involvement in lung carcinogenesis.[9,10]

Another *ERBB* family member, *HER2/neu*, is highly expressed (gene amplification rarely occurs in lung cancer) in about 30% of NSCLC, especially ADC.

The prognostic value of *EGFR* as well as *HER2/neu* overexpression in NSCLC remains controversial.[11–13] Clinical trials investigating monoclonal antibodies against *EGFR* (C225, ImClone) and *HER2/neu* (Herceptin) as well as tyrosine kinase inhibitors such as *EGFR* blocker ZD1839-Iressa, in combination with chemotherapy are in progress in lung cancer.[14,15] Recently, mutations in the tyrosine kinase domain of EGFR strongly associated with gefitinib and erlotinib sensitivity in NSCLC patients were identified. The incidence of EGFR mutations is only 10% in unselected populations, whereas they are more frequently found in tumors from never smokers, females adenocarcinomas and in patients of East Asian origin.[16]

At least 70% of small cell lung cancers express the *c-KIT* receptor tyrosine kinase and its ligand, stem cell factor (SCF). Numerous lines of evidence have demonstrated that this coexpression constitutes a functional autocrine loop, suggesting that inhibitors of Kit tyrosine kinase activity could have therapeutic efficacy in this disease. STI571, that was designed as an Abl tyrosine kinase inhibitor, but also has efficacy against the platelet-derived growth factor receptor and Kit in vitro, is an attractive novel therapeutic approach for this lethal subtype.[17]

The receptor tyrosine kinase *c-MET* has been implicated in various solid tumors, including SCLC, and is involved in mediating tumorigenesis, cell motility, scattering, invasion and metastasis.

Overexpression and activation of c-MET and its ligand hepatocyte growth factor/scatter factor has been detected in 25% of primary non-small-cell lung carcinomas[18] and in SCLC cell lines[19] demonstrating that the c-Met/HGF pathway is functional. Recently novel gain-of-function somatic mutations in the JM domain of c-MET have been reported in a small percentage of SCLC samples[20] but with significant implications in cytoskeletal functions and metastatic potentially associated with a more aggressive phenotype. These results suggest a role of c-MET signaling in SCLC thus making the inhibition of c-MET a possible therapeutic target against SCLC.[20]

Ras family

The ras family is composed of three subtypes encoded by different genes, H-, N-, and K-ras.[21] Point mutation of these genes is rather specific with regard to the organ or histological type of tumors. Mutations of the *K-ras* gene are seen in colorectal, pancreatic, endometrial and lung cancers.[22,23] In lung cancer, *K-ras* gene point mutations, which most frequently occur at codon 12, are restricted exclusively to adeno-carcinoma, with a frequency of 10–30%.[24]

Kras2 gene is causally linked with lung tumorigenesis, since somatic mutations of this gene cause lung tumor development in mice.[24] A gene-targeting procedure was used to create mouse strains carrying oncogenic alleles of Kras2 that can be activated only on a spontaneous recombination event in the whole animal. Mice carrying these mutations were highly predisposed to early-onset lung cancer.[25]

The wild-type Kras2 allele seems to have a tumor suppressor activity in mutant-ras driven lung tumorigenesis.[26] Indeed, a lung tumor bioassay showed that mice with a heterozygous Kras2 deficiency were highly susceptible to the chemical induction of lung tumors when compared to wild-type mice.[26] Allelic loss of wild-type Kras2 was found in 67–100% of chemically induced mouse lung adenocarcinomas that harbor a mutant Kras2 allele.[26] However, in contrast with the reported loss of heterozygosity of the wild-type Kras2 allele in mouse lung tumors,[26] we have recently found an almost perfect 1:1 ratio of the wild-type and mutated Kras2 alleles in lung tumors.[27] In mice, genomic Kras2 polymorphisms are tightly linked with genetic predisposition to lung cancer and with the Pas1 locus;[27] thus, we can hypothesize that these genomic polymorphisms might modulate gene mutability and, in turn, numbers of tumors after chemical carcinogen treatment.

MYC family

The MYC (MYCC, MYCN and MYCL) oncogene family shares many structural and functional similarities and encodes a group of nuclear phosphoproteins that plays a role in cell growth and in the development of human tumors. Depending on the cellular context, however, the MYC family of proteins is also known for its potent apoptotic properties.[28]

Alterations of MYC gene family members have been reported at various levels by a variety of methodologies. Distal 8q region, where MYCC is located, was gained by CGH in 65% of samples of both SCLC and NSCLC type (eight primary tumors and 15 cell lines) and low-level MYCC amplification was confirmed by FISH analysis.[29] Amplification of MYCC (more than four copies) was observed at a similar frequency in SCLC and NSCLC by PCR approaches.[30] High-level MYCC DNA amplification was not a frequent finding in NSCLC[29] but high-level amplification of regions containing MYCL and MYCN was reported in SCLC.[31] MYC family amplification occurs more commonly in specimens from chemotherapy-treated than -untreated SCLC patients.[32] A study that analyzed by FISH the copy number of MYCC with respect to centromeric signals in 31 NSCLC primary tumors showed that MYCC amplification occurred in about 50% of the patients with a significant difference between N0 and N2 tumors.[33]

In addition to amplification, MYCC overexpression has also been reported in lung cancer cell lines[34] and primary tumor samples.[35] Considering that MYC overexpression can also act as a potent stimulator of apoptosis it is interesting to note that MYC-amplified SCLC lines had significantly higher rates of loss of Death Inducing Signalling Complex (DISC) components than MYC-negative lines.[36] Although the mechanism of MYC action is not yet fully understood, MYC has been proposed to play a role in growth control and cell cycle progression by stimulating and repressing the expression of key cell cycle regulators.[37] Recent data point to MYC oncogenes as another potential molecular target for the development of novel drugs that can specifically regulate MYC-related cell cycle activity in lung cancer.[38]

ALTERATIONS IN APOPTOTIC PATHWAYS

Bax/Bcl2 apoptotic factors

Besides cell cycle deregulation, loss of suscepti-bility for apoptosis leads to cell accumulation and tumor growth. Bcl2 and Bax are respectively anti-apoptotic and apoptotic factors of the Bcl2 family of proteins. Their equilibrium in the cell cytoplasm at mitochondrial membrane is known to influence the susceptibility for apop-tosis.[39,40] Bcl2 overexpression has been demonstrated in about 30% of non-small-cell lung carcinoma (NSCLC),[41,42] as well as an inversion of Bax:Bcl2 ratio in favor of Bcl2 in precursor bronchial lesions of lung cancer.[43,44] Bax is one of the main target genes of p53 tran-scription for apoptosis along with Fas, IGF, BP3, TRAIL Receptor 5. Thus, the effect of wild-type p53 on apoptosis may be mediated in part through its effects on the expression on Bax and Bcl2 since wild-type p53 may induce the tran-scription of Bax and repress that of Bcl2.[45] When Bax and Bcl2 expression were immuno-histochemically assessed in preinvasive lung lesions,[43,46] Bcl2 overexpression and Bax down-regulation was observed in an increasing pro-portion of preinvasive lesions with their histological grade, with a Bcl2:Bax ratio deregu-lated in favor of Bcl2 in respectively 3% of meta-plasia, 25% of mild dysplasia, 67% of moderate dysplasia, 78% of severe dysplasia and 53% of CIS. It is worthwhile to mention that the highest frequency of Bcl2 overexpression in NSCLC was of only 30%, which provides support to the concept that susceptibility to apoptosis during the preneoplastic states related to Bcl2 and Bax ratio is more mandatory during the clonal selection of preinvasion lesions, than after invasion and clonal selection against multiple apoptotic pathways.

ALTERATIONS OF NEGATIVE GROWTH SIGNALS: TUMOR SUPPRESSOR GENES

Loss of heterozygosity (LOH)

In lung cancer it has long been shown that chromosome arms 3p (*FHIT* locus and several other sites), 13q (Rb locus) and 17p (p53 locus) have the most frequent LOH in both SCLC (>90%) and NSCLC (>70%).[47–51] A high-resolution (10 cM) genome-wide search using 399 markers evenly spaced across the genome performed in 36 lung cancer cell lines showed 22 regions with more than 60% LOH, 13 with a preference for SCLC, seven for NSCLC and two affecting both tumor types, confirming and extending the previous results obtained on primary tumors. The chromosomal arms with the most frequent LOH were: 1p, 3p, 4p, 4q, 5q, 8p, 9p, 9q, 10p, 10q, 13q, 15q, 17p, 18q, 19p, Xp, Xq.[52]

Human bronchial carcinoma is thought to develop through progressive stages from basal cell hyperplasia to squamous metaplasia, dys-plasia, carcinoma in situ, and finally invasive cancer. Loss of heterozygosity of chromosomes 3p14.2, 3p21, 5q21, 9p21 and 17p13 was examined by several authors at each stage of the epithelial progression to invasive cancers.[2,50,53–56] LOH frequency and size increased significantly from the lowest to the highest grade lesions, showing evidence of accumulation of genetic damage. The molecular follow-up analysis showed that the same genomic alteration can persist in a given dysplastic bronchial area for several months or years, and that the persis-tence or the regression of the molecular abnor-mality is well correlated with the evolution of the disease on follow-up.[56,57] In addition mul-tiple small clonal or subclonal patches contain-ing LOH are present in normal or slightly abnormal bronchial epithelium of disease-free current or former smokers[1,2] and in patients with lung cancer.[3,56] Longitudinal prospective trials are needed in order to determine if the presence of LOH in biological samples just reflect smoking related lung damage or truly indicate an increased risk of neoplastic transformation.

Promoter hypermethylation

Promoter hypermethylation is recognized as an important epigenetic mechanism for silencing the expression of a tumor suppressor gene (TSG). Hypermethylation of certain gene promoters has a relevance in a context of early detection for several reasons. In contrast to genetic markers, in which mutations occur at multiple sites and can be of very different types, promoter hypermethylation occurs only within CpG islands. Furthermore, hypermethylation is a positive signal that can be observed even in a high background of normal cells whereas genetic changes such as loss of heterozygosity and homozygous deletions, cannot be detected easily. Several papers attempted to define the DNA methylation signature (also called 'methylotype') of lung cancer trying to identify which markers are always unmethylated in normal cells and can be used for methylation profiling of lung cancer cells in biological fluids. In particular the following tumor suppressor genes have been reported as frequently methylated in lung cancer: $p16^{INK4}$,[59–61] $RARB$,[62,63] $FHIT$,[63] $RASSF1$,[64,65] MGM,[66] $DAPK$,[67] APC,[68,69] $CDH1$.[63] For these studies various technical approaches have been developed, the most promising, in a context of early detection, being a nested-methylation specific PCR (MSP) assay that allows distinguishing methylated from unmethylated CpG by means of a differential PCR amplification with specific primers after conversion of unmethylated cytosines into thymidines and quantitative assays such as real-time-PCR. The promoter hypermethylation in

tumor suppressor genes occurs early in tumorigenesis but the presence of aberrant methylation alone does not necessarily indicate an invasive cancer since premalignant or precursor lesions (especially those more exposed to carcinogens) can also carry this epigenetic markers.[66,70,71] This finding has implications for early detection, especially in high-risk individuals. In fact, aberrant DNA methylation has been found up to 3 years before diagnosis of lung cancer in exposed individuals.[66]

Reactivation of the promoter of methylated genes is now being developed both as a therapeutic approach or as chemopreventive treatment as in the case of restoring sensitivity to retinoic acid through demethylation of RARB promoter.

FHIT and chromosome 3p genes

Chromosome 3p deletions are the most frequent genetic abnormalities observed in lung cancer with almost 100% of SCLC and 90% of NSCLC showing loss of at least a portion of this chromosomal arm in a detailed deletion mapping analysis of micro-dissected samples.[50] These deletions occur very early in lung cancer development, being present in almost 80% of preinvasive bronchial lesions and in histologically normal epithelium from smokers but not from never smokers[50] and are also very common in many other major cancers of epithelial origin indicating that chromosome 3p may harbor tumor suppressor genes (TSGs) that play an early and fundamental role in epithelial carcinogenesis.[72] Functional support for this hypothesis has also initially been obtained by microcell fusion experiments that demonstrated tumor suppressor activity of several 3p regions[73] and then by targeted reintroduction in deleted cells of some of the many candidate TSGs identified in this area. The techniques used to study 3p deletions ranged over the years from microsatellite amplification for loss of heterozygosity detection (LOH) to genome-wide comparative genomic hybridization (CGH), or more recently to single nucleotide polymorphism (SNP) analysis: the pattern of deletion that emerges from the many different studies that have investigated this genomic region in NSCLC is very complex, with evidence of many areas of discontinuous loss of genetic material. Although some of the discrepancies in the results from different studies may be explained with technical problems due to contamination from normal tissue, biased detection of LOH in certain alleles[74] or imprecise mapping of some of the polymorphic markers, it now appears clear that there are distinct regions on 3p-containing genes with tumor suppressive properties.

Together with the complex pattern of deletions the hunt for TSGs on chromosome 3p has also been complicated by the fact that for many of the candidates studied the loss-of-function mechanism did not seem to fit the classical two-hit hypothesis formulated by Knudson. Recent attention to the relevance of epigenetic mechanisms in TSG inactivation such as transcriptional repression through promoter hypermethylation has changed this perspective as many of the genes mapping to chromosome 3p seem to be silenced in this way rather than through point mutations. Furthermore some of the genes may suffer from haploinsufficiency and therefore a rearrangement targeting only one allele could be sufficient to promote neoplastic growth. These peculiar inactivation mechanisms have generated substantial controversy on the evidences needed to validate the tumor suppressor function of the isolated genes.[75]

In conclusion, many areas of deletion on 3p have been identified and numerous putative TSGs were isolated from these regions,[76] but many of these lack sufficient support to be classified as bona fide TSG involved in lung carcinogenesis. The following description will therefore concentrate on some of the most extensively characterized from a functional point of view and on those for which a mouse model is available. Many of the most promising candidates were isolated from areas of homozygous deletions that have helped to pinpoint some hotspots for the rearrangements in particular at 3p12, 3p14.2 and 3p21.3.

ROBO1/DUTT1 (3p12)

The ROBO1 gene exemplifies the problems related to the validation of a candidate 3p TSG. It resides in a region on 3p12 frequently involved in homozygous deletions in lung, renal and breast cancer and it was demonstrated that the chromosome 3p12-p14 region could suppress the tumorigenic phenotype in a renal cell carcinoma (RCC) cell line.[77] The gene codes for a 1615 amino acid (aa) protein homologous to the Drosophila Roundabout, a receptor with similarities to NCAM which has been implicated in the guidance and migration of axons, myoblasts and leukocytes in vertebrates.[78,79] Although its location and function made it a very attractive candidate as a TSG, mutation analysis in lung, breast and renal cancers did not reveal any alteration and promoter hypermethylation was reported in 19% of primary breast carcinomas, 18% of primary CC-RCC, but only 4% (1/26) of NSCLC.[80] On the other hand, the mouse model displays a very interesting phenotype of delayed lung maturation: many nullizygous mice die of respiratory failure and the survivors show bronchial hyperplasia indicating a possible intriguing link between a chromosome 3p gene and bronchial function.[81] In conclusion there are some interesting indications on the possible relevance of ROBO1/DUTT1 in early lung cancer from functional studies but its relevance as a TSG for NSCLC still has to be confirmed.

FHIT (3p14.2)

The chromosomal region around 3p14.2 has been the site of thorough investigation for the presence of a TSG since the description of a family with a t(3;8)(p14.2;q24.1) translocation predisposing to renal cell cancer.[82] Analysis of the breakpoint area on chromosome 3p led to the identification of the FHIT (fragile histidine triad) gene, covering 1.8 Mb on 3p14.2 and encoding for a small protein of 147 aa with homology to the highly conserved Histidine Triad Superfamily of proteins, involved in the metabolism of diadenosine polyphosphates.[83] Within the FHIT gene is also contained FRA3B, the most active among the aphidicolin inducible fragile sites in the human genome, and it has been suggested that this localization could contribute to the rearrangements observed in cancer by making this gene particularly susceptible to the damage induced by carcinogenic substances. Altered expression of FHIT mRNA has been reported in several human cancers including gastric, esophageal, cervical and lung carcinomas (reviewed in[84]) and the gene seems to be preferentially inactivated by large scale rearrangements or discontinuous biallelic deletions and not by mutations.[85] Promoter hypermethylation has also been shown to contribute to gene silencing in 37% of primary NSCLC and 65% of lung cancer cell lines.[63] Strong support for the importance of Fhit loss-of-function in the development of cancer comes from two lines of investigation: protein expression analyses and functional studies of the mouse model and of the effect of Fhit reintroduction in Fhit-negative cell lines. In the largest immunohistochemical analysis described so far (474 cases of NSCLC) reduced or lost Fhit expression was reported in 73% of primary tumors and 93% of preinvasive lesions, indicating an early and central role of Fhit in lung carcinogenesis.[86] In particular the percentage of Fhit-negative tumors was higher

in smokers than in non-smokers (75% vs 39%, $P < 0.0005$) confirming the possibility that the gene is a direct target of carcinogenic damage. Reintroduction of FHIT in lung cancer cell lines has been shown to slow growth, induce apoptosis and reduce in vivo tumorigenicity using both plasmid[87] and adenoviral vectors[88,89] as shown in Figure 6.1. Furthermore Fhit-deficient mice are susceptible to both spontaneous tumors of different types and carcinogen-induced tumors of the forestomach[90] and protection from induced tumors could be achieved by administration of viral vectors expressing the Fhit protein.[91] Interestingly the tumor spectrum in these mice is similar for heterozygous (+/−) and homozygous (−/−) animals, indicating that the gene may be haploinsufficient. The reduced or absent Fhit expression often observed in bronchial dysplasias could then indicate the transition from normal epithelium to a preneoplastic state characterized by resistance to apoptotic stimuli and the consequent possibility of accumulation of genetic damage.

3p21.3 (LUCA region)

The 3p21.3 region is the most frequently targeted by deletions and rearrangements in lung cancers, possesses tumor suppressor activity in vivo[92] and has long been thought to contain gene(s) playing a central role in lung cancer development. Conversely, this region is extremely gene rich, making it difficult to understand the role of single candidate genes in the oncogenic transformation. A minimal region of deletion of 630 Kb named LUCA (lung cancer TSG region) was defined by the analysis of nested homozygous deletions in various cancer cell lines and over 20 different genes have been isolated from this region.[93] Many of these genes showed reduced expression in lung cancer specimens but none of them displayed a high mutation rate (>10%), indicating that if they are

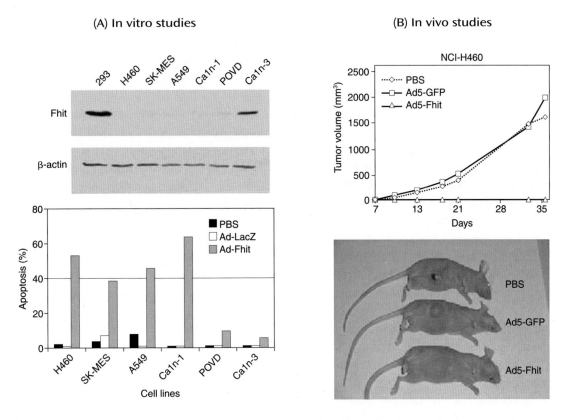

Figure 6.1
Oncosuppressive effects of restoration of FHIT expression in lung cancer cell lines. (A) In vitro
studies. Lack of expression of the Fhit protein in most lung cancer cell lines (upper panel) and pro-
apoptotic effect of adenoviral-mediated Fhit transfer in Fhit-negative cell lines (lower panel). (B) In
vivo studies. Reduction of the tumorigenic potential in the nude mouse of NCI-H460 lung cancer
cells after in vitro transfer of the FHIT gene.

TSG they may be inactivated by alternative
mechanisms (i.e. methylation) or be haploinsufficient. In fact, promoter methylation has been
described frequently with some reports also
showing independent methylation of the
different genes, thus excluding a global regional
alteration of the epigenetic status.

Some of the genes have been evaluated functionally and shown to possess tumor suppressor
properties. The CACNA2D2 gene, that encodes
a functional calcium channel auxiliary subunit,
has been shown to induce apoptosis in NSCLC

cell lines possibly through disruption of mitochondrial membrane integrity[94] and expression
of the BLU gene (methylated in 19% of primary
NSCLC) results in reduced colony formation
ability of the H1299 cell line.[95] Similar functional results were obtained also for FUS1,
101F6 and NPRL2 that were introduced into
adenoviral vectors and shown to inhibit tumor
cell growth by inducing apoptosis and altering
the cycling properties of lung cancer cells.[96] The
same vectors (and also the adenoviral vector
expressing HYAL2, another gene from the

LUCA region) also suppressed tumorigenicity in vivo of H1299 and A549 xenografts.

More data are available on two other putative TSGs from 3p21.3: RASSF1A and SEMA3B. RASSF1A (Ras ASSociation domain Family 1A) is a soluble cytoplasmic protein that contains a Ras association domain and may be involved in the regulation of the Ras signaling pathway. It is frequently inactivated in lung and other cancers by methylation (over 90% of SCLC and 30–40% of NSCLC) and has growth suppressive and anti-tumorigenic properties on lung cancer cell lines.[64,65] Furthermore, promoter methylation was found to correlate with reduced patient survival.[65] This protein has been shown to interfere with cell cycle progression through interaction with the Rb-pathway culminating with inhibition of cyclin D1 accumulation[97] and very recently it was suggested that it may control mitosis by inhibiting the APC-Cdc20[98] complex. It seems therefore likely that RASSF1A could play an important role in the neoplastic transformation by controlling key steps of cellular proliferation.

Semaphorins are a family of secreted transmembrane and membrane-associated proteins initially identified as regulators of nerve growth cone guidance and then found to be potentially involved in cell migration, metastasis, apoptosis and angiogenesis (reviewed in[99]). Two members of the family (SEMA3B and SEMA3F) map to the LUCA region and methylation of the SEMA3B promoter has been found in 40% of primary NSCLC.[100] SEMA3B re-expression in the negative H1299 cell line resulted in apoptosis and strongly reduced colony formation[101] and SEMA3F expression levels seem to correlate with higher-stage disease.[102] In addition, the signaling pathway VEGF/SEMA3F/NP has been shown to be altered early in lung cancer progression[103] indicating that semaphorins should be further investigated as lung cancer TSGs.

RARβ (3p24-p26)

Retinoic acid (RA) plays an important role in lung development and differentiation exerting its action through interaction with its nuclear receptors encoded by the RARβ gene. The observation that RARβ expression is often down-regulated in lung cancer suggests therefore the possibility that the retinoic acid pathway could be involved in lung tumorigenesis and RA analogs have long been tested as chemopreventive agents.[104] Most lung cancer cell lines were also shown to be resistant to the growth-suppression properties of RA as compared to normal lung tissue.[105] Although mutations in the RARβ gene have not been detected in lung cancers, epigenetic inactivation was reported in 72% of SCLC and 41% of NSCLC[62,106] and expression of RARβ2 (the putative tumor suppressor isoform) inhibits Calu-1 cell growth in vitro.[107,108] Finally, it is noteworthy that 60% of the transgenic mice expressing antisense RARβ2 transcripts develop lung tumors with a twofold higher incidence in homozygous versus hemizygous mice[109] confirming the relevance of this pathway in bronchial neoplasias.

The p53 pathway

p53 is a tumor suppressor gene that plays multiple roles in the cells. In response to DNA damage the expression of high levels of wild-type p53 has basically two outcomes: cell cycle arrest, allowing DNA repair and cellular differentiation, and apoptosis, protecting the genome from accumulating excess of mutations.[110] Consistent with this notion, cells lacking p53 seem to be genetically unstable and thus more prone to transformation.

p53 gene is located on chromosome 17p13 and encodes a 53 kDa nuclear phosphoprotein able to bind DNA and acting as a transcription factor. In normal cells p53 is a labile protein with a half-life ranging from 5–30 min,[111] and is present at very low cellular levels, due to continuous degradation mediated by HDM2, the human homologue of the murine double minute 2 (MDM2) oncogene. Upon binding with p53, HDM2 decreases p53 protein levels by enhancing its proteasome-dependent degradation, thus reducing its function as activator of transcription.[112]

Conversely, several cellular stress pathways such as DNA damaging, hypoxia or telomere shortening, lead to a rapid stabilization of *p53* through a block of its degradation. This mechanism is also regulated by another important upstream gene identified as an alternative reading frame gene (ARF) of the p16[INK4A] locus at chromosome 9p21, p14[ARF] (p19[ARF] in mouse). p19[ARF] protein binds MDM2 inhibiting its nuclear export and sequestering this protein into the nucleosome.[113] This mechanism blocks MDM2-induced p53 degradation, stabilizing p53 protein. Thus, downregulation of p14[ARF] results functionally equivalent to loss of p53 function.

Downstream, *p53* induces the expression of *p21*[waf1] that binds cyclin-dependent kinase complexes, blocking the kinase activity. This mechanism prevents the phosphorylation of substrates critical for cell cycle progression and causes, therefore, a G1 phase block, confirming the important role of p53 as a major cell-cycle regulator factor.[114]

Mutations in p53 gene are currently the most commonly identified genetic changes associated with sporadic and hereditary human cancer.[115] Inherited germline *p53* mutations in humans, (Li-Fraumeni syndrome) as well as genetic disruption of this gene in mice, confer a markedly increased susceptibility to cancer. For this reason p53 is considered to be one of the most important genetic biomarkers and it has been extensively studied for its diagnostic/prognostic value and as a possible therapeutic target in different types of cancer, particularly lung cancer. Mutations of p53 gene have been reported in a meta-analysis study as occurring in 75–100% of small-cell lung cancer (SCLC) and in 47% of 4684 non-small-cell lung cancers (NSCLCs), with frequencies around 39% for adenocarcinoma, 51% for squamous-cell carcinoma, and 54% for large-cell carcinoma.[116] Concerning its prognostic value, even though the data published in literature are often controversial, a meta-analysis study, that included more than 1000 patients demonstrated a negative prognostic effect of p53 mutations in patients with lung adenocarcinoma but not in those with squamous-cell carcinoma.[117] In addition a recent prospective study in 188 NSCLC patients suggested that tumor p53 mutations are significant predictors of poor outcome in patients with stage I NSCLC.[118]

Somatic mutations of p53 gene have been identified in highly evolutionary conserved regions, principally from exon 5 to exon 8, which encode the DNA binding domains. Among the somatic mutations, 70–80% are of missense type that results in prolonged half-life of the p53 protein; however small deletions, insertions and splicing errors, which are not detectable at immunohistochemical level, are reported.[119] It has been suggested that only missense mutations, but not the null mutations are associated with negative impact on prognosis.[120]

The mutational spectrum of p53 gene can give information on particular carcinogen exposure or biological mechanism associated with lung cancer formation: p53 mutations linked to cigarette smoking and certain tobacco carcinogens,[121] result in an increased frequency of G to T transversions[122] whereas the spectrum found in non-smokers, is dominated by G to A transitions. Benzopyrene, the major cigarette smoke carcinogen, has been shown to bind and form adducts preferentially at guanine positions at codons 157, 248 and 273, which are important p53 mutational hotspots in bronchial epithelial cells.[123]

p53 alterations are an early event in lung carcinogenesis and the frequency of abnormalities increases with the severity of the lesions. Immuhistochemical studies showed that nuclear p53 protein was present in 0% of normal mucosa, 3–6% of squamous metaplasias, 30–50% of mild dysplasias, 30% of moderate dysplasias, 60–80% of severe dysplasias and 60% of carcinoma in situ.[46,124]

An alternative mechanism of functional inactivation of p53 pathway is also associated with a deregulation of the major important regulators of p53, already described above: p14[ARF], HDM2 and p21[WAF1]. Alterations of p14[ARF] gene, through homozygous deletions or promoter hypermethylation have been reported in 20% of NSCLC,[125] overexpression of the HDM2 is found in about 25% of NSCLCs,[126] whereas overexpression of p21 protein was reported in 40–70% of NSCLCs.[127]

All these evidences indicate p53 as a suitable target for novel biological therapies. In fact p53 is a prototypic model for gene-therapy approaches in lung cancer. Preclinical and phase I studies showed that plasmid or retroviral-mediated restoration of p53 function induces apoptosis in lung cancer p53-deficient cells with an initial evidence of regression of the treated lesions in patients.[128] Phase II and III clinical trials have proceeded with adenoviral vectors transducing p53 and injected directly intratumor. No evidence of additional benefit in NSCLC patients treated with adjuvant chemotherapy regimens were reported,[129] whereas a recent study by Swisher et al[130] demonstrated pathological regression at the locoregional adeno-p53 injected areas in NSCLC patients receiving concomitant radiation therapy.

The RB and p16[INK4A] pathway

The tumor suppressor gene Rb acts as a cell cycle regulator producing arrest of the cycle at G1, and inactivation of Rb functions is an essential step in tumor progression.[131] G1 arrest is achieved by the hypophosphorylated form of Rb which forms a stable complex with E2F1, thus repressing E2F1 transcriptional activities. Cyclin D1, along with cyclins D2 and D3, complex with cyclin-dependent kinase (cdk) 4 and 6 in G1, resulting in phosphorylation of Rb. Hyperphosphorylation of Rb, completed by cyclin E–cdk2 complexes results in release of E2F transcription factors, triggering G1–S transition and subsequent cell cycle progression. Cyclin D1 overexpression produces persistent hyperphosphorylation of Rb with resultant evasion of cell cycle arrest and shortening of G1 phase length.[132,133] Conversely, p16[INK4a] inhibits cdk4 and cdk6 activity by replacing cyclin D1 in the binary cdk–cyclin D1 complex.[131] This inhibition negatively regulates phosphorylation of Rb by the cyclin D1–cdk complex, inhibiting cell cycle progression. Therefore, inactivation of p16[INK4a] results in loss of inhibition of Rb phosphorylation, thereby disrupting the control of G1 cell cycle arrest.[131–134]

In non-small-cell carcinomas (NSCLCs), inactivation of the Rb pathway occurs more frequently via p16[INK4a] loss[135–140] or cyclin D1 overexpression[135,141–143] than by direct loss of Rb.[135–138] Cyclin E overexpression is also a mechanisms of Rb aberrant phosphorylation observed frequently in NSCLC.[144]

The mechanisms of p16[INK4] inactivation in non-small-cell lung cancers have been investigated.[145] Strikingly, homozygous deletion has been described with higher frequency for these tumor suppressor genes in lung cancer than for any other tumor suppressor genes in any other tumor type. Indeed, FISH is the most reliable method to discriminate between normal and tumoral cells to overcome contamination by normal or stromal cells. p16^{INK4a} homozygous deletion as assessed by FISH occurs in 30–40% of NSCLC. It is likely that it prevails in established tumor as a late event, in contrast with methylation of the 5′ CpG island of the promoter associated with transcriptional silencing of p16^{INK4}. This mechanism occurs in 25–33% of lung cancers in large series.[59,66,145] In contrast, only 10–15% of non-small-cell lung carcinoma disclose a frameshift or a missense mutation in the p16^{INK4a} gene sequence.[145–148] Taken together the deregulation of the p16^{INK4a} gene locus is a frequently occurring event in non-small-cell lung carcinoma and it was shown that immunohistochemistry is the most rapid and simplest way to screen p16^{INK4a} gene inactivation that results in loss of protein expression, since 95% of the tumors with p16^{INK4} negative immunostaining carry one of the three alternative genetic or epigenetic alterations.[145] The redundancy of Rb and p16^{INK4a} inactivation on a common p16^{INK4a}/Rb pathway for G1 arrest control is supported by the observation of an inverse correlation between alterations in the expression of both proteins in several tumor types including lung cancer.[135,145,149,150]

Cyclin D1 overexpression is another frequent event in NSCLC as routinely observed using immunohistochemistry monitored in order to obtain a negative immunostaining on genetically normal and stromal cells. Cyclin D1 overexpression in several studies was shown between 37–47%.[135,141–143] Again a direct correlation between cyclin D1 overexpression and normal Rb expression was repeatedly reported in NSCLC[135,143,151] corroborating the hypothesis that p16^{INK4a} and Rb, and cyclin D1 and Rb, function in a common regulatory pathway of tumor suppression. The prognostic value of Rb, p16^{INK4a} and cyclin D1 abnormalities has been questioned but their isolated or combined influence on survival was not convincingly demonstrated.[135]

Alteration of the Rb pathway (Rb, p16^{INK4a}, cyclin D1) largely precedes invasion.[152,153] Indeed p16 alterations are relied on a rather difficult immunohistochemistry on paraffin embedded tissues and only two reports have documented this lack of expression in early preinvasive lesions.[46,135] In contrast, there are several reports documenting the early methylation of p16^{INK4a} in lung cancer which appears to be a much earlier phenomenon than that of homozygous deletion.[60,66,70,154] Cyclin D1 and E are frequent in bronchial preneoplasia.[39,144]

When several molecular abnormalities including Rb pathway (Rb, p16^{INK4a}, cyclin D1) and p53 pathway (p53, Bax and Bcl2) were gathered in preinvasive bronchial lesions, the cumulative index of immunohistochemical abnormalities reflecting alterations of these pathways was predictive of and related to the occurrence of a NSCLC in the bronchial tree independent of the histopathological grade of the dysplasia.[46]

GENOTYPIC AND SOMATIC MARKERS

Biomarkers for early detection in circulating plasma DNA/RNA

Only a small percentage (around 10%) of lung cancer patients can be cured and benefit from long-term survival due to the absence of early detection plans, the frequency of metastases at diagnosis and poor responsiveness to chemotherapy. However, survival of patients undergoing lung resection for small intrapulmonary cancers is greater than 80%.[155] As a consequence, there is a need to develop new tests that may facilitate earlier diagnosis and more effective treatment. Low-dose spiral CT scan of the chest has been very effective in detecting small tumors, with a high proportion of resectable (96%) and stage I (80%) disease.[156,157]

On the other hand, increased knowledge of molecular pathogenesis of lung cancer offers a basis for the use of molecular markers in biological fluids for early detection as well as identification of higher-risk smokers.

A non-invasive blood test able to detect sporadic cancer has been seen as something of a holy grail by clinicians with an interest in cancer. For this reason the detection of cell-free circulating DNA in the plasma and serum of cancer patients, already reported in the early 1970s, raised a substantial interest but it was not until the late 1990s that circulating DNA was shown to exhibit genetic changes identical to those present in the primary tumors (K-ras and p53 mutations, microsatellite alterations, hypermethylation of several genes, mitochondrial DNA mutations, EBV DNA).[158] Circulating DNA appears to be an ubiquitous finding across the cancer spectrum with over 200 publications

in the literature that include solid and hematological tumors. Nowadays, nucleic acids circulating in plasma/serum are considered a suitable source for development of non invasive diagnostic, prognostic and follow-up tests for cancer.

In particular, the establishment of sensitive molecular techniques able to detect small amounts of altered DNA/RNA, was a crucial step in order to allow the detection in the plasma/serum samples of lung cancer patients of tumor-like molecular changes. These studies can be divided into studies measuring DNA markers including (a) methylation patterns,[69,159-161] (b) microsatellite changes,[162-167] (c) mutations in K-ras and p53 genes[160,161,165,168] (Table 6.2).

The frequencies of these changes in plasma/serum in the various series of patients analyzed ranged around 35–50% for methylation markers and 30–40% (NSCLC) and 60–70% (SCLC), for microsatellite changes. K-ras mutations were studied in two papers only that reported discrepant results. Bearzatto et al did not identify

Table 6.2 Frequency of plasma/serum biomarkers in lung cancer series

Markers	Frequency	Reference
DNA methylation markers (p16^{ink4A}, DAPK, GST1, MGMT, APC, TMS1, RASSF1)	34–50% NSCLC	69, 159, 160, 161
Microsatellite changes (LOH/MIN)	30–40% NSCLC 60–70% SCLC	160, 162, 163, 164, 165, 166, 167
K-ras mutations	0–24%	160, 161
p53 mutations	73% NSCLC 86% SCLC	165, 168
DNA total amounts	36–69%	172, 174, 175
RNA expression markers (5T4, RNPB1, HER2)	39–78% NSCLC	169, 170

K-ras mutations in any of the plasma samples analyzed in 35 patients that were instead detected at 33% frequency in their corresponding tumors[160] whereas Ramirez et al reported a paradoxical finding of a higher frequency of Kras mutation in serum samples compared to tumor samples with only one type of nucleotide substitution (TGT) at codon 12 that was not found (except in one case) in the corresponding tumor samples.[161]

More concordant results were reported for p53 mutations that were detected in six or seven plasma samples of SCLC patients[165] whereas the same p53 mutation identified in the corresponding tumor was found in 19 of 26 (73.1%) plasma DNA in NSCLC patients[168] (Figure 6.2).

Only two studies so far have reported the analysis of circulating serum mRNA for tumor markers (5T4, RNPB1, HER2) in lung cancer patients at a frequency ranging from 40% to 78%.[169,170]

Interestingly, an increased frequency of genetic changes in circulating DNA was observed in SCLC with respect to NSCLC patients for most of the markers so far reported. This finding could lead to speculation that more aggressive tumor phenotypes with greater access to the vasculature have increased the potential to release DNA into blood.

Several studies have also demonstrated the presence of significantly higher amounts of total circulating DNA in the plasma of patients with primary or recurrent lung cancer.[171–174] The largest published study,[175] both in number of cases and controls, using real-time quantitative PCR of the human telomerase reverse transcriptase (hTERT) gene reported elevated circulating DNA levels in 69% of 100 cases and 2% of 100 asymptomatic chronic smokers as controls with a receiver operator characteristic value of 0.94. This report has the best sensitivity and specificity for detecting

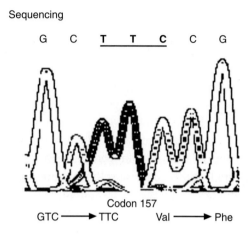

Sequencing

G   C   **T   T   C**   C   G

Codon 157

GTC ⟶ TTC   Val ⟶ Phe

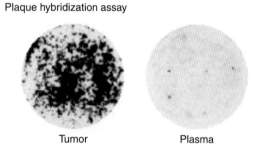

Plaque hybridization assay

Tumor   Plasma

Figure 6.2
Analysis of p53 mutations in plasma of lung cancer patients. Example of detection of mutations in the p53 gene by DNA sequencing in lung tumors (upper panel). The same mutation detected in the tumor DNA can also be identified by plaque hybridization assay in plasma-circulating DNA from the affected individual, acting as a molecular biomarker of the disease (lower panel).

cases among all the series so far reported in literature. Thus quantification of the amount of circulating plasma DNA might implement other more accurate molecular characterization of tumor-like rearrangements in early detection and screening programs. To this purpose large, matched case-control studies would be of considerable value.

Genetic factors of susceptibility to lung cancer

Lung cancer is a major cause of cancer death in Western countries. The disease has a poor prognosis, and few early diagnostic and therapeutic tools are available. Recent estimates in the European population indicate elevated odds ratios (ORs; 23.9 among men and 8.7 among women) attributed to cigarette smoke.[176] However, not all heavy smokers will develop a lung cancer, and lung cancer may also develop in non-smokers. It is therefore possible that additional risk factors, including genetic factors, play a role in lung cancer risk. Several epidemiological studies support the role of genetic factors in lung cancer risk as rare clustering of lung cancer cases in families have been reported, suggesting inherited predisposition to lung cancer in these families; in addition, the relative risk to develop a lung cancer in first-degree relatives of lung cancer patients is 2–5-fold higher than that of the general population. Thus, complex genetic factors, together with exposure to environmental carcinogens (e.g., tobacco smoke, radon, asbestos) may confer a high risk of developing lung cancer.[177] Epidemiological studies of lung cancer families supported the involvement of a 'major' gene interacting with tobacco smoking in the risk and early onset of lung cancer.[177,178] The difficulties in dissecting the genetic risk factors directly in humans make the use of experimental models attractive.

Inbred strains of mice differ in their susceptibility to spontaneous and chemically induced lung tumors. Some strains show high or intermediate propensity to these tumors, while others are almost completely resistant. Typically, mouse lung tumors may be classified as adenomas or adenocarcinomas, and they may be considered the experimental counterpart of human lung adenocarcinomas. Indeed, tumors of the two species share a common morphology and also common biochemical markers and molecular alterations.[179,180]

Genetic analysis of different crosses allowed the mapping of the major locus responsible for inherited predisposition to lung cancer in mice, the pulmonary adenoma susceptibility 1 (*Pas1*) locus.[181] Linkage disequilibrium (LD) analysis in 21 inbred strains of known susceptibility/resistance to lung cancer indicated that the *Pas1* susceptibility allele (*Pas1*^{s}) derives from an ancestral mouse and maps in a 1.5-Mb region.[182] Mice carrying the susceptibility allele at this locus may display a high or intermediate susceptibility to lung tumorigenesis, depending on the presence of additional lung cancer modifier loci,[183] whereas mice carrying the resistance allele at the *Pas1* locus (*Pas1*^{r}) do not or rarely develop lung cancer.[179,182] More recent results delimited the *Pas1* locus to a minimal region of 468 kb containing six genes. That region defined a core *Pas1* haplotype, including intragenic polymorphisms in five genes (*Bcat1*, *Lrmp*, *Las1*, *Ghiso*, and *Kras2*) and amino acid changes in three genes (*Lrmp*, *Las1*, *Lmna-rs1*). The amino acid and genomic polymorphisms of the six putative cancer modifier genes may operate together to confer susceptibility or resistance to lung tumorigenesis.[27] Observations in other models suggest or demonstrate that the functional activities of several Quantitative Trait Loci are mediated by a cluster of genes with related functions.[184–186]

In humans, population-based association studies have implicated the homologous *Pas1* locus region as a potential cancer modifier,[187–189] although these studies cannot be considered conclusive.

To identify transcriptional alterations in normal lungs associated with lung cancer risk, we analyzed the gene expression profile of 16 mouse inbred strains characterized for their susceptibility/resistance to lung tumorigenesis and *Pas1* allele status. From the 19K RIKEN array, 91

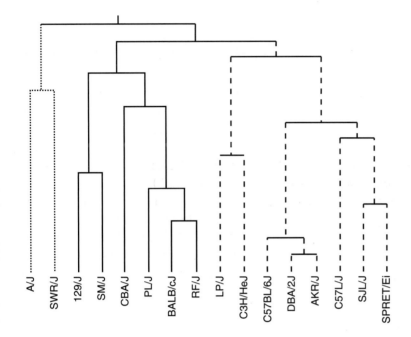

Figure 6.3
Analysis of genetic susceptibility in mice. Dendrogram of genetic relatedness of 16 mouse inbred strains on the basis of their gene expression profile in normal lungs. The analysis included 91 genes whose expression levels showed a correlation coefficient $|r| \geq 0.6$ with the strain lung tumor multiplicity (N) (expressed as $\log(N + 1)$ units).[190]

cDNA clones showed a correlation between strain-specific expression profile and lung tumor susceptibility of the strain (Figure 6.3). These results indicate that mouse inbred strains can be grouped according to lung tumor susceptibility phenotype based on their gene expression profile in normal lungs, suggesting that the gene expression profile of normal lung tissue is predictive of the genetic predisposition to lung tumorigenesis in mice.[190] If these results could be extended to humans to identify a gene expression profile of normal lungs predictive of genetic risk of lung tumor development, it could be possible, in principle, to develop new diagnostic markers to estimate the individual risk of lung cancer.

REFERENCES

1. Mao L, Lee JS, Kurie JM, et al, Clonal genetic alterations in the lungs of current and former smokers. J Natl Cancer Inst 1997; 89:857–62.

2. Wistuba II, Lam S, Behrens C, et al, Molecular damage in the bronchial epithelium of current and former smokers. J Natl Cancer Inst 1997; 89:1366–73.

3. Park IW, Wistuba II, Maitra A, et al, Multiple clonal abnormalities in the bronchial epithelium of patients with lung cancer. J Natl Cancer Inst 1999; 91:1863–8.

4. Amos CI, Xu W, Spitz MR, Is there a genetic basis for lung cancer susceptibility? Recent Results Cancer Res 1999; 151:3–12.

5. Garber ME, Troyanskaya OG, Schluens K, et al, Diversity of gene expression in adenocarcinoma of the lung. Proc Natl Acad Sci USA 2001; 98:13784–9.

6. Bhattacharjee A, Richards WG, Staunton J, et al, Classification of human lung carcinomas by mRNA expression profiling reveals distinct adenocarcinoma subclasses. Proc Natl Acad Sci USA 2001; 98:13790–5.

7. Wigle DA, Jurisica I, Radulovich N, et al, Molecular profiling of non-small cell lung cancer and correlation with disease-free survival. Cancer Res 2002; 62:3005–8.

8. Franklin WA, Veve R, Hirsch FR, Helfrich BA, Bunn PA Jr, Epidermal growth factor receptor family in lung cancer and premalignancy. Semin Oncol 2002; 29:3–14.

9. Rusch V, Klimstra D, Venkatraman E, et al, Aberrant p53 expression predicts clinical resistance to cisplatin-based chemotherapy in locally advanced non-small cell lung cancer. Cancer Res 1995; 55:5038–42.

10. Piyathilake CJ, Frost AR, Manne U, et al, Differential expression of growth factors in squamous cell carcinoma and precancerous lesions of the lung. Clin Cancer Res 2002; 8:734–44.

11. Pastorino U, Andreola S, Tagliabue E, et al, Immunocytochemical markers in stage I lung cancer: relevance to prognosis. J Clin Oncol 1997; 15:2858–65.

12. Nicholson RI, Gee JM, Harper ME, EGFR and cancer prognosis. Eur J Cancer 2001; 37 (Suppl 4):S9–15.

13. Brabender J, Danenberg KD, Metzger R, et al, Epidermal growth factor receptor and HER2-neu mRNA expression in non-small cell lung cancer is correlated with survival. Clin Cancer Res 2001; 7:1850–5.

14. Baselga J, New therapeutic agents targeting the epidermal growth factor receptor. J Clin Oncol 2000; 18:54S–9S.

15. Agus DB, Bunn PA Jr, Franklin W, Garcia M, Ozols RF, HER-2/neu as a therapeutic target in non-small cell lung cancer, prostate cancer, and ovarian cancer. Semin Oncol 2000; 27:53–63.

16. Pao W, Miller VA, Epidermal growth factor receptor mutatious small-molecule kinase inhibitors, and non-small-cell lung cancer: current knowledge and future directions. J Clin Oncol 2005; 23:1–13.

17. Krystal GW, Honsawek S, Kiewlich D, et al, Indolinone tyrosine kinase inhibitors block Kit activation and growth of small cell lung cancer cells. Cancer Res 2001; 61:3660–8.

18. Olivero M, Rizzo M, Madeddu R, et al, Over-expression and activation of hepatocyte growth factor/scatter factor in human non-small-cell lung carcinomas. Br J Cancer 1996; 74:1862–8.

19. Maulik G, Kijima T, Ma PC, et al, Modulation of the c-Met/hepatocyte growth factor pathway in small cell lung cancer. Clin Cancer Res 2002; 8:620–7.

20. Ma PC, Kijima T, Maulik G, et al, c-MET mutational analysis in small cell lung cancer: novel juxtamembrane domain mutations regulating cytoskeletal functions. Cancer Res 2003; 63:6272–81.

21. Barbacid M, ras genes. Annu Rev Biochem 1987; 56:779–827.

22. Bos JL, ras oncogenes in human cancer: a review. Cancer Res 1989; 49:4682–9.

23. Minamoto T, Mai M, Ronai Z, K-ras mutation: early detection in molecular diagnosis and risk assessment of colorectal, pancreas, and lung cancers – a review. Cancer Detect Prev 2000; 24:1–12.

24. Ellis CA, Clark G, The importance of being K-Ras. Cell Signal 2000; 12:425–34.

25. Johnson L, Mercer K, Greenbaum D, et al, Somatic activation of the K-ras oncogene causes early onset lung cancer in mice. Nature 2001; 410:1111–16.

26. Zhang Z, Wang Y, Vikis HG, et al, Wildtype Kras2 can inhibit lung carcinogenesis in mice. Nat Genet 2001; 29:25–33.

27. Manenti G, Galbiati F, Giannì Barrera R, et al, Haplotype sharing suggests that a genomic segment containing six genes accounts for the pulmonary adenoma susceptibility 1 (Pas1) locus activity in mice. Oncogene 2004; 23: 4495–504.

28. Prendergast GC, Mechanisms of apoptosis by c-Myc. Oncogene 1999; 18:2967–87.

29. Luk C, Tsao MS, Bayani J, Shepherd F, Squire JA, Molecular cytogenetic analysis of non-small cell lung carcinoma by spectral karyotyping and comparative genomic hybridization. Cancer Genet Cytogenet 2001; 125:87–99.

30. Mitani S, Kamata H, Fujiwara M, et al, Analysis of c-myc DNA amplification in non-small cell lung carcinoma in comparison with small cell lung carcinoma using polymerase chain reaction. Clin Exp Med 2001; 1:105–11.

31. Lui WO, Tanenbaum DM, Larsson C, High level amplification of 1p32–33 and 2p22–24 in small cell lung carcinomas. Int J Oncol 2001; 19:451–7.

32. Brennan J, O'Connor T, Makuch RW, et al, myc family DNA amplification in 107 tumors and tumor cell lines from patients with small cell lung cancer treated with different combination chemotherapy regimens. Cancer Res 1991; 51:1708–12.

33. Kubokura H, Tenjin T, Akiyama H, et al, Relations of the c-myc gene and chromosome 8 in non-small cell lung cancer: analysis by fluorescence in situ hybridization. Ann Thorac Cardiovasc Surg 2001; 7:197–203.

34. Bernasconi NL, Wormhoudt TA, Laird-Offringa IA, Post-transcriptional deregulation of myc genes in lung cancer cell lines. Am J Respir Cell Mol Biol 2000; 23:560–5.

35. Broers JL, Viallet J, Jensen SM, et al, Expression of c-myc in progenitor cells of the bronchopulmonary epithelium and in a large number of non-small cell lung cancers. Am J Respir Cell Mol Biol 1993; 9:33–43.

36. Shivapurkar N, Reddy J, Matta H, et al, Loss of expression of death-inducing signaling complex (DISC) components in lung cancer cell lines and the influence of MYC amplification. Oncogene 2002; 21:8510–14.

37. Nasi S, Ciarapica R, Jucker R, Rosati J, Soucek L, Making decisions through Myc. FEBS Lett 2001; 490:153–62.

38. Zajac-Kaye M, Myc oncogene: a key component in cell cycle regulation and its implication for lung cancer. Lung Cancer 2001; 34 (Suppl 2): S43–6.

39. Krajewski S, Krajewska M, Shabaik A, et al, Immunohistochemical determination of in vivo distribution of Bax, a dominant inhibitor of Bcl-2. Am J Pathol 1994; 145:1323–36.

40. Krajewski S, Chatten J, Hanada M, Reed JC, Immunohistochemical analysis of the Bcl-2 oncoprotein in human neuroblastomas. Comparisons with tumor cell differentiation and N-Myc protein. Lab Invest 1995; 72:42–54.

41. Pezzella F, Turley H, Kuzu I, et al, bcl-2 protein in non-small-cell lung carcinoma. N Engl J Med 1993; 329:690–4.

42. Fontanini G, Vignati S, Bigini D, et al, Bcl-2 protein: a prognostic factor inversely correlated to p53 in non-small-cell lung cancer. Br J Cancer 1995; 71:1003–7.

43. Brambilla E, Gazzeri S, Lantuejoul S, et al, p53 mutant immunophenotype and deregulation of p53 transcription pathway (Bcl2, Bax, and Waf1) in precursor bronchial lesions of lung cancer. Clin Cancer Res 1998; 4:1609–18.

44. Walker C, Robertson L, Myskow M, Dixon G, Expression of the BCL-2 protein in normal and dysplastic bronchial epithelium and in lung carcinomas. Br J Cancer 1995; 72:164–9.

45. Miyashita T, Krajewski S, Krajewska M, et al, Tumor suppressor p53 is a regulator of bcl-2 and bax gene expression in vitro and in vivo. Oncogene 1994; 9:1799–805.

46. Jeanmart M, Lantuejoul S, Fievet F, et al, Value of immunohistochemical markers in preinvasive bronchial lesions in risk assessment of lung cancer. Clin Cancer Res 2003; 9:2195–203.

47. Kishimoto Y, Sugio K, Hung JY, et al, Allele-specific loss in chromosome 9p loci in preneoplastic lesions accompanying non-small-cell lung cancers. J Natl Cancer Inst 1995; 87:1224–9.

48. Sozzi G, Veronese ML, Negrini M, et al, The FHIT gene 3p14.2 is abnormal in lung cancer. Cell 1996; 85:17–26.

49. Virmani AK, Fong KM, Kodagoda D, et al, Allelotyping demonstrates common and distinct patterns of chromosomal loss in human lung cancer types. Genes Chromosomes Cancer 1998; 21:308–19.

50. Wistuba II, Behrens C, Virmani AK, et al, High resolution chromosome 3p allelotyping of human lung cancer and preneoplastic/preinvasive bronchial epithelium reveals multiple, discontinuous sites of 3p allele loss and three regions of frequent breakpoints. Cancer Res 2000; 60:1949–60.

51. Liloglou T, Maloney P, Xinarianos G, Fear S, Field JK, Sensitivity and limitations of high

throughput fluorescent microsatellite analysis for the detection of allelic imbalance: application in lung tumors. Int J Oncol 2000; 16: 5–14.

52. Girard L, Zochbauer-Muller S, Virmani AK, Gazdar AF, Minna JD, Genome-wide allelotyping of lung cancer identifies new regions of allelic loss, differences between small cell lung cancer and non-small cell lung cancer, and loci clustering. Cancer Res 2000; 60:4894–906.

53. Sundaresan V, Ganly P, Hasleton P, et al, p53 and chromosome 3 abnormalities, characteristic of malignant lung tumours, are detectable in preinvasive lesions of the bronchus. Oncogene 1992; 7:1989–97.

54. Sozzi G, Miozzo M, Donghi R, et al, Deletions of 17p and p53 mutations in preneoplastic lesions of the lung. Cancer Res 1992; 52: 6079–82.

55. Hung J, Kishimoto Y, Sugio K, et al, Allele-specific chromosome 3p deletions occur at an early stage in the pathogenesis of lung carcinoma. JAMA 1995; 273:1908.

56. Thiberville L, Payne P, Vielkinds J, et al, Evidence of cumulative gene losses with progression of premalignant epithelial lesions to carcinoma of the bronchus. Cancer Res 1995; 55:5133–9.

57. Sozzi G, Oggionni M, Alasio L, et al, Molecular changes track recurrence and progression of bronchial precancerous lesions. Lung Cancer 2002; 37:267–70.

58. Sozzi G, Miozzo M, Tagliabue E, et al, Cytogenetic abnormalities and overexpression of receptors for growth factors in normal bronchial epithelium and tumor samples of lung cancer patients. Cancer Res 1991; 51:400–4.

59. Merlo A, Herman JG, Mao L, et al, 5′ CpG island methylation is associated with transcriptional silencing of the tumour suppressor p16/CDKN2/MTS1 in human cancers. Nat Med 1995; 1:686–92.

60. Belinsky SA, Nikula KJ, Palmisano WA, et al, Aberrant methylation of p16(INK4a) is an early event in lung cancer and a potential biomarker for early diagnosis. Proc Natl Acad Sci USA 1998; 95:11891–6.

61. Kim DH, Nelson HH, Wiencke JK, et al, p16(INK4a) and histology-specific methylation of CpG islands by exposure to tobacco smoke in non-small cell lung cancer. Cancer Res 2001; 61:3419–24.

62. Virmani AK, Rathi A, Zochbauer-Muller S, et al, Promoter methylation and silencing of the retinoic acid receptor-beta gene in lung carcinomas. J Natl Cancer Inst 2000; 92:1303–7.

63. Zochbauer-Muller S, Fong KM, Maitra A, et al, 5′ CpG island methylation of the FHIT gene is correlated with loss of gene expression in lung and breast cancer. Cancer Res 2001; 61: 3581–5.

64. Dammann R, Li C, Yoon JH, et al, Epigenetic inactivation of a RAS association domain family protein from the lung tumour suppressor locus 3p21.3. Nat Genet 2000; 25:315–19.

65. Burbee DG, Forgacs E, Zochbauer-Muller S, et al, Epigenetic inactivation of RASSF1A in lung and breast cancers and malignant phenotype suppression. J Natl Cancer Inst 2001; 93:691–9.

66. Palmisano WA, Divine KK, Saccomanno G, et al, Predicting lung cancer by detecting aberrant promoter methylation in sputum. Cancer Res 2000; 60:5954–8.

67. Kim DH, Nelson HH, Wiencke JK, et al, Promoter methylation of DAP-kinase: association with advanced stage in non-small cell lung cancer. Oncogene 2001; 20:1765–70.

68. Virmani AK, Rathi A, Sathyanarayana UG, et al, Aberrant methylation of the adenomatous polyposis coli (APC) gene promoter 1A in breast and lung carcinomas. Clin Cancer Res 2001; 7:1998–2004.

69. Usadel H, Brabender J, Danenberg KD, et al, Quantitative adenomatous polyposis coli promoter methylation analysis in tumor tissue, serum, and plasma DNA of patients with lung cancer. Cancer Res 2002; 62:371–5.

70. Kersting M, Friedl C, Kraus A, et al, Differential frequencies of p16(INK4a) promoter hypermethylation, p53 mutation, and K-ras mutation

in exfoliative material mark the development of lung cancer in symptomatic chronic smokers. J Clin Oncol 2000; 18:3221–9.

71. Belinsky SA, Palmisano WA, Gilliland FD, et al, Aberrant promoter methylation in bronchial epithelium and sputum from current and former smokers. Cancer Res 2002; 62:2370–7.

72. Braga E, Pugacheva E, Bazov I, et al, Comparative allelotyping of the short arm of human chromosome 3 in epithelial tumors of four different types. FEBS Lett 1999; 454:215–19.

73. Shimizu M, Yokota J, Mori N, et al, Introduction of normal chromosome 3p modulates the tumorigenicity of a human renal cell carcinoma cell line YCR. Oncogene 1990; 5:185–94.

74. Liu J, Zabarovska VI, Braga E, et al, Loss of heterozygosity in tumor cells requires re-evaluation: the data are biased by the size-dependent differential sensitivity of allele detection. FEBS Lett 1999; 462:121–8.

75. Baylin SB, Herman JG, Promoter hypermethylation – can this change alone ever designate true tumor suppressor gene function? J Natl Cancer Inst 2001; 93:664–5.

76. Zabarovsky ER, Lerman MI, Minna JD, Tumor suppressor genes on chromosome 3p involved in the pathogenesis of lung and other cancers. Oncogene 2002; 21:6915–35.

77. Sanchez Y, El Naggar A, Pathak S, Killary AM, A tumor suppressor locus within 3p14-p12 mediates rapid cell death of renal cell carcinoma in vivo. Proc Natl Acad Sci USA 1994; 91:3383–7.

78. Sundaresan V, Roberts I, Bateman A, et al, The DUTT1 gene, a novel NCAM family member is expressed in developing murine neural tissues and has an unusually broad pattern of expression. Mol Cell Neurosci 1998; 11:29–35.

79. Kidd T, Brose K, Mitchell KJ, et al, Roundabout controls axon crossing of the CNS midline and defines a novel subfamily of evolutionarily conserved guidance receptors. Cell 1998; 92: 205–15.

80. Dallol A, Forgacs E, Martinez A, et al, Tumour specific promoter region methylation of the human homologue of the Drosophila Round-

about gene DUTT1 (ROBO1) in human cancers. Oncogene 2002; 21:3020–8.

81. Xian J, Clark KJ, Fordham R, et al, Inadequate lung development and bronchial hyperplasia in mice with a targeted deletion in the Dutt1/Robo1 gene. Proc Natl Acad Sci USA 2001; 98:15062–6.

82. Cohen AJ, Li FP, Berg S, et al, Hereditary renal-cell carcinoma associated with a chromosomal translocation. N Engl J Med 1979; 301:592–5.

83. Ohta M, Inoue H, Cotticelli MG, et al, The FHIT gene, spanning the chromosome 3p14.2 fragile site and renal carcinoma-associated t(3;8) breakpoint, is abnormal in digestive tract cancers. Cell 1996; 84:587–97.

84. Huebner K, Croce CM, Cancer and the FRA3B/FHIT fragile locus: it's a HIT. Br J Cancer 2003; 88:1501–6.

85. Druck T, Hadaczek P, Fu TB, et al, Structure and expression of the human FHIT gene in normal and tumor cells. Cancer Res 1997; 57:504–12.

86. Sozzi G, Pastorino U, Moiraghi L, et al, Loss of FHIT function in lung cancer and preinvasive bronchial lesions. Cancer Res 1998; 58:5032–7.

87. Sard L, Accornero P, Tornielli S, et al, The tumor-suppressor gene FHIT is involved in the regulation of apoptosis and in cell cycle control. Proc Natl Acad Sci USA 1999; 96:8489–92.

88. Ji L, Fang B, Yen N, et al, Induction of apoptosis and inhibition of tumorigenicity and tumor growth by adenovirus vector-mediated fragile histidine triad (FHIT) gene overexpression. Cancer Res 1999; 59:3333–9.

89. Roz L, Gramegna M, Ishii H, Croce CM, Sozzi G, Restoration of fragile histidine triad (FHIT) expression induces apoptosis and suppresses tumorigenicity in lung and cervical cancer cell lines. Proc Natl Acad Sci USA 2002; 99: 3615–20.

90. Zanesi N, Fidanza V, Fong LY, et al, The tumor spectrum in FHIT-deficient mice. Proc Natl Acad Sci USA 2001; 98:10250–5.

91. Dumon KR, Ishii H, Fong LY, et al, FHIT gene therapy prevents tumor development in

Fhit-deficient mice. Proc Natl Acad Sci USA 2001; 98:3346–51.

92. Killary AM, Wolf ME, Giambernardi TA, Naylor SL, Definition of a tumor suppressor locus within human chromosome 3p21-p22. Proc Natl Acad Sci USA 1992; 89:10877–81.

93. Lerman MI, Minna JD. The 630-kb lung cancer homozygous deletion region on human chromosome 3p21.3: identification and evaluation of the resident candidate tumor suppressor genes. The International Lung Cancer Chromosome 3p21.3 Tumor Suppressor Gene Consortium. Cancer Res 2000; 60:6116–33.

94. Carboni GL, Gao B, Nishizaki M, et al, CACNA2D2-mediated apoptosis in NSCLC cells is associated with alterations of the intracellular calcium signaling and disruption of mitochondria membrane integrity. Oncogene 2003; 22:615–26.

95. Agathanggelou A, Dallol A, Zochbauer-Muller S, et al, Epigenetic inactivation of the candidate 3p21.3 suppressor gene BLU in human cancers. Oncogene 2003; 22:1580–8.

96. Ji L, Nishizaki M, Gao B, et al, Expression of several genes in the human chromosome 3p21.3 homozygous deletion region by an adenovirus vector results in tumor suppressor activities in vitro and in vivo. Cancer Res 2002; 62:2715–20.

97. Shivakumar L, Minna J, Sakamaki T, Pestell R, White MA, The RASSF1A tumor suppressor blocks cell cycle progression and inhibits cyclin D1 accumulation. Mol Cell Biol 2002; 22:4309–18.

98. Song MS, Song SJ, Ayad NG, et al, The tumour suppressor RASSF1A regulates mitosis by inhibiting the APC–Cdc20 complex. Nat Cell Biol 2004; 6:129–37.

99. Roche J, Drabkin HA, The role of semaphorins in lung cancer. Clin Lung Cancer 2001; 3:145–50.

100. Kuroki T, Trapasso F, Yendamuri S, et al, Allelic loss on chromosome 3p21.3 and promoter hypermethylation of semaphorin 3B in non-small cell lung cancer. Cancer Res 2003; 63:3352–5.

101. Tomizawa Y, Sekido Y, Kondo M, et al, Inhibition of lung cancer cell growth and induction of apoptosis after reexpression of 3p21.3 candidate tumor suppressor gene SEMA3B. Proc Natl Acad Sci USA 2001; 98:13954–9.

102. Brambilla E, Constantin B, Drabkin H, Roche J, Semaphorin SEMA3F localization in malignant human lung and cell lines: A suggested role in cell adhesion and cell migration. Am J Pathol 2000; 156:939–50.

103. Lantuejoul S, Constantin B, Drabkin H, et al, Expression of VEGF, semaphorin SEMA3F, and their common receptors neuropilins NP1 and NP2 in preinvasive bronchial lesions, lung tumours, and cell lines. J Pathol 2003; 200:336–47.

104. van Zandwijk N, Hirsch FR, Chemoprevention of lung cancer: current status and future prospects. Lung Cancer 2003; 42 (Suppl 1):S71–9.

105. Geradts J, Chen JY, Russell EK, et al, Human lung cancer cell lines exhibit resistance to retinoic acid treatment. Cell Growth Differ 1993; 4:799–809.

106. Zochbauer-Muller S, Fong KM, Virmani AK, et al, Aberrant promoter methylation of multiple genes in non-small cell lung cancers. Cancer Res 2001; 61:249–55.

107. Houle B, Rochette-Egly C, Bradley WE, Tumor-suppressive effect of the retinoic acid receptor beta in human epidermoid lung cancer cells. Proc Natl Acad Sci USA 1993; 90:985–9.

108. Toulouse A, Morin J, Dion PA, Houle B, Bradley WE, RARbeta2 specificity in mediating RA inhibition of growth of lung cancer-derived cells. Lung Cancer 2000; 28:127–37.

109. Berard J, Laboune F, Mukuna M, et al, Lung tumors in mice expressing an antisense RARbeta2 transgene. FASEB J 1996; 10:1091–7.

110. Levine AJ. p53, the cellular gatekeeper for growth and division. Cell 1997; 88:323–31.

111. Lahav G, Rosenfeld N, Sigal A, et al, Dynamics of the p53-Mdm2 feedback loop in individual cells. Nat Genet 2004; 36:147–50.

112. Momand J, Zambetti GP, Olson DC, George D,

Levine AJ, The mdm-2 oncogene product forms a complex with the p53 protein and inhibits p53-mediated transactivation. Cell 1992; 69:1237–45.

113. Tao W, Levine AJ, P19(ARF) stabilizes p53 by blocking nucleo-cytoplasmic shuttling of Mdm2. Proc Natl Acad Sci USA 1999; 96:6937–41.

114. Harper JW, Adami GR, Wei N, Keyomarsi K, Elledge SJ, The p21 Cdk-interacting protein Cip1 is a potent inhibitor of G1 cyclin-dependent kinases. Cell 1993; 75:805–16.

115. Hainaut P, Hollstein M, p53 and human cancer: the first ten thousand mutations. Adv Cancer Res 2000; 77:81–137.

116. Tammemagi MC, McLaughlin JR, Bull SB, Meta-analyses of p53 tumor suppressor gene alterations and clinicopathological features in resected lung cancers. Cancer Epidemiol Biomarkers Prev 1999; 8:625–34.

117. Mitsudomi T, Hamajima N, Ogawa M, Takahashi T, Prognostic significance of p53 alterations in patients with non-small cell lung cancer: a meta-analysis. Clin Cancer Res 2000; 6:4055–63.

118. Ahrendt SA, Hu Y, Buta M, et al, p53 mutations and survival in stage I non-small-cell lung cancer: results of a prospective study. J Natl Cancer Inst 2003; 95:961–70.

119. Casey G, Lopez ME, Ramos JC, et al, DNA sequence analysis of exons 2 through 11 and immunohistochemical staining are required to detect all known p53 alterations in human malignancies. Oncogene 1996; 13:1971–81.

120. Tomizawa Y, Kohno T, Fujita T, et al, Correlation between the status of the p53 gene and survival in patients with stage I non-small cell lung carcinoma. Oncogene 1999; 18:1007–14.

121. Ahrendt SA, Chow JT, Yang SC, et al, Alcohol consumption and cigarette smoking increase the frequency of p53 mutations in non-small cell lung cancer. Cancer Res 2000; 60:3155–9.

122. Pfeifer GP, Hainaut P, On the origin of G→T transversions in lung cancer. Mutat Res 2003; 526:39–43.

123. Denissenko MF, Pao A, Tang M, Pfeifer GP, Preferential formation of benzo[a]pyrene adducts at lung cancer mutational hotspots in P53. Science 1996; 274:430–2.

124. Bennett WP, Colby TV, Travis WD, et al, p53 protein accumulates frequently in early bronchial neoplasia. Cancer Res 1993; 53: 4817–22.

125. Nicholson SA, Okby NT, Khan MA, et al, Alterations of p14ARF, p53, and p73 genes involved in the E2F-1-mediated apoptotic pathways in non-small cell lung carcinoma. Cancer Res 2001; 61:5636–43.

126. Higashiyama M, Doi O, Kodama K, et al, MDM2 gene amplification and expression in non-small-cell lung cancer: immunohistochemical expression of its protein is a favourable prognostic marker in patients without p53 protein accumulation. Br J Cancer 1997; 75: 1302–8.

127. Vonlanthen S, Heighway J, Kappeler A, et al, p21 is associated with cyclin D1, p16INK4a and pRb expression in resectable non-small cell lung cancer. Int J Oncol 2000; 16:951–7.

128. Roth JA, Nguyen D, Lawrence DD, et al, Retrovirus-mediated wild-type p53 gene transfer to tumors of patients with lung cancer. Nat Med 1996; 2:985–91.

129. Schuler M, Herrmann R, De Greve JL, et al, Adenovirus-mediated wild-type p53 gene transfer in patients receiving chemotherapy for advanced non-small-cell lung cancer: results of a multicenter phase II study. J Clin Oncol 2001; 19:1750–8.

130. Swisher SG, Roth JA, Nemunaitis J, et al, Adenovirus-mediated p53 gene transfer in advanced non-small-cell lung cancer. J Natl Cancer Inst 1999; 91:763–71.

131. Sherr CJ, Cancer cell cycles. Science 1996; 274:1672–7.

132. Resnitzky D, Gossen M, Bujard H, Reed SI, Acceleration of the G1/S phase transition by expression of cyclins D1 and E with an inducible system. Mol Cell Biol 1994; 14: 1669–79.

133. Quelle DE, Ashmun RA, Shurtleff SA, et al, Overexpression of mouse D-type cyclins accelerates G1 phase in rodent fibroblasts. Genes Dev 1993; 7:1559–71.

134. Michalides R, van Veelen N, Hart A, et al, Overexpression of cyclin D1 correlates with recurrence in a group of forty-seven operable squamous cell carcinomas of the head and neck. Cancer Res 1995; 55:975–8.

135. Brambilla E, Moro D, Gazzeri S, Brambilla C, Alterations of expression of Rb, p16(INK4A) and cyclin D1 in non-small cell lung carcinoma and their clinical significance. J Pathol 1999; 188:351–60.

136. Kamb A, Gruis NA, Weaver-Feldhaus J, et al, A cell cycle regulator potentially involved in genesis of many tumor types. Science 1994; 264:436–40.

137. Lukas J, Parry D, Aagaard L, et al, Retinoblastoma-protein-dependent cell-cycle inhibition by the tumour suppressor p16. Nature 1995; 375:503–6.

138. Kratzke RA, Greatens TM, Rubins JB, et al, Rb and p16INK4a expression in resected non-small cell lung tumors. Cancer Res 1996; 56:3415–20.

139. Kinoshita I, Dosaka-Akita H, Mishina T, et al, Altered p16INK4 and retinoblastoma protein status in non-small cell lung cancer: potential synergistic effect with altered p53 protein on proliferative activity. Cancer Res 1996; 56: 5557–62.

140. Sakaguchi M, Fujii Y, Hirabayashi H, et al, Inversely correlated expression of p16 and Rb protein in non-small cell lung cancers: an immunohistochemical study. Int J Cancer 1996; 65:442–5.

141. Betticher DC, Heighway J, Hasleton PS, et al, Prognostic significance of CCND1 (cyclin D1) overexpression in primary resected non-small-cell lung cancer. Br J Cancer 1996; 73: 294–300.

142. Mate JL, Ariza A, Aracil C, et al, Cyclin D1 overexpression in non-small cell lung carcinoma: correlation with Ki67 labelling index and poor cytoplasmic differentiation. J Pathol 1996; 180:395–9.

143. Nishio M, Koshikawa T, Yatabe Y, et al, Prognostic significance of cyclin D1 and retinoblastoma expression in combination with p53 abnormalities in primary, resected non-small cell lung cancers. Clin Cancer Res 1997; 3:1051–8.

144. Lonardo F, Rusch V, Langenfeld J, Dmitrovsky E, Klimstra DS, Overexpression of cyclins D1 and E is frequent in bronchial preneoplasia and precedes squamous cell carcinoma development. Cancer Res 1999; 59:2470–6.

145. Gazzeri S, Gouyer V, Vour'ch C, Brambilla C, Brambilla E, Mechanisms of p16INK4A inactivation in non small-cell lung cancers. Oncogene 1998; 16:497–504.

146. Cairns P, Mao L, Merlo A, et al, Rates of p16 (MTS1) mutations in primary tumors with 9p loss. Science 1994; 265:415–17.

147. Rusin MR, Okamoto A, Chorazy M, et al, Intragenic mutations of the p16(INK4), p15(INK4B) and p18 genes in primary non-small-cell lung cancers. Int J Cancer 1996; 65:734–9.

148. Okamoto A, Hussain SP, Hagiwara K, et al, Mutations in the p16INK4/MTS1/CDKN2, p15INK4B/MTS2, and p18 genes in primary and metastatic lung cancer. Cancer Res 1995; 55:1448–51.

149. Geradts J, Kratzke RA, Niehans GA, Lincoln CE. Immunohistochemical detection of the cyclin-dependent kinase inhibitor 2/multiple tumor suppressor gene 1 (CDKN2/MTS1) product p16INK4A in archival human solid tumors: correlation with retinoblastoma protein expression. Cancer Res 1995; 55: 6006–11.

150. Shapiro GI, Park JE, Edwards CD, et al, Multiple mechanisms of p16INK4A inactivation in non-small cell lung cancer cell lines. Cancer Res 1995; 55:6200–9.

151. Schauer IE, Siriwardana S, Langan TA, Sclafani RA. Cyclin D1 overexpression vs. retinoblastoma inactivation: implications for growth

control evasion in non-small cell and small cell lung cancer. Proc Natl Acad Sci USA 1994; 91:7827–31.

152. Brambilla E, Gazzeri S, Moro D, et al, Alterations of Rb pathway (Rb-p16INK4-cyclin D1) in preinvasive bronchial lesions. Clin Cancer Res 1999; 5:243–50.

153. Alle KM, Henshall SM, Field AS, Sutherland RL, Cyclin D1 protein is overexpressed in hyperplasia and intraductal carcinoma of the breast. Clin Cancer Res 1998; 4:847–54.

154. Ahrendt SA, Chow JT, Xu LH, et al, Molecular detection of tumor cells in bronchoalveolar lavage fluid from patients with early stage lung cancer. J Natl Cancer Inst 1999; 91:332–9.

155. Patz EF Jr, Rossi S, Harpole DH Jr, Herndon JE, Goodman PC, Correlation of tumor size and survival in patients with stage IA non-small cell lung cancer. Chest 2000; 117:1568–71.

156. Henschke CI, McCauley DI, Yankelevitz DF, et al, Early Lung Cancer Action Project: overall design and findings from baseline screening. Lancet 1999; 354:99–105.

157. Pastorino U, Bellomi M, Landoni C, et al, Early lung-cancer detection with spiral CT and positron emission tomography in heavy smokers: 2-year results. Lancet 2003; 362: 593–7.

158. Anker P, Mulcahy H, Stroun M, Circulating nucleic acids in plasma and serum as a non-invasive investigation for cancer: time for large-scale clinical studies? Int J Cancer 2003; 103:149–52.

159. Esteller M, Sanchez-Cespedes M, Rosell R, et al, Detection of aberrant promoter hypermethylation of tumor suppressor genes in serum DNA from non-small cell lung cancer patients. Cancer Res 1999; 59:67–70.

160. Bearzatto A, Conte D, Frattini M, et al, p16(INK4A) hypermethylation detected by fluorescent methylation-specific PCR in plasmas from non-small cell lung cancer. Clin·Cancer Res 2002; 8:3782–7.

161. Ramirez JL, Sarries C, de Castro PL, et al, Methylation patterns and K-ras mutations in tumor and paired serum of resected non-small-cell lung cancer patients. Cancer Lett 2003; 193:207–16.

162. Chen XQ, Stroun M, Magnenat JL, et al, Microsatellite alterations in plasma DNA of small cell lung cancer patients. Nat Med 1996; 2:1033–5.

163. Sanchez-Cespedes M, Monzo M, Rosell R, et al, Detection of chromosome 3p alterations in serum DNA of non-small-cell lung cancer patients. Ann Oncol 1998; 9:113–16.

164. Sozzi G, Musso K, Ratcliffe C, et al, Detection of microsatellite alterations in plasma DNA of non-small cell lung cancer patients: a prospect for early diagnosis. Clin Cancer Res 1999; 5:2689–92.

165. Gonzalez R, Silva JM, Sanchez A, et al, Microsatellite alterations and TP53 mutations in plasma DNA of small-cell lung cancer patients: follow-up study and prognostic significance. Ann Oncol 2000; 11:1097–104.

166. Cuda G, Gallelli A, Nistico A, et al, Detection of microsatellite instability and loss of heterozygosity in serum DNA of small and non-small cell lung cancer patients: a tool for early diagnosis? Lung Cancer 2000; 30: 211–14.

167. Bruhn N, Beinert T, Oehm C, et al, Detection of microsatellite alterations in the DNA isolated from tumor cells and from plasma DNA of patients with lung cancer. Ann NY Acad Sci 2000; 906:72–82.

168. Andriani F, Conte D, Mastrangelo T, et al, Detecting lung cancer in plasma with the use of multiple genetic markers. Int J Cancer 2004; 108:91–6.

169. Kopreski MS, Benko FA, Gocke CD, Circulating RNA as a tumor marker: detection of 5T4 mRNA in breast and lung cancer patient serum. Ann NY Acad Sci 2001; 945:172–8.

170. Fleischhacker M, Beinert T, Ermitsch M, et al, Detection of amplifiable messenger RNA in the serum of patients with lung cancer. Ann NY Acad Sci 2001; 945:179–88.

171. Leon SA, Shapiro B, Sklaroff DM, Yaros MJ,

Free DNA in the serum of cancer patients and the effect of therapy. Cancer Res 1977; 37:646–50.

172. Fournie GJ, Courtin JP, Laval F, et al, Plasma DNA as a marker of cancerous cell death. Investigations in patients suffering from lung cancer and in nude mice bearing human tumours. Cancer Lett 1995; 91:221–7.

173. Jahr S, Hentze H, Englisch S, et al, DNA fragments in the blood plasma of cancer patients: quantitations and evidence for their origin from apoptotic and necrotic cells. Cancer Res 2001; 61:1659–65.

174. Sozzi G, Conte D, Mariani L, et al, Analysis of circulating tumor DNA in plasma at diagnosis and during follow-up of lung cancer patients. Cancer Res 2001; 61:4675–8.

175. Sozzi G, Conte D, Leon M, et al, Quantification of free circulating DNA as a diagnostic marker in lung cancer. J Clin Oncol 2003; 21:3902–8.

176. Simonato L, Agudo A, Ahrens W, et al, Lung cancer and cigarette smoking in Europe: an update of risk estimates and an assessment of inter-country heterogeneity. Int J Cancer 2001; 91:876–87.

177. Sellers TA, Weaver TW, Phillips B, Altmann M, Rich SS, Environmental factors can confound identification of a major gene effect: results from a segregation analysis of a simulated population of lung cancer families. Genet Epidemiol 1998; 15:251–62.

178. Yang P, Schwartz AG, McAllister AE, Swanson GM, Aston CE, Lung cancer risk in families of nonsmoking probands: heterogeneity by age at diagnosis. Genet Epidemiol 1999; 17:253–73.

179. Malkinson AM, The genetic basis of susceptibility to lung tumors in mice. Toxicology 1989; 54:241–71.

180. Dragani TA, Manenti G, Pierotti MA, Genetics of murine lung tumors. Adv Cancer Res 1995; 67:83–112.

181. Gariboldi M, Manenti G, Canzian F, et al, A major susceptibility locus to murine lung carcinogenesis maps on chromosome 6. Nat Genet 1993; 3:132–6.

182. Manenti G, Stafford A, De Gregorio L, et al, Linkage disequilibrium and physical mapping of Pas1 in mice. Genome Res 1999; 9:639–46.

183. Manenti G, Gariboldi M, Elango R, et al, Genetic mapping of a pulmonary adenoma resistance (Par1) in mouse. Nat Genet 1996; 12:455–7.

184. Darvasi A, Pisante-Shalom A, Complexities in the genetic dissection of quantitative trait loci. Trends Genet 2002; 18:489–91.

185. Cormier RT, Bilger A, Lillich AJ, et al, The Mom1AKR intestinal tumor resistance region consists of Pla2g2a and a locus distal to D4Mit64. Oncogene 2000; 19:3182–92.

186. Steinmetz LM, Sinha H, Richards DR, et al, Dissecting the architecture of a quantitative trait locus in yeast. Nature 2002; 416:326–30.

187. Manenti G, De Gregorio L, Pilotti S, et al, Association of chromosome 12p genetic polymorphisms with lung adenocarcinoma risk and prognosis. Carcinogenesis 1997; 18:1917–20.

188. Dragani TA, Hirohashi S, Juji T, et al, Population-based mapping of pulmonary adenoma susceptibility 1 locus. Cancer Res 2000; 60:5017–20.

189. Yanagitani N, Kohno T, Sunaga N, et al, Localization of a human lung adenocarcinoma susceptibility locus, possibly syntenic to the mouse Pas1 locus, in the vicinity of the D12S1034 locus on chromosome 12p11.2-p12.1. Carcinogenesis 2002; 23:1177–83.

190. Gariboldi M, Spinola M, Milani S, et al, Gene expression profile of normal lungs predicts genetic predisposition to lung cancer in mice. Carcinogenesis 2003; 24:1819–26.

7 Proteomic strategies for the early detection of lung cancer

Pierre P Massion, Pinar B Yildiz, David P Carbone

Contents Introduction • Methodological approaches • Application of these proteomic methods to lung cancer • Integration of multiple molecular methods to early detection • Challenges ahead • Conclusions

INTRODUCTION

Proteins are responsible for biological systems to function and are favored targets for therapy. Application of cDNA microarrays to cancer aimed to generate new molecular-based classifications of disease and to identify new biomarkers of disease based on gene expression profiles. Preliminary results from these studies have confirmed the existence of gene expression profiles that correlate with lung cancer histopathology and clinical outcome and some aspects of biology.[1–5] Most studies have examined pathologically homogeneous sets of tumors to identify occult clinically relevant subtypes, pathologically distinct subtypes of tumors to identify molecular correlates. Studies using DNA microarrays in breast cancer have identified potential new classifications with striking molecular differences,[6–9] including powerful predictors of disease outcome.[10] Studies in lung cancer are less advanced, but have identified potentially important subgroups of lung adenocarcinoma.[1,11]

Comparisons of messenger RNA and protein levels for the same tumors reported for lung cancer demonstrated that only a small percentage of genes had a statistically significant correlation between the levels of their corresponding proteins and mRNAs;[12] thus the overall correlation between level of expression of the transcriptome and protein expression is relatively poor. This may not be entirely surprising and underscores the potential importance of proteomic analysis.

Most biological fluids contain cellular and non-cellular components. Proteomics has the greatest potential to uncover important biological information in this non-cellular component. In an effort to further characterize the molecular determinants of lung cancer, it is therefore critical that we probe these tissues with tools that address the biology of lung cancer directly at the protein level. As a result, there is substantial interest in developing technologies that allow the rapid and systematic analysis of thousands of proteins. In particular, the identification of novel biomarkers to differentiate tumor from normal cells and predict individuals likely to develop lung cancer represents a major clinical question.

The hypothesis behind protein-based early detection of lung cancer is that a transformed cancer cell and its clonal expansion results in up- or down-regulation of specific host- or tumor-derived proteins, some of which will be secreted. These proteins should be detectable in biological specimens, including airway samples, sputum, exhaled breath or other samples obtained by methods ranging from venopuncture, bronchial brushing, lavage or biopsy, transthoracic needle aspirates or surgical biopsy specimen. These proteins, including tumor antigens, can be detected by a variety of methods with different sensitivity and specificity. Historically, early detection has been most challenging because of the limited sensitivity of most tests applied to screening strategies and a molecular approach may address some of the limitations of more traditional imaging or histological-based approaches. Recently, studies have shown that cancer-specific 'fingerprints' can be obtained directly from tissue or serum and have great promise for the early diagnosis of cancer.[13–17] In this chapter we will review the proteomic methodologies applied to lung cancer specimens, review the original published data, and propose future directions.

METHODOLOGICAL APPROACHES

2D gel electrophoresis

Two-dimensional (2D) gel electrophoresis has been the primary method of comprehensive proteomic analysis of many tissue samples. In this method, proteins are separated on the basis of their charge through isoelectric focusing in one dimension and are further separated in a second dimension in a polyacrylamide gel on the basis of their molecular weight. When silver-staining techniques are used, approximately 3000 proteins can be visualized on a single gel. Stained gels are scanned with laser densitometers, and spot detection can be analyzed and quantified with software such as PDQUEST.[18]

A series of improvements have been brought to this technology to address the quality of information obtained from this technique. Immobilized pH gradients have greatly enhanced reproducibility in resolving the rather large spectrum of basic to acidic proteins and have allowed both analytical and preparative amounts of proteins to be resolved.[19–22] Narrow-range pH gradients are also increasing protein resolution and detection. A range of 1 pH unit was demonstrated to resolve 1000 protein spots.[23] Detection and quantitation of protein spots in 2D gels has been greatly improved by fluorescent dye labeling techniques to overcome some of the drawbacks of silver staining and make protein samples more amenable to mass spectrometric identification.[24,25]

Another development in 2D gels is the use of differential in-gel electrophoresis (DIGE), in which two pools of proteins are labeled with different fluorescent dyes.[26] The labeled proteins are mixed and analyzed in the same 2D gel. Differential in-gel electrophoresis (DIGE) provides a methodology that improves the reproducibility, sensitivity and quantitative aspects of 2D-gel analysis.[27,28]

2D-PAGE and related technologies have proven to be excellent tools for discovery of proteins associated with pathological states. However, only a small percentage of the proteome can be visualized by 2D-PAGE, and in spite of the improvement in proteomics technology, 2D gels remain a low-throughput approach that requires relatively large amounts of sample. 2-D gels are cumbersome to run, have a poor dynamic range, and are biased toward abundant and soluble proteins. The amount of sample required for analysis is particularly important for clinically applicable proteomics. Various tissue microdissection approaches can substantially reduce heterogeneity, but they further reduce the amount of sample available. Also, 2D gel analysis alone cannot provide the identity of the proteins that have been resolved.

Two-dimensional gel electrophoresis was very early on applied to the profiling of protein expression patterns, and when combined with mass spectrometry can lead to identification of discriminating protein spots.[19,20,29,30] When matrix-assisted laser desorption ionization mass spectrometry (MALDI-MS) is used after 2D gel-based protein separation, the samples are crystallized with a matrix which absorbs energy and ejects and ionizes the molecules into the gas phase. A strong electrical field accelerates the ions to reach a detector at a speed that is inversely proportional to their mass-to-charge (m/z) ratios.

Reducing sample complexity prior to analysis improves the reach of 2D gels or other separation techniques for the quantitative analysis of low-abundance proteins. Protein tagging enhances sensitivity and is currently being implemented for the comprehensive analysis of the cell surface proteome. A surface-protein biotinylation strategy coupled with the use of mass spectrometry have led to the detection and identification of many new proteins on the surface of cancer cells.[31]

Besides 2D gel separation, various techniques that rely on liquid-based separations of proteins or peptides, with or without tagging, will have utility for proteomic analysis, particularly given their potential for automation. Additionally, advances in microfluidics technology (the technology to move, mix, pump and control fluids on a microscopic level) will allow automated separation of proteins in complex lysates using much reduced sample amounts. Applications of this technology to protein separation, drug development, diagnostics and environmental monitoring are already being integrated with mass spectrometry for protein digestion and identification.[32]

Mass spectrometry techniques

Development of ionization techniques such as electrospray ionization (ESI), matrix-assisted laser-desorption ionization (MALDI), and surface-enhanced laser desorption ionization (SELDI), and using new analyzers such as TOF and quadrupole technologies, have facilitated the characterization of proteins by mass spectrometry (MS). These techniques transfer proteins into a gas phase, enabling analysis in the mass spectrometer. After separation through 2-DE or HPLC, digested peptide samples can be analyzed in a mass spectrometer through a 'nanoelectrospray', allowing for direct sequencing and identification of proteins. Recently, a MALDI quadrupole TOF instrument has been developed that allows a combination of peptide mapping with peptide sequencing.[33,34] This instrument allows identification of a protein either by peptide mass fingerprinting of the protein digest or from tandem mass spectra acquired by collision-induced dissociation of individual peptide precursors. A peptide mass map of the digest and tandem mass spectra of multiple peptide precursor ions can be acquired from the same sample in the course of a single experiment.

Improved mass spectrometric ionization sources such as ESI, MALDI and SELDI and analyzers such as TOF and quadrupole have enabled easy analysis of the proteome and with excellent sensitivity (Table 7.1). Using this technique, a spectrum is generated with the molecular mass of individual peptides and used to search databases to find matching proteins.

MALDI-MS/MS

MALDI-MS

Complex mixtures can be analyzed by MALDI mass spectrometry without fractionation.[34] This type of analysis allows the simultaneous determination of protein molecular masses from 1–40 kDa with excellent accuracy. The mass spectrum obtained does not require elaborate interpretation because there is no fragmentation of the ionized protein or peptide. Therefore, there is a one-to-one correspondence between

Table 7.1 Comparison of proteomic platforms

	2D-PAGE	ESI-MS (LC-MS/MS) MudPit	MALDI-TOF MS
Throughput	Relatively low; labor intensive Increased with automation	*Moderate* Single separations (reversed-phase) typically 70 minutes *Low* Multidimensional chromatographic fractionations (10–15 fractions)	*High* Increased with automation (hundreds of samples/day)
Sensitivity	Low for low abundance proteins, proteins with extreme pI, molecular weights, and hydrophobicity	Higher sensitivity; dependent upon fractionations to reduce sample complexity. Increased coverage of sample mixture	Typically high-abundant proteins are favored Low-abundant proteins suppressed unless fractionation techniques applied
Detection limits	Typically 10–100 kDa proteins Detection dependent upon stains used to visualize proteins: Coomassie = low µg Silver and Sypro Ruby = 1 ng 20% of loaded proteins visualized	Digested proteins analyzed rather than intact proteins Typical scan range 300–2000 Da Higher molecular weight proteins are observed as multiply charged ions Not compatible with non-volatile salts, buffer and detergents	Optimal range ≤25 kDa Resolution decreases at higher molecular weights
Quantitative analysis	2D-DIGE technology using fluorescent dyes – more reproducibility and accurate quantitative analysis Analysis of multiple samples on one gel	Isotopic labeling (ICAT) allows for quantitative analysis	Not commonly used for quantitative analysis

the peaks in the mass spectrum and the proteins/peptides present in the original mixture. The identification of these peaks remains more time consuming as it requires purification and sequencing by various methods.

One feature of MALDI-TOF MS which makes it especially promising for mass spectrometric analysis of biological samples is its ability to detect biomolecules in complex mixtures in the presence of large molar excesses of salts, buffers and other species. Because of these qualities, MALDI MS has been utilized to study proteins/peptides in serum, blood, urine, tissue extracts and whole cells. MALDI MS was also successfully applied to LCM captured cells, e.g. from the mammary epithelium or colon crypt.[36]

LC-MS, MS-MS (tandem MS)

Typically, a mixture of proteins is first digested with site-specific proteases, then the resulting peptides are separated by liquid chromatography (LC), and fractions are then analyzed by tandem MS (MS/MS). In this procedure, a mixture of charged peptides is separated in the first MS according to their m/z ratios to create a list of the most intense peptide peaks. In the second MS analysis, the instrument is adjusted so that only a specific m/z species is directed into a collision cell that fractures these peptides into predictable 'daughter' ions derived from the 'parent' species. Using the appropriate collision energy, fragmentation occurs predominantly at the peptide bonds such that a ladder of fragments, each of which differs by the mass of a single amino acid, is generated. The daughter fragments are separated according to their m/z, and, since the mass spectrometer can identify amino acids by measuring the precise differences in molecular weight of these fragments, the sequence of the peptide can then be deduced from the resulting fragments. By comparison with predicted sequences in the

databases, the identity of the peptide is deduced.

The direct measurement of peptide mass enables an important aspect of MS-MS analysis to accurately identify post-translational modifications, such as phosphorylation and glycosylation, through the measurement of mass shifts.

The coupling of liquid chromatography (HPLC) with MS has had a great impact on small molecule and protein profiling, and on protein identification, and has proven to be an important alternative method to 2D gels.[37,38] Briefly, proteins in a complex mixture are separated by ionic or reverse phase column chromatography and identified with MS analysis by using various ionization methods, most widely ESI. This approach greatly complicates the analysis, but LC-MS has been applied to large-scale protein characterization and identification. Unlike the 2D/MS approaches, Yates group was able to show that even low-abundant proteins could be clearly identified.[37]

MALDI MS imaging

Imaging MS is a new technology for direct mapping and high-resolution imaging of biomolecules present in tissue sections.[39] In this system, frozen tissue sections or individual cells are mounted on a metal plate, spotted with droplets of matrix in a regular array spaced at 50–100 μm, mass spectra acquired from each 'pixel', and the spectrum from each pixel is then queried for the presence of specific mass spectral peaks. An image is then generated representing the intensity of a given peak in each pixel in the array. This yields a spatial image showing the distribution of individual masses across the tissue section. Imaging MS has been used in human glioblastoma and found to increase expression of several proteins in the proliferating area when compared to the healthy tissue.[39] Imaging MS shows potential for several applications, including biomarker discovery, biomarker tissue localization, understanding molecular complexity of tumor tissues, and assessment of surgical margins in resected tumors.[40] Recently it has become possible to analyze tissue sections directly on metallized but transparent glass slides after staining with MS-friendly staining protocols instead of being applied onto gold plates. This allows careful histological review of the very same samples and regions from which MS profiles are obtained.[41]

MALDI-MS advantages

Due to the pulsed nature of most lasers, ions are formed in discrete events. Therefore, MALDI can achieve very high levels of sensitivity, often providing data from sub-femtomole ($<1 \times 10{-}15$ moles) amounts of sampling loading. Another advantage of MALDI MS lies in the fact that singly charged analytes are usually generated. When coupled with certain mass analyzers (TOF), MALDI can be used to rapidly provide molecular weight information for one or more peptides/proteins. Throughput issues are beginning to be addressed by loading sample plates with ~100 different samples, and instrumentation improvements are allowing data acquisition in a matter of minutes. Another practical advantage of MALDI is its relatively high tolerance to salts and buffers common in biological samples. Unlike ESI, high-quality spectra can be generated from MALDI MS using samples that contain physiological levels of salts.[42]

MALDI-MS limitations

Because of the pulsed nature of the technique, only certain mass spectrometers are easily coupled with MALDI. Although matrix can facilitate ionization, it causes a large degree of chemical noise to be observed at m/z ratios below 500 Da. In fact, samples with low molecular weights are usually difficult to analyze by MALDI. Recent variations of MALDI, in particular the desorption/ionization on silicon (DIOS) technique, seem promising for enabling the analyses of low-molecular-weight compounds without the chemical background at low m/z ratios.[43,44]

SELDI

Surface-enhanced laser desorption-ionization (SELDI), described by Hutchens and Yip[45] uses MALDI MS on affinity-captured species through the use of specific surfaces or chips. Affinity surfaces retain proteins based on their physical or chemical characteristics (i.e., hydrophobic, cationic, anionic, hydrophilic). This MS technology enables both biomarker discovery and protein profiling directly from complex samples without using any separation techniques or with very simple ones. A great amount of work has been done in the analysis of serum biomarkers. Recently published reports describe distinction between disease and controls based on 'signature protein patterns' of the serum generated by SELDI-TOF MS, e.g. cancer patients from cancer-free individuals.[14–16] Besides discovery and protein-profiling applications, SELDI can also be used in an immunoassay platform. In this application, specific antibodies are bound to the chip array to capture protein antigens for analysis.[46]

ESI

Electrospray ionization is a technique by which peptides and proteins in solution are converted into multiply charged ions in a gas phase for analysis in a mass spectrometer. These gas phase ions move to the analyzer under the influence of varying pressures and electric fields at the boundary leading to the mass analyzer.[47] The multiple charges on the gas phase peptides bring the mass-to-charge ratio down to a few thousand from a molecular weight of tens of thousands. Since mass spectrometers directly measure mass per charge, this method allows measurement of large molecules without going over the largest-mass limit of the detector (usually about 2000 atomic mass unit). Generally ESI is coupled with a triple quadrupole, ion trap or hybrid TOF MS. The ability to conduct tandem MS after electrospray ionization has revolutionized proteomics since this MS-MS method can be used to directly obtain amino acid sequence information.[48]

Compared with MALDI, ESI presents significant advantages in the ease of coupling to separation techniques such as liquid chromatography (LC) and high-pressure LC (HPLC), allowing high throughput and on-line analysis of protein or peptide mixtures.

Protein arrays

Unlike cDNA microarrays, which provide one measure of gene expression (mRNA levels), there is a need to implement protein microarray strategies that address the many different expression profiles and functions of proteins that are altered in disease. Protein microarray technology provides an in vitro way to study function as reflected in protein alterations. For this application, the proteins themselves are arrayed on a solid support. Protein microarrays can be used to study function in this way on a genome-wide basis.[49]

In protein microarrays, the spots may consist of antibodies, cell or phage lysates, nucleic acids, drugs or recombinant proteins or peptides.[50-53] Detection of the array is achieved by probing with a tagged antibody, ligand or serum/cell lysate. The signal generates a pattern of positive and negative spots. The signal intensity of each spot is proportional to the quantity of applied tagged molecules bound to the molecule. Significant difficulties in this technology

relate to the detection of low abundance proteins with adequate sensitivity and specificity – the ability to block endogenous molecules such as peroxidases, biotin or immunoglobulins, and which may be important due to ability to interfere with the detection amplification chemistries.

Autoantibodies can be particularly useful for studying cell-surface antigens on cancer cells and could become a powerful tool for screening large numbers of antigens by protein microarray.[54] In lung cancer patients, the protein PGP9.5 has been found to be a circulating tumor biomarker with potential clinical use in screening and diagnosis.[55]

A reverse-phase protein array approach that immobilizes the whole repertoire of a tissue's proteins has been developed.[56,57] Using this approach, Paweletz et al showed an association between cancer progression and increased phosphorylation of the serine/threonine kinase Akt, suppression of apoptosis pathways, and decreased phosphorylation of extracellular signal-regulated kinase (ERK).[56]

Knezevic et al analyzed protein expression in tissue derived from squamous cell carcinomas of the oral cavity by using an antibody microarray approach for high-throughput proteomic analysis.[58] Differential expression of multiple proteins was found in stromal cells surrounding and adjacent to regions of diseased epithelium that correlated directly with tumor progression of the epithelium. Most of the proteins identified were involved in signal transduction pathways.

In addition to several advantages, protein microarray technology has some limitations. This technology requires high-quality and comprehensive expression libraries and methods that allow the robust analysis of a large number of functionally active proteins. Lack of availability of high-affinity and high-specificity antibodies for gene products and post-translationally modified proteins is one of the major current limitations of this technology.[59] Besides protein microarrays, peptide microarray technology is of great interest for functional analysis. This methodology could analyze substrate interactions and substrate specificity, enzyme–substrate interactions and can be applied to drug discovery.[60,61]

APPLICATION OF THESE PROTEOMIC METHODS TO LUNG CANCER

Lung tissue

A comprehensive analysis of the proteome in lung cancer is being pursued.[62] Hanash and colleagues have analyzed over 1000 lung cancer-related samples using 2D PAGE, in combination with mass spectrometry, and have constructed the lung proteomic database.[62] The aim of their studies is to identify biomarkers for the early detection of cancer, for developing novel classification of tumors, and for revealing novel targets for therapeutic intervention.[12,30,63] They performed parallel analysis of the transcriptome and of the proteome in lung tumors comparing mRNA and protein levels in the same tumors.[12] The integrated intensities of 165 protein spots representing protein products of 98 genes were analyzed in 76 lung adenocarcinomas and nine unaffected lung tissues using 2D PAGE. For the same 85 samples, mRNA levels were determined using oligonucleotide microarrays. Only 21 out of the 98 genes analyzed (21.4%) showed a statistically significant correlation between protein and mRNA levels. This does not mean that microarray studies are uninformative, rather that they convey additional information with only partial overlap with proteomic data.

Recently, the Michigan group identified a battery of genes and related proteins validated

using a training and independent testing set associated with survival of adenocarcinoma of the lung.[64] Using 2D gel analysis, the same group identified five CK7 cleavage products best associated with patient survival, a subset of which correlated to gene expression (Figure 7.1).[63] Using two-dimensional PAGE and mass spectrometry, Chen et al identified and characterized several lung-cancer-specific protein markers of lung adenocarcinomas such as Antioxidant enzyme AOE372, ATP synthase subunit d(ATP5D), beta1,4-galactosyltransferase, cytosolic inorganic pyrophosphatase, glucose-regulated M(r) 58000 protein, glutathione-S-transferase M4, prolyl 4-hydroxylase beta subunit, triosephosphate isomerase, and ubiquitin thiolesterase (UCHL1).[12] They went on to identify 33 of 46 survival-associated proteins by mass spectrometry. Expression of 12 candidate proteins was confirmed as tumor-derived with immunohistochemical analysis and tissue microarrays.[65] Two polypeptide markers, TAO1 and TAO2 were found expressed in approximately 90% of primary lung adenocarcinomas and found to be identical to napsin A, a recently described member of the aspartic proteinase family.[66–68]

Using a MALDI-MS technology, Bergman et al detected increases in the expression of Cathepsin D in lung adenocarcinoma.[18] Many of these proteins represent specific isoforms of known proteins and reflect post-translational modifications and potential degradation forms. They also confirmed these candidates by using both mRNA microarrays and tissue microarray (TMA).[64,65] As yet, none of those candidate biomarkers has an application in the clinic.

A proteomic approach has allowed the identification of endothelial cell surface proteins aminopeptidase-P and annexin A1, exhibiting restricted lung tissue distribution and overexpression in lung tumors. Radio-immunotherapy

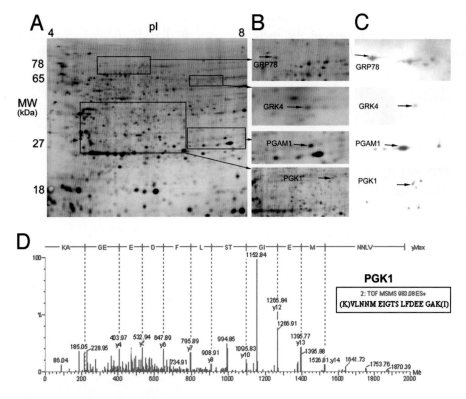

Figure 7.1
Two-dimensional PAGE image and 2D Western blots for selected survival-related proteins. (A) Two-dimensional gel image showing protein separation by molecular mass (MW) and isoelectric point (pI). (B) Two-dimensional separation of the regions that include GRP78, GRK4, PGAM1 and PGK1 isoforms. (C) Two-dimensional Western blot showing GRP78, PGAM1, GRK4, or PGK1 immunoreactive protein spots. The same isoforms for each protein are indicated with arrows for B and C. (D) Tandem mass spectrometry (ESI MS/MS) confirmation for the PGK1 protein spot shown in B. (From[64]. Reprinted by permission.)

to annexin A1 destroyed tumors and increased animal survival.[69]

With recent advances in mass spectrometry techniques, it is now possible to investigate protein expression profiles from small biological specimens over a wide range of molecular weights. Using this technology on tumor lysates, profiles of ten non small-cell lung cancer were analyzed, and two proteins, MMIF and cyclophilin A, were identified as biomarkers[70] and later found not to be prognostic markers of disease based on a 240 lung

cancer tissue microarray immunohistochemical analysis.[71]

We and others have recently demonstrated that proteomic profiling of lung tumors using MALDI-MS or 2D gel electrophoresis methods allows distinction between normal and cancer tissue, and may predict lymph node involvement or survival (Figure 7.2).[13,65] In a recent report we used conventional matrix-assisted laser desorption/ionization time-of-flight mass spectrometry (MALDI-MS) to generate protein profiles that accurately classify and predict histological sub-

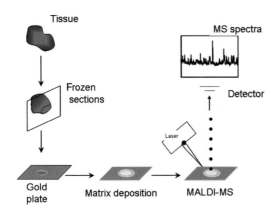

Figure 7.2
MALDI-MMS on tissue sections is performed by mounting frozen sections of the tissue directly on a stainless steel plate. A MALDI matrix is applied to the samples prior to analysis by TOF mass spectrometry.

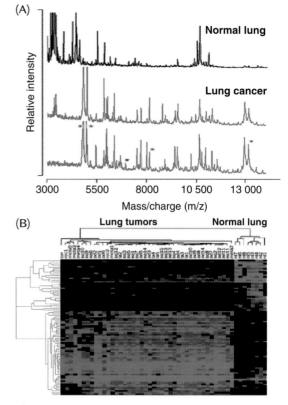

groups of lung cancer (Figure 7.3).[13] Using biostatistical methods to select differentially expressed peaks (MS signals) and after the development of a class prediction model,[72] 82 discriminatory signals were found to classify normal lung from lung cancer tissue samples in a derivation and validation study design with excellent accuracy. Other recent studies indicated the importance of using protein expression profiles as a diagnostic or prognostic biomarker for patients with early-stage lung cancer using surface-enhanced laser desorption/ionization (SELDI) technology.[73] Although preliminary, these studies stress the relevance of protein signatures for the diagnosis and the evaluation of response to therapy in lung cancer.

Most recently, a small series of surgically resected lung tumors was recently analyzed by 2D gel and MALDI MS to identify a series of proteins previously reported such as annexin II, cathepsin D, HSP27, stathmin and MnSOD, confirming the validity of this methodology to identify candidate biomarkers.[74]

Figure 7.3
Detection of the optimum discriminatory biomarker sets in lung tumors. (A) Representative MALDI-TOF-MS spectra obtained from tumor and normal lung tissue samples with molecular weight calculation (m/z values). Examples of the MS peaks identified by the statistical analyses as optimum discriminatory patterns between normal and tumor are indicated by asterisks. (B) Hierarchical cluster analysis of 42 lung tumors and eight normal lung tissues in the training cohort according to the protein expression patterns of 82 MS signals. Each row represents an individual proteomic signal, and each column represents an individual sample. The dendrogram at the top shows the similarity in protein expression profiles of the samples. Substantially raised (red) expression of the proteins is noted in individual tumor and normal lung tissue samples. AD = adenocarcinoma; SQ = squamous-cell carcinoma; LA = large-cell carcinoma; META = metastases to lung from other sites; REC = recurrent NSCLC; CAR = pulmonary carcinoid; NL = normal lung.[13]

Serum and plasma

Serum proteomic studies, although very challenging, have a great promise for the early detection of cancer, the monitoring of disease status, the discovery of new targets for therapy, and the assessment of response to therapy. This new approach is facing the difficulties of lack of standardization, continuously evolving technologies, limitations of bioinformatics tools, the complex nature and large dynamic range of the blood proteome, assay reproducibility and quantitation of candidate biomarkers. Proteomic studies using the blood as a source of proteins still have not resolved the question of whether analysis of serum or plasma is more informative. Arguments in favor of both approaches exist, and a systematic, rigorous and prospective collection protocol is essential to answering all of these questions.

The human plasma proteome project is an international collaboration to characterize proteins in the human serum and plasma. This organization is addressing in detail issues of protein identification, specimen collection, handling, storage, depletion of highly abundant proteins, fractionation and mass spectrometry instruments for the identification of peptides from digested proteins. They have already identified over 9500 proteins, 3000 of which have at least two peptide matches (http://211.32.65.137/hpp/hppp.htm). Their original reports are expected in mid 2005.

Another great argument revolves around the need for fractionation of the serum/plasma. The simple fact that 22 of these tens of thousands of proteins in serum constitute 99% of the total protein content in the serum and that there is a large concentration range of these proteins ($\sim 10^8$ fold) results in serious difficulties in the identification of tumor-specific markers, many of which are likely to be present in low abundance. Fractionation is intuitively more satisfy-

ing, reducing the complexity of the biological mixture, increasing the number of peaks obtained by MALDI MS, and increasing the likelihood of finding new biomarkers among lower-abundance proteins. However, disadvantages also exist since fractionation requires large sample amounts, is more time and cost consuming, and increases the risk of variability within and between samples, and these may preclude the use of the resulting proteomic patterns for diagnosis. A dual approach is probably worth emphasizing at the early stage of development of this proteomic strategy.

Analysis of the serum proteome assumes that tissue perfusion of tumors or host responses contributes to modification of circulating protein or peptide concentrations. Therefore, the proteins present in the serum are hypothesized to reflect the pathological state of the organism. Thus, what we are attempting to uncover is a discriminating pattern in a small subset of proteins among thousands that are useful for diagnostic purposes. Evaluation of the lower-molecular-weight protein profile can be accurately analyzed by a variety of methods, including surface-enhanced laser desorption ionization time-of-flight (SELDI-TOF), electron spray mass spectrometry (ES-MS), and MALDI MS and may correlate with these pathological states. It remains to be seen if there is sufficient information in this slice of the blood proteome.

Recently published studies have reported serum protein expression profiles that distinguish cancer patients with a variety of malignancies from controls using various mass spectrometry-related approaches SELDI-TOF[14–16,75–77] and MALDI MS.[17] In the latter publication, the authors identified a serum protein pattern in head and neck cancer patients that achieved a sensitivity of between 34–52% when applied to the serum of patients with lung cancer. Protein patterns were distinguished by using MALDI-TOF MS combined with a simple classification procedure, based on a *t*-test and linear discriminant analysis in tumor sera that included head and neck or lung cancer patients.[17] By using the optimal head and neck cancer model cutoff of 73% sensitivity and 90% specificity, they were able to discriminate squamous cell lung cancer with sensitivities of 52% (for adenocarcinoma it was 34%), and for large cell carcinoma it was 40%.[17] However, this study was not designed to address whether this protein profile can discriminate lung cancer patients from controls.

This is a unique study that generates proteomic profiles in serum by using MALDI-TOF-MS, a very simple, rapid, and inexpensive technology that requires only basic sample processing and shows potential to achieve practical early cancer detection in biological fluids. A single protein by itself may not be useful for early detection, but it is thought that the most informative biomarker may be a combination of markers into 'signature' protein profiles for the early diagnosis. These studies are very encouraging and demonstrate that MALDI fingerprint protein profiling, coupled with a learning algorithm, can be useful for early diagnosis of prostate, ovarian, breast, bladder and aerodigestive cancers by using only 1 μl of serum.

Our group recently generated protein expression profiles using MALDI-TOF-MS directly from 1 μl of unfractionated serum to define a discriminatory 'protein fingerprint' to distinguish patients with lung cancer from matched controls.[78] We found several proteins could discriminate early-stage lung cancer from controls; most of the proteins were in lower m/z ranges. Recently, automated tools for the discovery of serum markers have been developed. These apply small-volume robotics to serum fractionation and MALDI-MS analysis. This approach may provide better reproducibility, multidimensionality and high throughput to the analysis of biological specimens (Figure 7.4).[79] These approaches need to be validated in larger populations and from a number of institutions before the further translation of this tool into general clinical decision-making for the early diagnosis of lung cancer.

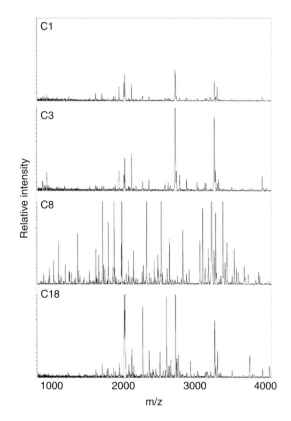

Figure 7.4
Effect of carbon chain length on serum peptide profiling using RP-derivatized, magnetic particles and MALDI-TOF-MS. Equal volumes of serum were incubated with fixed-weight amounts of SiMAG RP beads (K type) in separate experiments, beads washed and eluted with 50% MeCN, and the eluates analyzed, all as described in the Methodological Approaches section. Segments of the MALDI-TOF-MS corresponding to peptides in the 0.8–4-kDa mass range (assuming z = 1) are shown.[79] Reprinted by permission.

Using MALDI-TOF MS, Howard et al identified SAA (m/z 11702) in serum as a discriminant protein in the tumor from normal[80] and confirmed their finding by enzyme-linked immunosorbent assay. However, this protein alone does not provide the desired sensitivity or specificity for a clinically useful diagnostic test.

Hanash and colleagues have also searched for circulating tumor antigens by screening for auto-antibodies in lung cancer patients using Western blotting.[55] Briefly, 2D PAGE of the lung adenocarcinoma cell line (A549) was incubated with sera from patients with lung adenocarcinoma, other cancers, and no cancer controls. These studies found auto-antibodies against glycosylated annexins I and II in 60% of the patients with lung adenocarcinomas and 33% of patients with SCCs and that this was associated with high circulating levels of IL-6.[81] Similarly, studies involving sera from 64 newly diagnosed patients with lung cancer, 99 patients with other types of cancer, and 71 non-cancer controls revealed a tumor antigen, protein gene product 9.5 (PGP 9.5, a neurospecific protein) that induces a humoral response in lung cancer.[55]

In an effort to speed up the analysis of serum for auto-antibodies to lungs bearing antigens, Madoz-Gurpide et al have developed a novel approach that combines liquid phase protein separation with microarray technologies.[82] Whole-cell or tissue lysates are fractionated by isoelectric focusing and reverse phase chromatography into hundreds of fractions, which are then arrayed onto nitrocellulose-coated slides and incubated with the sera. Such biochips require low sample volume and provide a rapid procedure to molecularly profile the antibody response to tumor antigens in cancer. Circulating antibodies to tumor-associated proteins were also isolated from the serum of patients with lung cancer from cDNA T7

phage libraries, and 45 candidates were identified. Protein expression in serum is being confirmed by ELISA.[83]

Pleural effusions

Proteomics has the advantage of allowing the analysis of both tissue and biological fluids, the identification of proteins and protein post-translational modifications such as phosphorylation, glycosylation, sulfation, that could be specific for different tumor types. Nilsson et al analyzed pleural exudates by applying 2D gel electrophoresis, MALDI-TOF MS, and Western blotting.[84,85] They confirmed the identity of proteins of potential diagnostic value such as cystatin C. Although it is possible to obtain mass spectra of proteins in complex biological mixtures (e.g. pleural effusion, CSF) without previous purification steps,[35,86] simple fractionation often results in a dramatic improvement of the signal-to-noise ratio. Because larger volumes of low concentrations of proteins can be loaded onto analytical 2D gels, low abundance proteins in biological fluids such as pleural exudates may be enriched for further characterization by mass spectrometry.

Recently, Bard et al studied the presence of exosomes (membrane vesicles from endosomes) in cancerous pleural effusions and to identify their proteomic content.[87] They found the presence of antigen-presenting molecules, cytoskeletal proteins and signal transduction-involved proteins as well as SNX25, BTG1, PEDF and thrombospondin 2. A high concentration of antigen–antibody humoral immunity components in exosomes may be important as an antigen source for cancer immunotherapy.

Exhaled breath and sputum

Condensation of exhaled breath is a newly described non-invasive way to collect material originating from the lung, including the lower respiratory tract. To date, exhaled breath condensate samples have been mainly studied for NO metabolites,[88,89] 8-isoprostane,[90,91] hydrogen peroxide[92] and various inflammatory cytokines.[93] EBC and saliva proteins have been characterized by using 2DE electrophoresis,[94] but characterization of the methods as well as the specimens have not yet been completed. Looking at a set of volatile markers may enable recognition and diagnosis of diseases such as lung cancer. Recently, tumor suppressor gene p53 mutation was detected by PCR in exhaled breath condensate of patients with lung cancer.[95] Although very appealing, there are technical problems of sampling and analysis and a lack of normalization and standardization, huge variations exist between results of different studies.[96] To move the analysis of EBC to clinical practice is likely to be problematic.

The sputum represents an even more complex mixture than exhaled breath condensate to analyze by proteomic methods. Sputum induction using hypertonic saline has allowed minimally invasive assessment of airway inflammation.[97] Two-dimensional electrophoresis of sputum induction specimen is attractive, though specific alterations in protein composition upon lung disorders are not well characterized. The soluble and cellular components may represent useful and separate components to analyze by MALDI-MS. This work needs to be developed in the future.

Bronchial biopsies

In some preliminary studies we used MALDI-MS to identify specific patterns of protein expression of the airway epithelium of different histological stages of tumor progression. MALDI-MS data were acquired from 25 normal alveolar epithelium, 29 normal bronchial epithelium, 20 preinvasive and 36 invasive lung cancer tissues mainly from patients with and

without concomitant lung cancer. Statistical analysis and supervised hierarchical cluster analysis revealed that protein profiles are able to distinguish between groups with excellent accuracy.[98] We hope to validate these data in an independent set of tissues and select proteins expressed in invasive and preinvasive, but not histologically, in normal epithelium. Ultimately, these proteins may provide us with targets for diagnostic markers and therapeutic intervention.

Bronchioalveolar lavage (BAL)

BAL performed during fiberoptic bronchoscopy is a relatively safe technique which allows the collection of cells and a wide variety of soluble components including proteins from the human lung.[99] Due to the wide variety of origins for proteins present in BAL, as well as the huge diversity of proteins considered, analysis of the protein content of BAL is of outstanding potential interest to define biomarkers in many lung diseases. The potential for discovery of new lung disease markers in BAL via the 2-DE and proteomics approaches is significant. The first 2-DE map displaying the major soluble proteins present in lung lavage was published in 1979[100] and pattern matched with 2-DE maps of serum samples.[101] After many different technical improvements, current work still aims at the construction of a 2-DE reference database of BAL proteins and the understanding of the molecular processes involved in lung disease.[102]

Recently, the identification of proteins present in the BAL 2-DE map has been published.[103–105] The most important technical advancement that enabled BALF proteomic analysis was the improvement in the method used for isoelectric focusing (IEF). In 1990, Lenz et al used improved methods for IEF for the first-dimensional separation of proteins from dog BAL.[106] The BAL sample preparation (salt removal, sample concentration, fractionation), sample loading technique, the choice of pH range, and the second dimensional gel to be used are critical to obtain optimal resolution of the widest range of proteins present in BAL.[104,107] Several proteins have been identified related to lung inflammation, altered in the smokers, and specific for the different inflammatory conditions (sarcoidosis, IPF, hypersensitivity pneumonitis). This BAL technique has not been studied in detail in patients at risk of lung cancer.

INTEGRATION OF MULTIPLE MOLECULAR METHODS OF EARLY DETECTION

Integration of genomics and proteomics approaches will allow us to move closer to the goals of earlier detection. The rapid development of proteomic and genomic technologies has provided a large amount of novel information, comprehensive analysis of the molecular basis of disease, and is leading to the assembly of large protein inventories.[108] Functional proteomics is emerging as a powerful tool that uses proteomic technologies to investigate the interaction, integration and functions of proteins. This strategy couples proteomic information with biochemical and physiological analysis to advance our understanding of the functional role of proteins in normal and diseased organs.

Molecular profiling may assist in identifying high-risk populations and offers a unique opportunity to study early carcinogenesis and potentially to reduce cancer mortality through the available effective treatment modalities amenable to early cancer. Proteomics-based early-detection strategies for cancer diagnosis will include the analysis of complex mixtures such as tissue samples, serum, plasma, sputum and exhaled breath condensate.

The inherent analytical advantages of mass spectrometry, including sensitivity and speed, and combined with recent advances promises to make MS a mainstay of drug design and discovery. The development of ionization techniques, such as ESI and MALDI, now allows almost any compound to be studied by MS. In addition, MS/MS adds the capability for structural analysis of compounds that are present at low levels and/or are present in complex mixtures. The gentle nature of relatively new ionization techniques such as ESI and the structural analysis capability of MS should extend this technique into new areas. The optimal combinations depend on the desired goal, such as protein identification, de novo peptide sequencing, identification of post-translation modification and determination of protein–protein interactions.[42] Ultimately, we will need to integrate in our prediction models not only molecular markers e.g. proteomic, genetic and epigenetic but also epidemiological, pathological and imaging data elements.

CHALLENGES AHEAD

Standardization of methods

Proteomics studies use various methods for collecting, preparing and analyzing samples on the mass spectrometer; yet the optimal steps in sample collection, processing and analysis needs to be standardized.[109] One of the limitations of direct analysis of tissues or biological fluids by MALDI is the preferential detection of proteins of lower molecular mass and the difficulty in determining the identity of proteins precisely in a high-throughput manner. Because of the inherent instability of proteins, sample procurement and preservation issues will need to be addressed to make them compatible with proteomics analysis.

Bioinformatics issues

Databases do not agree on criteria necessary to assign a protein ID. The HUPO has over 9600 proteins identified according to internal criteria proposed but yet identification of proteins and statistical methods[110] leading to identification of proteins still are needed to reach agreement. The development of bioinformatics tools and optimization of biostatistical analysis is essential. Analyzing MALDI-MS data requires starting with a large number of variables (approximately 3000 peaks) to detect a small number of key disease-associated proteins. To extract as much information as possible from a limited number of samples and to avoid non-disease-related artifacts is a great challenge. Further, to make sample processing simple enough for a diagnostic test is an important goal of clinical proteomics. Obviously, the size of the datasets obtained after fractionation leads to difficulties in data analysis. The complex nature of the sample fractionation and data analysis also call for a major effort in mobilization of a process otherwise subject to a relatively high variability.

The integration of genomic with proteomic data represents a great challenge for the future. A large number of proteins that are expressed in different types of lung cancer have been identified and have been correlated with the expression measures for their corresponding genes at the RNA level. Because of the non-linear relationship between gene expression, translation to protein, and changes in function, it will be important to assay not only for protein overexpression but also their functional post-translational modifications.

Low-abundance proteins

When analyzing biological samples, it is desirable to avoid excessive purification steps, since a loss of material is unavoidable at each step. The analysis of biological samples is also complicated by the fact that the sample contains many proteins, many of them at a low concentration. The low abundance of proteins of interest in biological materials makes isolation of sufficient material for proteomic analysis problematic, particularly for 2D electrophoresis. The more we fractionate proteins, the more we have a risk of increasing variability.

Quantitation

Alterations in the proteome are dynamic rather than static and may occur in many different ways. A better understanding of those alterations will have a substantial impact in lung cancer research. Further technological innovations would be beneficial to increase sensitivity, reduce sample requirements, increase throughput, and more effectively uncover various types of protein alterations such as post-translational modifications. Quantitation of molecular species, in particular of candidate biomarkers, will be of critical importance. It is hoped that standard chemical assays, ELISA assays and mass spectrometric analysis will render the assays sensitive and reliable. Fluorescence-based and mass spectrometry-based methodologies are actively pursued, difference gel electrophoresis (DIGE),[26] multiplexed proteomics.[111,112] and isotope-coded affinity tagging (ICAT)[26,113] are being developed in part to this end.

The increased emphasis on proteomics for disease investigations is stimulating a reassessment of strategies for sample acquisition and preservation to render them compatible with proteomic analysis because of the inherent instability of proteins. Especially in biological fluids, there is a need to reduce handling-related protein degradation and other forms of artifactual protein modifications that may substantially alter protein content and interfere with global profiling.

CONCLUSIONS

Proteomic analysis has the potential to profile differences between lung tumor and no tumor, between different stages and histology of cancer and between different cancer samples at the same stage of progression. The ability to identify important proteins involved in the transformation process may lead to early markers for detection of specific types of cancers and treatments based upon the molecular profile of lung cancer. In the past decade, lung cancer treatment has become increasingly target-oriented. However all targets have been identified in late invasive and metastatic disease, thereby limiting the success of treatment. If specific targets important in the earliest stage of the tumor can be identified, then application of these treatments early in the course of disease or premalignancy is likely to be more successful than attempting to treat late-stage tumors. Screening methods that combine features of high sensitivity and high specificity for early-stage lung cancer, hopefully non-invasive, affordable and safe, are urgently needed. While measurements of chromosomal aberrations, point mutations, and loss of heterozygosity can be obtained from a series of biological specimens,[113] the integration of these data with proteomic analysis will be critical in the years to come to bring to the clinic better tools for early detection and management of lung cancer as a whole.

REFERENCES

1. Garber ME, Troyanskaya OG, Schluens K, et al, Diversity of gene expression in adenocarcinoma of the lung. Proc Natl Acad Sci USA 2001; 98(24):13784–9.
2. Bhattacharjee A, Richards WG, Staunton J, et al, Classification of human lung carcinomas by mRNA expression profiling reveals distinct adenocarcinoma subclasses. Proc Natl Acad Sci USA 2001; 98(24):13790–5.
3. Wigle DA, Jurisica I, Radulovich N, et al, Molecular profiling of non-small cell lung cancer and correlation with disease-free survival. Cancer Res 2001; 62(11):3005–8.
4. Yamagata N, Shyr Y, Yanagisawa K, et al, A training-testing approach to the molecular classification of resected non-small cell lung cancer. Clin Cancer Res 2003; 9(13): 4695–704.
5. Massion PP, Kuo WL, Stokoe D, et al, Genomic copy number analysis of non-small cell lung cancer using array comparative genomic hybridization: implications of the phosphatidylinositol 3-kinase pathway. Cancer Res 2002; 62(13):3636–40.
6. Perou CM, Sorlie T, Eisen MB, et al, Molecular portraits of human breast tumours. Nature 2000; 406(6797):747–52.
7. Brenton JD, Aparicio SA, Caldas C, Molecular profiling of breast cancer: portraits but not physiognomy. Breast Cancer Res 2001; 3(2): 77–80.
8. Sorlie T, Perou CM, Tibshirani R, et al, Gene expression patterns of breast carcinomas distinguish tumor subclasses with clinical implications. Proc Natl Acad Sci USA 2001; 98(19): 10869–74.
9. Gruvberger S, Ringner M, Chen Y, et al, Estrogen receptor status in breast cancer is associated with remarkably distinct gene expression patterns. Cancer Res 2001; 61(16):5979–84.
10. van de Vijver MJ, He YD, van't Veer LJ, et al, A gene-expression signature as a predictor of survival in breast cancer. N Engl J Med 2002; 347(25):1999–2009.
11. Beer DG, Kardia CC, Huang TJ, et al, Gene-expression profiles predict survival of patients with lung adenocarcinoma. Nat Med 2002; 8(8): 816–24.
12. Chen G, Gharib TG, Huang CC, et al, Proteomic analysis of lung adenocarcinoma: identification of a highly expressed set of proteins

in tumors. Clin Cancer 2002; Res 8(7): 2298–305.

13. Yanagisawa K, Shyr Y, Xu BJ, et al, Proteomic patterns of tumour subsets in non-small-cell lung cancer. Lancet 2003; 362(9382):433–9.

14. Petricoin EF, Ardekani AM, Hitt BA, et al, Use of proteomic patterns in serum to identify ovarian cancer. Lancet 2002; 359(9306): 572–7.

15. Petricoin EF 3rd, Ornstein DK, Paweletz CP, et al, Serum proteomic patterns for detection of prostate cancer. J Natl Cancer Inst 2002; 94(20):1576–8.

16. Adam BL, Qu Y, Davis JW, et al, Serum protein fingerprinting coupled with a pattern-matching algorithm distinguishes prostate cancer from benign prostate hyperplasia and healthy men. Cancer Res 2002; 62(13):3609–14.

17. Sidransky D, Irizarry R, Califano JA, et al, Serum protein MALDI profiling to distinguish upper aerodigestive tract cancer patients from control subjects. J Natl Cancer Inst 2003; 95(22):1711–17.

18. Bergman AC, Benjamin T, Alaiya A, et al, Identification of gel-separated tumor marker proteins by mass spectrometry. Electrophoresis 2000; 21(3):679–86.

19. Gorg A, Obermaier C, Boguth G, et al, The current state of two-dimensional electrophoresis with immobilized pH gradients. Electrophoresis 2000; 21(6):1037–53.

20. Hanash SM, Biomedical applications of two-dimensional electrophoresis using immobilized pH gradients: current status. Electrophoresis 2000; 21(6):1202–9.

21. Hoving S, Gerrits B, Voshol H, et al, Preparative two-dimensional gel electrophoresis at alkaline pH using narrow range immobilized pH gradients. Proteomics 2002; 2(2):127–34.

22. Zuo X, Speicher DW, Comprehensive analysis of complex proteomes using microscale solution isoelectrofocusing prior to narrow pH range two-dimensional electrophoresis. Proteomics 2002; 2(1):58–68.

23. Tonella L, Walsh BJ, Sanchez JC, et al, '98

Escherichia coli SWISS-2DPAGE database update. Electrophoresis 1998; 19(11):1960–71.

24. Chambers G, Lawrie L, Cash P, et al, Proteomics: a new approach to the study of disease. J Pathol 2000; 192(3):280–8.

25. Steinberg TH, Jones LJ, Haugland RP, et al, SYPRO orange and SYPRO red protein gel stains: one-step fluorescent staining of denaturing gels for detection of nanogram levels of protein. Anal Biochem 1996; 239(2):223–37.

26. Patton WF, Detection technologies in proteome analysis. J Chromatogr B Analyt Technol Biomed Life Sci 2002; 771(1–2):3–31.

27. Unlu M, Morgan ME, Minden JS, Difference gel electrophoresis: a single gel method for detecting changes in protein extracts. Electrophoresis 1997; 18(11):2071–7.

28. Zhou G, Li H, DeCamp D, et al, 2D differential in-gel electrophoresis for the identification of esophageal scans cell cancer-specific protein markers. Mol Cell Proteomics 2002; 1(2):117–24.

29. Li G, Waltham M, Anderson NL, et al, Rapid mass spectrometric identification of proteins from two-dimensional polyacrylamide gels after in gel proteolytic digestion. Electrophoresis 1997; 18(3–4):391–402.

30. Hanash S, 2-D or not 2-D – is there a future for 2-D gels in proteomics? Insights from the York proteomics meeting. Proteomics 2001; 1(5): 635–7.

31. Shin BK, Wang H, Yim AM, et al, Global profiling of the cell surface proteome of cancer cells uncovers an abundance of proteins with chaperone function. J Biol Chem 2003; 278(9): 7607–16.

32. Brivio M, Fokkens RH, Verboom W, et al, Integrated microfluidic system enabling (bio)chemical reactions with on-line MALDI-TOF mass spectrometry. Anal Chem 2002; 74(16):3972–6.

33. Krutchinsky AN, Zhang W, Chait BT, Rapidly switchable matrix-assisted laser desorption/ ionization and electrospray quadrupole-time-of-flight mass spectrometry for protein identifi-

cation. J Am Soc Mass Spectrom 2000; 11(6):493–504.

34. Merchant M, Weinberger SR, Recent advancements in surface-enhanced laser desorption/ionization-time of flight-mass spectrometry. Electrophoresis 2000; 21(6):1164–77.

35. Beavis RC, Chait BT, Rapid, sensitive analysis of protein mixtures by mass spectrometry. Proc Natl Acad Sci USA 1990; 87(17):6873–7.

36. Xu BJ, Caprioli RM, Sanders ME, Direct analysis of laser capture microdissected cells by MALDI mass spectrometry. J Am Soc Mass Spectrom 2002; 13(11):1292–7.

37. McCormack AL, Schieltz DM, Goode B, et al, Direct analysis and identification of proteins in mixtures by LC/MS/MS and database searching at the low-femtomole level. Anal Chem 1997; 69(4):767–76.

38. Peng J, Elias JE, Thoreen CC, et al, Evaluation of multidimensional chromatography coupled with tandem mass spectrometry (LC/LC-MS/MS) for large-scale protein analysis: the yeast proteome. J Proteome Res 2003; 2(1): 43–50.

39. Stoeckli M, Chaurand P, Hallahan DE, Caprioli RM, Imaging mass spectrometry: a new technology for the analysis of protein expression in mammalian tissues. Nat Med 2001; 7(4): 493–6.

40. Chaurand P, Fouchecourt S, DaGue BB, et al, Profiling and imaging proteins in the mouse epididymis by imaging mass spectrometry. Proteomics 2003; 3(11):2221–39.

41. Chaurand P, Schwartz SA, Billheimer D, et al, Integrating histology and imaging mass spectrometry. Anal Chem 2004; 76(4):1145–55.

42. Glish GL, Vachet RW, The basics of mass spectrometry in the twenty-first century. Nat Rev Drug Discov 2003; 2(2):140–50.

43. Shen Z, Thomas JJ, Averbuj C, et al, Porous silicon as a versatile platform for laser desorption/ionization mass spectrometry. Anal Chem 2001; 73(3):612–19.

44. Thomas JJ, Shen Z, Crowell JE, Finn MG, Siuzdak G, Desorption/ionization on silicon (DIOS): a diverse mass spectrometry platform for protein characterization. Proc Natl Acad Sci USA 2001; 98(9):4932–7.

45. Yip TT, Hutchens TW, Immobilized metal ion affinity chromatography. Methods Mol Biol 1996; 59:197–210.

46. Wang S, Diamond DL, Hass GM, Sokoloff R, Vessella RL, Identification of prostate specific membrane antigen (PSMA) as the target of monoclonal antibody 107-1A4 by proteinchip; array, surface-enhanced laser desorption/ionization (SELDI) technology. Int J Cancer 2001; 92(6):871–6.

47. Kebarle P, A brief overview of the present status of the mechanisms involved in electrospray mass spectrometry. J Mass Spectrom 2000; 35(7):804–17.

48. Roepstorff P, Mass spectrometry in protein studies from genome to function. Curr Opin Biotechnol 1997; 8(1):6–13.

49. Zhu H, Bilgin M, Bangham R, et al, Global analysis of protein activities using proteome chips. Science 2001; 293(5537):2101–5.

50. Zhu H, Snyder M, Protein chip technology. Curr Opin Chem Biol 2003; 7(1):55–63.

51. MacBeath G, Schreiber SL, Printing proteins as microarrays for high-throughput function determination. Science 2000; 289(5485): 1760–3.

52. Schaeferling M, Schiller S, Paul H, et al, Application of self-assembly techniques in the design of biocompatible protein microarray surfaces. Electrophoresis 2002; 23(18): 3097–105.

53. Weng S, Gu K, Hammond PW, et al, Generating addressable protein microarrays with PROfusion covalent mRNA–protein fusion technology. Proteomics 2002; 2(1):48–57.

54. Robinson WH, DiGennaro C, Hueber W, et al, Autoantigen microarrays for multiplex characterization of autoantibody responses. Nat Med 2002; 8(3):295–301.

55. Brichory F, Beer D, Le Naour F, Giordano T, Hanash S, Proteomics-based identification of protein gene product 9.5 as a tumor antigen

that induces a humoral immune response in lung cancer. Cancer Res 2001; 61(21): 7908–12.

56. Paweletz CP, Charboneau L, Bichsel VE, et al, Reverse phase protein microarrays which capture disease progression show activation of pro-survival pathways at the cancer invasion front. Oncogene 2001; 20(16):1981–9.

57. Grubb RL, Calvert VS, Wulkuhle JD, Signal pathway profiling of prostate cancer using reverse phase protein arrays. Proteomics 2003; 3(11):2142–6.

58. Knezevic V, Leethanakul C, Bichsel VE, et al, Proteomic profiling of the cancer microenvironment by antibody arrays. Proteomics 2001; 1(10):1271–8.

59. Espina V, Mehta AI, Winters ME, et al, Protein microarrays: molecular profiling technologies for clinical specimens. Proteomics 2003; 3(11): 2091–100.

60. Houseman BT, Huh JH, Kron SJ, Mrksich M, Peptide chips for the quantitative evaluation of protein kinase activity. Nat Biotechnol 2002; 20(3):270–4.

61. Lizcano JM, Deak M, Morrice N, et al, Molecular basis for the substrate specificity of NIMA-related kinase-6 (NEK6). Evidence that NEK6 does not phosphorylate the hydrophobic motif of ribosomal S6 protein kinase and serum- and glucocorticoid-induced protein kinase in vivo. J Biol Chem 2002; 277(31): 27839–49.

62. Oh JM, Brichory F, Puravs E, et al, A database of protein expression in lung cancer. Proteomics 2001; 1(10):1303–19.

63. Gharib TG, Chen G, Wang H, et al, Proteomic analysis of cytokeratin isoforms uncovers association with survival in lung adenocarcinoma. Neoplasia 2002; 4(5):440–8.

64. Beer DG, Kardia SL, Huang CC, et al, Gene-expression profiles predict survival of patients with lung adenocarcinoma. Nat Med 2002; 8(8):816–24.

65. Chen G, Gharib TG, Wang H, et al, 2003. Protein profiles associated with survival in lung

adenocarcinoma. Proc Natl Acad Sci USA 2003; 100(23):13537–42.

66. Okuzawa K, Franzen B, Lindholm J, et al, Characterization of gene expression in clinical lung cancer materials by two-dimensional polyacrylamide gel electrophoresis. Electrophoresis 1994; 15(3–4):382–90.

67. Hirano T, Fujioka K, Franzen B, et al, Relationship between TA01 and TA02 polypeptides associated with lung adenocarcinoma and histocytological features. Br J Cancer 1997; 75(7): 978–85.

68. Chuman Y, Bergman A, Ueno T, et al, Napsin A, a member of the aspartic protease family, is abundantly expressed in normal lung and kidney tissue and is expressed in lung adenocarcinomas. FEBS Lett 1999; 462(1–2):129–34.

69. Oh P, Li Y, Yu J, et al, Subtractive proteomic mapping of the endothelial surface in lung and solid tumours for tissue-specific therapy. Nature 2004; 429(6992):629–35.

70. Campa MJ, Wang MZ, Howard B, Fitzgerald MC, Patz EF Jr, Protein expression profiling identifies macrophage migration inhibitory factor and cyclophilin a as potential molecular targets in non-small cell lung cancer. Cancer Res 2003; 63(7):1652–6.

71. Howard BA, Zheng Z, Campa MJ, et al, Translating biomarkers into clinical practice: prognostic implications of cyclophilin A and macrophage migratory inhibitory factor identified from protein expression profiles in non-small cell lung cancer. Lung Cancer 2004; 46(3):313–23.

72. Shyr Y, Kim K, Weighted flexible compound covariate method for classifying microarray data. In: Berrar D (ed.) A Practical Approach to Microarray Data Analysis. Kluwer Academic, NY, 2003; pp. 186–200.

73. Zhukov TA, Johanson RA, Cantor AB, Clark RA, Tockman MS, Discovery of distinct protein profiles specific for lung tumors and pre-malignant lung lesions by SELDI mass spectrometry. Lung Cancer 2003; 40(3):267–79.

74. Alfonso P, Catala M, Rico-Morales ML, et al,

Proteomic analysis of lung biopsies: Differential protein expression profile between peritumoral and tumoral tissue. Proteomics 2004; 4(2):442–7.

75. Li J, Zhang Z, Rosenzweig J, Wang YY, Chan DW, Proteomics and bioinformatics approaches for identification of serum biomarkers to detect breast cancer. Clin Chem 2002; 48(8):1296–304.

76. Banez LL, Prasanna P, Sun L, et al, Diagnostic potential of serum proteomic patterns in prostate cancer. J Urol 2003; 170(2 Pt 1): 442–6.

77. Mobley JA, Lam YW, Lau KM et al, Monitoring the serological proteome: the latest modality in prostate cancer detection. J Urol 2004; 172(1): 331–7.

78. Yildiz P, Shyr Y, Rahman S, et al, Diagnosis of lung cancer from serum protein profile analysis. AACR Proceedings 2004; 45:A3335.

79. Villanueva J, Philip J, Entenberg D, et al, Serum peptide profiling by magnetic particle-assisted, automated sample processing and MALDI-TOF mass spectrometry. Anal Chem 2004; 76(6): 1560–70.

80. Howard BA, Wang MZ, Campa MJ, et al, Identification and validation of a potential lung cancer serum biomarker detected by matrix-assisted laser desorption/ionization-time of flight spectra analysis. Proteomics 2003; 3(9):1720–4.

81. Brichory FM, Misek DE, Yim AM, et al, An immune response manifested by the common occurrence of annexins I and II autoantibodies and high circulating levels of IL-6 in lung cancer. Proc Natl Acad Sci USA 2001; 98(17): 9824–9.

82. Madoz-Gurpide J, Wang H, Misek DE, Brichory F, Hanash SM, Protein based microarrays: a tool for probing the proteome of cancer cells and tissues. Proteomics 2001; 1(10):1279–87.

83. Zhong L, Peng X, Hidalgo GE, et al, Identification of circulating antibodies to tumor-associated proteins for combined use as markers of non-small cell lung cancer. Proteomics 2004; 4(4):1216–25.

84. Nilsson CL, Brodin E, Ekman R, Substance P and related peptides in porcine cortex: whole tissue and nuclear localization. J Chromatogr A 1998; 800(1):21–7.

85. Nilsson CL, Puchades M, Westman A, Blennow K, Davidsson P, Identification of proteins in a human pleural exudate using two-dimensional preparative liquid-phase electrophoresis and matrix-assisted laser desorption/ionization mass spectrometry. Electrophoresis 1999; 20(4–5):860–5.

86. Westman A, Nilsson CL, Ekman R, Matrix-assisted laser desorption/ionization time-of-flight mass spectrometry analysis of proteins in human cerebrospinal fluid. Rapid Commun Mass Spectrom 1998; 12(16):1092–8.

87. Bard MP, Hegmans JP, Hemmes A, et al, Proteomic analysis of exosomes isolated from human malignant pleural effusions. Am J Respir Cell Mol Biol 2004; 31(1):114–21.

88. Balint B, Donnelly LE, Hanazawa T, Kharitonov SA, Barnes PJ, Increased nitric oxide metabolites in exhaled breath condensate after exposure to tobacco smoke. Thorax 2001; 56(6): 456–61.

89. Corradi M, Montuschi P, Donnelly LE, et al, Increased nitrosothiols in exhaled breath condensate in inflammatory airway diseases. Am J Respir Crit Care Med 2001; 163(4):854–8.

90. Carpenter CT, Price PV, Christman BW, Exhaled breath condensate isoprostanes are elevated in patients with acute lung injury or ARDS. Chest 1998; 114(6):1653–9.

91. Montuschi P, Collins JV, Ciabattoni G, et al, Exhaled 8-isoprostane as an in vivo biomarker of lung oxidative stress in patients with COPD and healthy smokers. Am J Respir Crit Care Med 2000; 162(3 Pt 1):1175–7.

92. Dekhuijzen PN, Aben KK, Dekker I, et al, Increased exhalation of hydrogen peroxide in patients with stable and unstable chronic obstructive pulmonary disease. Am J Respir Crit Care Med 1996; 154(3 Pt 1):813–16.

93. Scheideler L, Manke HG, Schwulera U, Inacker O, Hammerle H, Detection of nonvolatile

macromolecules in breath. A possible diagnostic tool? Am Rev Respir Dis 1993; 148(3): 778–84.

94. Griese M, Noss J, Bredow CCv, Protein pattern of exhaled breath condensate and saliva. Proteomics 2002; 2(6):690–6.

95. Gessner C, Kuhn H, Toepfer K, et al, Detection of p53 gene mutations in exhaled breath condensate of non-small cell lung cancer patients. Lung Cancer 2004; 43(2):215–22.

96. Chanin TD, Merrick DT, Franklin WA, Hirsch FR, Recent developments in biomarkers for the early detection of lung cancer: perspectives based on publications 2003 to present. Curr Opin Pulm Med 2004; 10(4):242–7.

97. Jones PD, Hankin R, Simpson J, Gibson PG, Henry RL, The tolerability, safety, and success of sputum induction and combined hypertonic saline challenge in children. Am J Respir Crit Care Med 2001; 164(7):1146–9.

98. Rahman S, Yildiz P, Gonzalez A, et al, Proteomic patterns of preinvasive bronchial lesions. Am J Respir Crit Care Med 2005; In press.

99. Reynolds HY, Use of bronchoalveolar lavage in humans – past necessity and future imperative. Lung 2000; 178(5):271–93.

100. Bell DY, Hook GE, Pulmonary alveolar proteinosis: analysis of airway and alveolar proteins. Am Rev Respir Dis 1979; 119(6):979–90.

101. Bell DY, Haseman JA, Spock A, McLennan G, Hook GE, Plasma proteins of the bronchoalveolar surface of the lungs of smokers and nonsmokers. Am Rev Respir Dis 1981; 124(1): 72–9.

102. Noel-Georis I, Bernard A, Falmagne P, Wattiez R, Database of bronchoalveolar lavage fluid proteins. J Chromatogr B Analyt Technol Biomed Life Sci 2002; 771(1–2):221–36.

103. Wattiez R, Hermans C, Bernard A, Lesur O, Falmagne P, Human bronchoalveolar lavage fluid: two-dimensional gel electrophoresis, amino acid microsequencing and identification of major proteins. Electrophoresis 1999; 20(7): 1634–45.

104. Lindahl M, Stahlbom B, Tagesson C, Two-dimensional gel electrophoresis of nasal and bronchoalveolar lavage fluids after occupational exposure. Electrophoresis 1995; 16(7): 1199–204.

105. Wattiez R, Falmagne P, Proteomics of bronchoalveolar lavage fluid. J Chromatogr B Analyt Technol Biomed Life Sci 2005; 815(1–2): 169–78.

106. Lenz AG, Meyer B, Weber H, Maier K, Two-dimensional electrophoresis of dog bronchoalveolar lavage fluid proteins. Electrophoresis 1990; 11(6):510–13.

107. Sabounchi-Schutt F, Astrom J, Eklund A, Grunewald J, Bjellqvist B, Detection and identification of human bronchoalveolar lavage proteins using narrow-range immobilized pH gradient DryStrip and the paper bridge sample application method. Electrophoresis 2001; 22(9):1851–60.

108. Pandey A, Mann M, Proteomics to study genes and genomes. Nature 2000; 405(6788): 837–46.

109. Baggerly KA, Morris JS, Wang J, et al, A comprehensive approach to the analysis of matrix-assisted laser desorption/ionization-time of flight proteomics spectra from serum samples. Proteomics 2003; 3(9):1667–72.

110. Fenyo D, Beavis RC, A method for assessing the statistical significance of mass spectrometry-based protein identifications using general scoring schemes. Anal Chem 2003; 75(4): 768–74.

111. Templin MF, Stoll D, Bachmann J, Joos TO, Protein microarrays and multiplexed sandwich immunoassays: what beats the beads? Comb Chem High Throughput Screen 2004; 7(3): 223–9.

112. Steinberg TH, Agnew BJ, Gee KR, et al, Global quantitative phosphoprotein analysis using Multiplexed Proteomics technology. Proteomics 2003; 3(7):1128–44.

113. Gygi SP, Rist B, Griffin TJ, Eng J, Aebersold R, Proteome analysis of low-abundance proteins using multidimensional chromatography and isotope-coded affinity tags. J Proteome Res 2002; 1(1):47–54.

114. Sidransky D, Nucleic acid-based methods for the detection of cancer. Science 1997; 278(5340):1054–9.

8 Sputum cytology and biomarkers

Melvyn S Tockman

Contents Introduction • Morphologic targets in sputum • Molecular targets in sputum • Conclusion

INTRODUCTION

Exfoliated cancer cells have been described in the sputum of lung cancer patients since the 1930s.[1] Papanicolaou and Saccomanno, pioneers of exfoliative cytology, demonstrated that premalignant cytological changes could be detected several years before a clinical diagnosis of lung cancer in high-risk people.[2,3] From the time of the initial report, it took almost 40 years to begin a systematic randomized evaluation of exfoliated sputum morphology as a screening test for lung cancer. Surprisingly, these NCI Collaborative Lung Cancer Screening Trials found no mortality benefit from morphologic screening of sputum specimens, and they were underpowered to detect a small benefit of chest X-ray screening.[4] The NCI trials established that frankly malignant cytology specimens are often associated with roentgenographically occult central lesions, most of which are squamous cell carcinomas.[5–7] Roentgenographically occult squamous cell lung cancer detected by cytology often (over 80%) is early cancer (stage 0 or stage 1), where the actual 5-year cure by surgery is excellent.[8] However, even in a screened population, only 14% of lung cancers are roentgenographically occult squamous cell tumors detectable only by cytology.[9] A recent evaluation of sputum morphology confirmed a relative risk of 3.3 for carcinoma in individuals with moderate sputum atypia or worse when compared to matched controls with normal sputum cytology.[10] Although insensitive to the majority of lung cancers, sputum atypia remains a standard of practice against which molecular methods should be compared. Subsequently, microscopic imaging and molecular biology have been applied to improve the sensitivity of this easily collected material for lung cancer screening.[11,12]

Today, there is a growing interest in the early identification of asymptomatic lung cancer by chest computerized tomography (CT). This interest may have resulted from the initial report of the Early Lung Cancer Action Project (ELCAP), which detected a lung cancer prevalence of 2.7% in asymptomatic heavy smokers over the age of 60; most of these lesions were early stage.[13] This represents a clear improvement over chest X-ray screening where the low density of up to 77% of surgically curable lesions detectable by CT would have caused them to be missed by chest X-ray.[14] Nevertheless, the improved sensitivity of helical CT comes at the cost of a lowered specificity (higher false-positive rate). New, non-calcified nodules are seen in up to 50% of screening helical CT examinations, increasing in frequency with thinner CT slices and decreasing with follow-up examinations.[15–19] Up to 90% of the abnormalities detected on the initial CT examination are not malignant.[13] Further, the CT scan may be insensitive to superficial, pre-invasive/microinvasive cancers in the central airways that may be manifest in sputum.[11] Within 5 years, the NCI has initiated a new randomized trial of lung cancer screening to determine whether low-radiation-dose spiral CT (LDCT) scanning can lead to reduced lung cancer mortality.[20] This multicenter NCI Lung Screening Study of helical CT screening will require another 6 years to complete. Although no new sputum tests were sufficiently validated to perform contemporaneously during this trial, NCI-LSS sputum specimens have been collected and stored for future evaluation of a sputum screening test. This discussion will consider candidate sputum tests that might be considered for evaluation as complementary to helical CT screening for lung cancer.

MORPHOLOGIC TARGETS IN SPUTUM

Automated sputum cytometry

Returning to slides saved from the NCI Cooperative Early Lung Cancer Study, Payne et al made measurements of nuclear features of epithelial cells found in sputum. These investigators restained 73 sputum slides from the original Mayo investigation using a modified Feulgen method followed by automated image cytometry.[21] The distribution of chromatin DNA, stoichiometrically stained by Feulgen-Thionin, is measured in several thousands of epithelial cell nuclei using a fully automated, high-resolution image cytometer.[22] The investigators examined 40 slides from nine patients in whom squamous carcinoma developed and 33 slides from 11 patients in whom no cancer developed during a follow-up of at least 5 years. Obtaining images of epithelial nuclei and measuring features based on DNA distribution, 74% correct classi-

fication of nuclei was possible without human review of the material and without the use of visually abnormal nuclei. A receiver operating characteristic (ROC) curve demonstrated 40% sensitivity at 90% specificity. This method is based on the observation that even in the absence of any frankly malignant cells in the sputum, it is possible to detect subjects with early lung cancers. In this preliminary work, these investigators detected a substantial proportion of patients with squamous cell cancer in 20-year-old slides without requiring a physician to recognize visually abnormal nuclei.[21]

Most recently this group of investigators conducted a prospective study to evaluate whether automated quantitative image cytometry (AQC) of sputum cells could be conducted prior to helical CT to improve the lung cancer detection rate.[11] They surveyed a total of 561 volunteer current or former smokers 50 years of age or older, with a smoking history of more than or equal to 30 pack-years. Among these, 423 were found to have sputum atypia defined as five cells or more with abnormal DNA content using AQC. Of the 14 lung cancers, AQC detected 13 in subjects with sputum atypia (sensitivity 92.8%). CT alone detected one cancer and ten cancers were detected by both modes (CT sensitivity 71.4%). However, in identifying 410 with atypia out of the 547 without lung cancer, AQC has a specificity of only 25%.[11] While a high sensitivity is necessary, it is not sufficient for lung cancer screening. Modification of the AQC technique or the subsequent management algorithm is required either to improve its specificity or to subject a smaller proportion of 'positives' to a follow-up examination by fiberoptic bronchoscopy. Perhaps a combination of AQC with other sputum tests (below) might be considered. While lung cancer is the most frequently lethal cancer in the United States, its annual incidence is only 1–3% in heavy smokers.[23] With such a low prior probability, a positive lung cancer screening test is far more likely to be falsely positive,[24] as is seen here (false-positive rate 75%).

Aneuploidy

Colorado Lung Cancer SPORE investigators evaluated whether chromosomal instability could be detected in sputum specimens and used as a biomarker for lung cancer risk.[25] They used a multi-target DNA FISH assay (LAVysion, Abbott/Vysis) to investigate the occurrence of chromosomal aneusomy in sputum from 33 cases and controls matched on age, gender and date of sample collection. Subjects had chronic obstructive pulmonary disease and at least 30 pack-years of tobacco use. In specimens collected within 12 months prior to the lung cancer diagnosis, aneusomy was more frequent among the cases (41%) than the controls (6%; $P = 0.04$). Aneusomy had no significant association with cytologic atypia, which might indicate that molecular and morphological changes could be independent markers of tumorigenesis. Combining both tests, abnormality was found in 83% of the cases and 20% of the controls ($P = 0.0004$) suggesting that FISH may improve the sensitivity of cytologic atypia as a predictor of lung cancer.[26]

MOLECULAR TARGETS IN SPUTUM

Loss of heterozygosity

A complex biology modifies the airway of chronic smokers. Slaughter first noted the widespread damage (field cancerization) that persists in the aerodigestive tract of current and former smokers.[27] From completely sectioned autopsy specimens, Auerbach recognized three progressive grades of histologic abnormality in the epithelium of 'uninvolved bronchi' surrounding lung tumors; hyperplasia (an increase in the number of cell rows), metaplasia (loss of cilia) and dysplasia (presence of atypical cells).[28,29] He also reported an increased frequency of carcinoma-in-situ associated with a higher frequency of smoking, from 0% in non-smokers to 11% in men who smoked $\geq$2 packs per day.[28] Field cancerization implies that detection of premalignant or malignant lesions in one area of the pulmonary epithelium identifies an epithelium at increased risk of developing neoplastic lesions in other areas.[30] Perhaps as a result of widespread, persistent epithelial injury (field cancerization), patients with a successfully resected first primary lung cancer have a high annual incidence (2–5%) of second primary lung cancer,[31] and approximately half of newly diagnosed lung cancers occur in individuals who no longer smoke.[32]

Progressive histopathological abnormality preceding cancer is thought to reflect an underlying accumulation of specific genetic changes in proto-oncogenes and tumor suppressor genes.[33-35] These genetic changes result in functional dysregulation of critical pathways (e.g. growth/anti-growth, invasion/metastases, replication, angiogenesis, evasion of apoptosis).[36] Changes that cannot be repaired and do not trigger a program of cell death (apoptosis) may lead to a cellular growth advantage. Many of these genetic changes are acquired prior to and during the earliest stages of clonal expansion and are retained by daughter cells through the course of carcinogenesis and malignancy. Wistuba et al observed that increasing severity of histopathological changes in lung squamous carcinoma is associated with a progression of genetic changes (increasing frequency of loss of heterozygosity, LOH).[37] Regions of chromosomal loss are suspected to have contained tumor suppressor genes, the losses of which would be advantageous for growth. This genetic damage is widespread throughout the airway even in areas of normal-appearing epithelium, and persists long after removal of the insult. If detected during the pre-malignant period, these genetic changes could serve as markers of carcinogenesis and indicate the need for chemoprevention.

Microsatellite markers are small repeating DNA sequences found in the introns (non-coding regions) of a gene. PCR amplification of these repeat sequences provides a rapid method for assessment of LOH and facilitates mapping of tumor suppressor genes.[38,39] Yet microsatellites can provide additional information. Expansion or deletion of these repeating elements is called microsatellite alteration. These microsatellite alterations, acquired during division of a single transformed cell, are passed on to daughter cells during clonal expansion. Since they are not transcribed, microsatellite alterations provide no growth advantage to the cell. However, detection of microsatellite alterations in histological specimens is equivalent to the detection of neoplastic (clonal) cell populations. Although detection of microsatellite alterations does not indicate the specific genetic change in the tumor, detection of clonal cell populations might serve as a cancer screening marker.[40]

Widespread microsatellite instability was first reported in colorectal tumors.[41] In hereditary non-polyposis colorectal carcinoma (HNPCC), mutations of mismatch repair genes are probably responsible for microsatellite alterations at multiple locations in the genome.[42] However, in non-HNPCC-associated tumors, including lung cancer, there is not a similar widespread loss of mismatch repair, indicating that another, as yet unknown, mechanism is responsible for somatic alterations of repeat sequences.[43]

The pattern of microsatellite alterations and LOH may be specific for different types of cancer. The high incidence of these changes on chromosomes 3, 5, 8, 9, 10, 11, 17 and 20 have been described in lung cancer specimens,[44,45] although the role of these changes in carcinogenesis is not yet known. Perhaps it is the cumulative effect of these genetic injuries that is important. We have already shown that microsatellite alterations are clonal markers for the detection of human lung cancer, and we, along with others, have shown microsatellite alterations at selected loci can be recognized in sputum cells prior to clinical lung cancer.[46]

Microsatellite DNA markers have successfully detected LOH and genomic instability in bladder cancer.[47] In a blinded study, microsatellite changes matching those in the tumor were detected in the urine sediment of 19 of the 20 patients (95%) who were diagnosed with bladder cancer, whereas standard urine cytopathology detected cancer cells in only nine of 18 (50%) samples. The specificity was 100% (in five non-cancer cases). The NCI Early Detection Research Network is currently validating microsatellite analysis for detection of bladder cancer in a multicenter trial.

Unfortunately, the results show a lower sensitivity when sputum is examined for microsatellites indicative of lung cancer, perhaps due to dilution by the large numbers of inflammatory cells frequently seen in the sputum of smokers. European investigators have reported success by analyzing sputum LOH in terms of the fractional allelic loss.[48,49]

Specific oncogene activation (*RAS*)

Three closely related genes, *H-RAS*, *N-RAS* and *K-RAS* make up the *RAS* family of oncogenes which code for a superfamily of GTPase signal proteins that act as molecular switches regulating cellular proliferation and apoptosis in response to extracellular signals.[50,51] Mutation of the *K-RAS2* oncogene is one of the most commonly occurring genetic lesions in colorectal cancer,[52] and is frequently mutated in lung cancer.[53] The Johns Hopkins Lung Project archive of preclinical sputum linked to tumor outcome allowed us to demonstrate that specific mutations could be detected in non-malignant sputum specimens in advance of clinical lung cancer.[54] This study demonstrated that eight of 15 patients (53%) with adenocarcinoma or large cell carcinoma of the lung could be detected by mutations in sputum cells from 1–13 months prior to clinical diagnosis. The ability to identify specific gene abnormalities is limited by the need to know the specific mutation sequence with which to probe the sputum specimens. In this pilot study, the mutation sequence was determined from the resected tumor. This approach is obviously not practical for screening undiagnosed individuals at present. Perhaps with future advances in gene chip technology, it might become feasible to probe for all possible mutations of common oncogenes and tumor suppressor genes in sputum specimens of asymptomatic individuals.

Recently, Dammann et al cloned a novel gene, *RAS*-association domain family 1 (*RASSF1*) which functions as an alternative mechanism for *RAS* suppression.[55] The *RASSF1* gene is located in the chromosomal segment of 3p21.3 and its protein seems to silence *RAS* and to signal apoptosis.[50,55] At least two forms of *RASSF1* are present in normal human cells. Methylated *RASSF1A* isoform is epigenetically inactivated in lung, breast, ovarian, kidney, prostate, thyroid and several other carcinomas. Loss of this negative effector is seen in 40–60% and 100% of non-small-cell and small-cell lung cancers, respectively.[56] *RASSF1A* inactivation and *K-RAS* activation seem to be mutually exclusive events in the development of certain carcinomas.[50] Re-expression of *RASSF1A* reduced the growth of human cancer cells supporting a role for *RASSF1* as a tumor suppressor gene. Thus, *RASSF1A* methylation could serve

as a useful marker for the prognosis of cancer patients and might be a marker for lung cancer early detection.[12]

Abnormal methylation

A 5′ methyl group added to a cytosine located 5′ to a guanosine in a CpG dinucleotide within a gene promoter-1st exon region results in gene transcription failure.[57] Transcriptional silencing due to promoter hypermethylation may be as common in cancer as the disruption of classic tumor-suppressor genes. Genes that are silenced by inappropriate promoter hypermethylation can be relatively easily reactivated by treatment with DNA-methylation inhibitors, such as 5-aza nucleosides.[57] As described by Belinsky, the rapid advance in the study of gene-promoter methylation in cancer was facilitated by two important discoveries.[12] The first demonstrated that an important tumor-suppressor gene, *CDKN2A* – which encodes INK4A (also known as p16) and ARF (also known as p14) – is silenced in many cancers through aberrant promoter hypermethylation.[58] The second advance was the development of the methylation-specific PCR (MSP) assay that allows for rapid detection of methylation in genes through the selective amplification of methylated alleles within a specific gene promoter.[59]

Belinsky et al recently measured hypermethylation of the CpG islands of the *p16* gene in the sputum of lung cancer patients and demonstrated a high correlation with the early stages of NSCLC.[60] These investigators suggest that detection of *p16* CpG island hypermethylation might be useful in the prediction of individuals who might develop lung cancer. Investigators from the Johns Hopkins and Colorado Lung Cancer SPOREs are conducting a nested, case-control study to determine whether a panel of methylation markers could be developed to predict risk and/or early detection of lung cancer. Methylation of the *p16*, *MGMT*, *RASSF1A*, *H-cadherin*, *PAX5 α*, *PAX5 β*, *GATA5* and *DAPK* genes was assessed in sputum specimens. Individual odds ratios ranged from 1.0–2.2 for detecting methylation of a specific gene in cases versus controls. These studies suggest that while the presence of any one of these methylation markers in sputum confers a marked increase in the relative risk (OR = 4.0) for lung cancer, that investigators are unlikely to be able to detect promoter hypermethylation within the developing tumor through the analysis of sputum.[12] The greater potential for sputum methylation markers will be to assess the relative risk of cancer by detecting field cancerization through quantifying the number of hypermethylated loci rather than detect cancer by recognizing hypermethylation of specific genes.

CONCLUSION

These sputum tests offer great promise to determine both the molecular risk and the molecular diagnosis of lung cancer far in advance of clinical presentation. Any or all of these tests could be incorporated into the routine management of individuals at risk of developing primary or second primary lung cancer. However, several issues must be considered before these tests are ready for clinical application. First, test performance characteristics (sensitivity, specificity, predictive value) must be confirmed in prospective trials. The archives of sputum specimens collected during helical CT lung cancer screening trials provide an opportunity for both sputum test validation and comparison with the test performance of LDCT. Second, the development of a management and intervention strategy appropriate to the stage at which lung cancer is detected will be needed. The ability to detect

lung cancer at the stage of clonal expansion, well in advance of malignant invasion of the basement membrane, suggests that non-invasive, chemoprevention might be appropriate in such patients. Preliminary studies of chemopreventive agents are now being sponsored by the NCI. Finally, the larger public health issues of cost and accessibility of lung cancer screening must be considered before these advances in sputum screening can reach their potential.

REFERENCES

1. Barrett N, Examination of the sputum for malignant cells and particles of malignant growth. J Thorac Surg 1938; 8:169–83.
2. Cromwell HA, Papanicolaou GN, Use of the cytologic method in industrial medicine with special reference to tumors of the lung and the bladder. AMA Arch Ind Hyg Occup Med 1952; 5(3):232–3.
3. Saccomanno G, Saunders RP, Ellis H, et al, Concentration of carcinoma or atypical cells in sputum. Acta Cytol 1963; 63:305–10.
4. Fontana RS, Sanderson DR, Woolner LB, et al, Screening for lung cancer. A critique of the Mayo Lung Project. Cancer 1991; 67(4 Suppl):1155–64.
5. Frost JK, Ball WC Jr, Levin ML, et al, Early lung cancer detection: results of the initial (prevalence) radiologic and cytologic screening in the Johns Hopkins study. Am Rev Respir Dis 1984; 130(4):549–54.
6. Flehinger BJ, Melamed MR, Zaman MB, et al, Early lung cancer detection: results of the initial (prevalence) radiologic and cytologic screening in the Memorial Sloan-Kettering study. Am Rev Respir Dis 1984; 130(4):555–60.
7. Fontana RS, Sanderson DR, Taylor WF, et al, Early lung cancer detection: results of the initial (prevalence) radiologic and cytologic screening in the Mayo Clinic study. Am Rev Respir Dis 1984; 130(4):561–5.

8. Bechtel JJ, Kelley WR, Petty TL, Patz DS, Saccomanno G, et al, Outcome of 51 patients with roentgenographically occult lung cancer detected by sputum cytologic testing: a community hospital program. Arch Intern Med 1994; 154(9):975–80.

9. Tockman M, Survival and mortality from lung cancer in a screened population: the Johns Hopkins Study. Chest 1986; 89(Suppl):324S–5S.

10. Prindiville SA, Byers T, Hirsch FR, et al, Sputum cytological atypia as a predictor of incident lung cancer in a cohort of heavy smokers with airflow obstruction. Cancer Epidemiol Biomarkers Prev 2003; 12(10):987–93.

11. McWilliams A, Mayo J, MacDonald S, et al, Lung cancer screening: a different paradigm. Am J Respir Crit Care Med 2003; 168(10):1167–73.

12. Belinsky SA, Gene-promoter hypermethylation as a biomarker in lung cancer. Nat Rev Cancer 2004; 4(9):707–17.

13. Henschke CI, McCauley DI, Yankelevitz DF, et al, Early Lung Cancer Action Project: overall design and findings from baseline screening. Lancet 1999; 354(9173):99–105.

14. Sone S, Li F, Yang ZG, et al, Characteristics of small lung cancers invisible on conventional chest radiography and detected by population based screening using spiral CT. Br J Radiol 2000; 73(866):137–45.

15. Sone S, Li F, Yang ZG, et al, Results of three-year mass screening programme for lung cancer using mobile low-dose spiral computed tomography scanner. Br J Cancer 2001; 84(1):25–32.

16. Henschke CI, Naidich DP, Yankelevitz DF, et al, Early lung cancer action project: initial findings on repeat screenings. Cancer 2001; 92(1):153–9.

17. Sobue T, Moriyama N, Kaneko M, et al, Screening for lung cancer with low-dose helical computed tomography: anti-lung cancer association project. J Clin Oncol 2002; 20(4):911–20.

18. Swensen SJ, Moriyama N, Kaneko M, et al, Screening for lung cancer with low-dose spiral computed tomography. Am J Respir Crit Care Med 2002; 165(4):508–13.

19. Diederich S, Wormanns D, Semik M, et al, Screening for early lung cancer with low-dose spiral CT: prevalence in 817 asymptomatic smokers. Radiology 2002; 222(3):773–81.

20. Gohagan J, Marcus P, Fagerstrom R, et al, Baseline findings of a randomized feasibility trial of lung cancer screening with spiral CT scan vs chest radiograph: the Lung Screening Study of the National Cancer Institute. Chest 2004; 126(1):114–21.

21. Payne PW, Sebo TJ, Doudkine A, et al, Sputum screening by quantitative microscopy: a reexamination of a portion of the National Cancer Institute Cooperative Early Lung Cancer Study. Mayo Clin Proc 1997; 72(8):697–704.

22. Zhang Y, LeRiche JC, Jackson SM, Garner D, Palcic B, et al, An automated image cytometry system for monitoring DNA ploidy and other cell features of radiotherapy and chemotherapy patients. Radiat Med 1999; 17(1):47–57.

23. Jemal A, Tiwari RC, Murray T, et al, Cancer statistics 2004. CA Cancer J Clin 2004; 54(1):8–29.

24. Vecchio TJ, Predictive value of a single diagnostic test in unselected populations. N Engl J Med 1966; 274(21):1171–3.

25. Romeo MS, Sokolova IA, Morrison LE, et al, Chromosomal abnormalities in non-small cell lung carcinomas and in bronchial epithelia of high-risk smokers detected by multi-target interphase fluorescence in situ hybridization. J Mol Diagn 2003; 5(2):103–12.

26. Varella-Garcia M, Kittelson J, Schulte AP, et al, Multi-target interphase fluorescence in situ hybridization assay increases sensitivity of sputum cytology as a predictor of lung cancer. Cancer Detect Prev 2004; 28(4):244–51.

27. Slaughter DP, Southwick HW, Smejkal W, Field cancerization in oral stratified squamous epithelium; clinical implications of multicentric origin. Cancer 1953; 6(5):963–8.

28. Auerbach O, Hammond EC, Garfinkel L, Changes in bronchial epithelium in relation to cigarette smoking, 1955–1960 vs. 1970–1977. N Engl J Med 1979; 300(8):381–5.

29. Auerbach O, Stout AP, Hammond EC, Garfinkel L, Changes in bronchial epithelium in relation to cigarette smoking and in relation to lung cancer. N Engl J Med 1961; 265:253–67.

30. Khuri FR, Lippman SM, Lung cancer chemoprevention. Semin Surg Oncol 2000; 18(2): 100–5.

31. Grover FL, Piantadosi S, Recurrence and survival following resection of bronchioloalveolar carcinoma of the lung – The Lung Cancer Study Group experience. Ann Surg 1989; 209(6): 779–90.

32. Tong L, Spitz MR, Fueger JJ, Amos CA, et al, Lung carcinoma in former smokers. Cancer 1996; 78(5):1004–10.

33. Fearon ER, Vogelstein B, A genetic model for colorectal tumorigenesis. Cell 1990; 61(5): 759–67.

34. Bishop JM, The molecular genetics of cancer. Science 1987; 235(4786):305–11.

35. Weinberg RA, Oncogenes, antioncogenes, and the molecular bases of multistep carcinogenesis. Cancer Res 1989; 49(14):3713–21.

36. Hanahan D, Weinberg RA, The hallmarks of cancer. Cell 2000; 100(1):57–70.

37. Wistuba II, Behrens C, Milchgrub S, et al, Sequential molecular abnormalities are involved in the multistage development of squamous cell lung carcinoma. Oncogene 1999; 18(3):643–50.

38. Gonzalez-Zulueta M, Ruppert JM, Tokino K, et al, Microsatellite instability in bladder cancer. Cancer Res 1993; 53(23):5620–3.

39. van der Riet P, Nawroz H, Hruban RH, et al, Frequent loss of chromosome 9p21-22 early in head and neck cancer progression. Cancer Res 1994; 54(5):1156–8.

40. Mao L, Lee DJ, Tockman MS, et al, Microsatellite alterations as clonal markers for the detection of human cancer. Proc Natl Acad Sci USA 1994; 91(21):9871–5.

41. Peinado MA, Malkosyan S, Velazquez A, Peracho M, et al, Isolation and characterization of allelic losses and gains in colorectal tumors by arbitrarily primed polymerase chain reaction. Proc Natl Acad Sci USA 1992; 89(21):10065–9.

42. Leach FS, Nicolaides NC, Papadopoulos N, et al, Mutations of a mutS homolog in hereditary nonpolyposis colorectal cancer. Cell 1993; 75(6):1215–25.

43. Merlo A, Mabry M, Gabrielson E, et al, Frequent microsatellite instability in primary small cell lung cancer. Cancer Res 1994; 54(8):2098–101.

44. Xu LH, Wu L, Ahrent S, et al, Identification of frequently altered microsatellite markers for clinical detection of non-small cell lung cancer. Proc Amer Assoc Cancer Res 1997; 38:329.

45. Mao L, Lee JS, Kurie JM, et al, Clonal genetic alterations in the lungs of current and former smokers. J Natl Cancer Inst 1997; 89(12): 857–62.

46. Tockman MS, Mulshine JL, The early detection of occult lung cancer. Chest Surg Clin N Am 2000; 10(4):737–49.

47. Mao L, Schoenberg MP, Scicchitano M, et al, Molecular detection of primary bladder cancer by microsatellite analysis. Science 1996; 271(5249):659–62.

48. Arvanitis DA, Papadakis E, Zafiropoulos A, Spandidos DA, et al, Fractional allele loss is a valuable marker for human lung cancer detection in sputum. Lung Cancer 2003; 40(1): 55–66.

49. Nunn J, Scholes AG, Liloglou T, et al, Fractional allele loss indicates distinct genetic populations in the development of squamous cell carcinoma of the head and neck (SCCHN). Carcinogenesis 1999; 20(12):2219–28.

50. Dammann R, Schagdarsurengin U, Strunnikova M, et al, Epigenetic inactivation of the Ras-association domain family 1 (RASSF1A) gene and its function in human carcinogenesis. Histol Histopathol 2003; 18(2):665–77.

51. Campbell SL, Khosravi-Far R, Rossman KL, et al, Increasing complexity of Ras signaling. Oncogene 1998; 17(11 Reviews):1395–413.

52. Bos JL, Fearon ER, Hamilton SR, et al, Prevalence of ras gene mutations in human colorectal cancers. Nature 1987; 327(6120):293–7.

53. Rodenhuis S, Slebos RJ, Clinical significance of ras oncogene activation in human lung cancer. Cancer Res 1992; 52(9 Suppl):2665s–9s.

54. Mao L, Hruban RH, Boyle JO, et al, Detection of oncogene mutations in sputum precedes diagnosis of lung cancer. Cancer Res 1994; 54(7):1634–7.

55. Dammann R, Li C, Yoon JH, et al, Epigenetic inactivation of a RAS association domain family protein from the lung tumour suppressor locus 3p21.3. Nat Genet 2000; 25(3):315–19.

56. Burbee DG, Forgacs E, Zochbauer-Muller S, et al, Epigenetic inactivation of RASSF1A in lung and breast cancers and malignant phenotype suppression. J Natl Cancer Inst 2001; 93(9): 691–9.

57. Jones PA, Baylin SB, The fundamental role of epigenetic events in cancer. Nat Rev Genet 2002; 3(6):415–28.

58. Merlo A, Herman JG, Mao L, et al, 5′ CpG island methylation is associated with transcriptional silencing of the tumour suppressor p16/CDKN2/MTS1 in human cancers. Nat Med 1995; 1(7):686–92.

59. Herman JG, Graff JR, Mychanen S, et al, Methylation-specific PCR: a novel PCR assay for methylation status of CpG islands. Proc Natl Acad Sci USA 1996; 93(18):9821–6.

60. Belinsky SA, Nikula KJ, Palmisano WA, et al, Aberrant methylation of p16(INK4a) is an early event in lung cancer and a potential biomarker for early diagnosis. Proc Natl Acad Sci USA 1998; 95(20):11891–6.

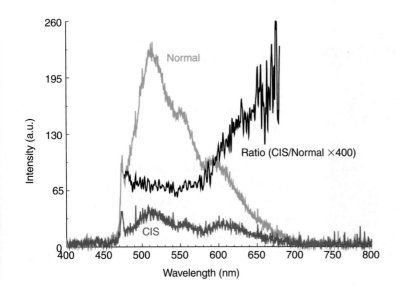

Figure 9.2
In-vivo autofluorescence spectra from normal bronchial tissue and an area of carcinoma in-situ (CIS) upon illumination of the bronchial surface with blue light. CIS shows a significant decrease in fluorescence intensity in the green region of the emission spectrum but comparatively less reduction in the red. As a result, the red to green ratio is significantly higher in CIS compared to normal.

and oxygenation may also alter the fluorescence quantum yield, spectral peak positions and line widths.[22] The extent to which these metabolic and morphologic changes will alter the fluorescence signal depends on the excitation and emission wavelengths used for illumination and detection in fluorescence imaging devices used clinically in bronchoscopy. The excitation wavelengths producing the highest tumor to normal tissue contrasts are between 400 nm and 480 nm with a peak at 405 nm.[17,23] The spectral differences between 500 nm and 700 nm in normal, pre-malignant and malignant tissues serve as the basis for the design of several autofluorescence endoscopic imaging devices for localization of early lung cancer in the bronchial tree.

Although white light bronchoscopy is the simplest imaging technique, less than 40% of carcinoma in-situ is detectable by standard white-light bronchoscopy.[24,25] This clinical problem, combined with the improvement of endoscopic technology, has driven the development and evaluation of fluorescence bronchoscopy for the localization of pre-invasive lung cancer.[14,17,25–27]

AUTOFLUORESCENCE BRONCHOSCOPY DEVICES

A number of devices have been developed for commercial use including the LIFE-Lung device (Xillix Technologies, Richmond, BC, Canada), Storz D-light (Karl Storz GmbH, Tuttlingen, Germany), and SAFE-1000 (Pentax, Japan). The first device, the LIFE-Lung system, uses a He-Cd laser (442 nm) for illumination.[26,28,29] A second-generation device, the LIFE-Lung II uses a filtered Xe lamp to produce the blue light.[25,30] Two image-intensified CCD sensors are used to capture the emitted fluorescence, one in the green region (480–520 nm) and the other in the red region ($\geq$625 nm). The red and green images are then combined. Because pre-malignant and malignant lesions lose more green autofluorescence than red, these lesions appear reddish-brown against a greenish normal background (Figure 9.3). The original LIFE-Lung device has separate light sources for the white light and fluorescence examinations and requires manual change of light source between examinations. In LIFE-Lung II, a filtered arc

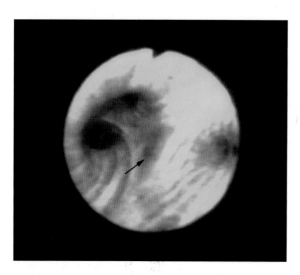

Figure 9.3
Autofluorescence image of a carcinoma in-situ lesion in the left upper lobe. The tumor area appears brownish red (arrow) against a normal green background. (Courtesy of LIFE-Lung II Device, Xillix Technologies Inc., Richmond, BC, Canada.)

lamp is used which allows rapid switching between the two examination modes. A unique design in LIFE-Lung II is its real time quantitative display of the red/green autofluorescence ratio to minimize human error of subjective color interpretation.[30]

The Pentax SAFE-1000 system uses a filtered Xe lamp in the 420–480 nm range to produce the excitation light, but only detects fluorescence in the green spectrum (490–590 nm) using a single image-intensified CCD sensor.[31]

The Wolf system is similar to the Xillix LIFE-Lung system with a filtered 300 W Xe lamp in the 'violet-blue' range (390–460 nm) and slightly different band-pass filters for detection: 500–590 nm (green region), and 600–700 nm (red region).[14,32]

The Storz system consists of a RGB CCD camera and a filtered Xe lamp (380–460 nm). It combines a fluorescence image with a blue

reflectance image.[27] The lesions appear purple against a bluish-green background. Frame averaging is used to amplify the weak autofluorescence.

The latest device by Xillix (Onco-LIFE, Richmond, Canada) also utilizes a combination of reflectance and fluorescence imaging.[31] A red reflectance image is used in combination with the green fluorescence image to enhance the contrast between malignant and normal tissues (Figure 9.4). Using reflected red light as a reference has the theoretical advantage over reflected blue light in that it is less absorbed by hemoglobin and hence less influenced by changes in vascularity associated with inflammation.

CLINICAL TRIALS

Most of the published clinical studies on autofluorescence bronchoscopy have been conducted with the Xillix LIFE-Lung devices with smaller studies in the other devices.[33–35] Over the last decade, a number of studies have been conducted in Canada, USA, Europe and Asia, using the LIFE-Lung devices involving more than 2000 patients.[10,21,25,26,28–30,36–58] In the majority of these trials, autofluorescence bronchoscopy was performed and evaluated as an adjunct to white light bronchoscopy. The relative sensitivity of autofluorescence bronchoscopy versus white-light examination alone in detecting high-grade dysplasia and carcinoma in-situ was found to increase by an average of two-fold (1.5–6.3-fold). Approximately 80% of the lesions (range 43–100%) can be localized by fluorescence examination compared to an average of 40% (range 9–78%) by white-light examination alone. A randomized study using a different bronchoscopist to perform either the white-light or the fluorescence examination also showed a significant increase in the relative

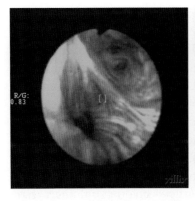 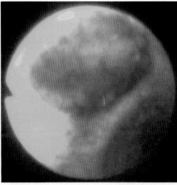

Figure 9.4
Fluorescence-reflectance image of an area with severe dysplasia (left) and an area with carcinoma in-situ (right). The lesion appears reddish in color against a normal green background. (Courtesy of Onco-LIFE Device, Xillix Technologies Inc., Richmond, BC, Canada.)

sensitivity of fluorescence examination versus white-light examination (68.8% versus 21.9%).[42] The improved sensitivity was associated with a lower specificity of an average of 60% compared to 81% by white-light examination. The wide range of sensitivity in both examinations most likely reflects the differences in study design and varying experience of endoscopists and pathologists in the interpretation of fluorescence images and bronchial biopsies.

The results of a multicenter trial of the Storz D-Light autofluorescence device involving 293 patients were recently reported.[33] Autofluorescence bronchoscopy improved the detection rate of pre-invasive lesions from 11% to 61%. The specificity of autofluorescence bronchoscopy and white-light bronchoscopy was 75% and 95%, respectively.

There has been only one report comparing the performance of the first LIFE-Lung device and the Storz D-light system.[36] Both systems gave comparable results although details of the cross-over design were not given in the report.

In the Xillix and Storz trials, most of the false-positive biopsies were found to be due to inflammation, goblet cell hyperplasia or metaplasia. However, areas with 'benign' pathology and abnormal fluorescence have been found to contain more genetic alterations on comparative genomic hybridization than areas with normal

fluorescence, suggesting that areas with abnormal fluorescence may represent higher-risk lesions.[59] Some areas with abnormal fluorescence and benign pathology have been shown to develop into carcinoma on bronchoscopic follow-up.[49,50] In addition, the presence of three or more sites of abnormal fluorescence was found to predict development of squamous cell carcinoma in high-risk patients.[48]

CLINICAL APPLICATIONS OF AUTOFLUORESCENCE BRONCHOSCOPY

Up until very recently, autofluorescence bronchoscopy in lung cancer diagnosis has been limited by equipment costs and availability, as well as the need for specialized training. Over the last decade, the principles behind exploiting both the reflectance and autofluorescence properties of bronchial tissues to improve the sensitivity of detecting pre-invasive lesions are becoming familiar to endoscopists. Commercial devices are cheaper and easier to use. Current devices using filtered lamps allow rapid switching between the white-light and fluorescence modes. The combined examination usually adds 5–10 minutes to a conventional white-light bronchoscopic procedure. The bronchoscopy is well tolerated by patients under local anesthesia and conscious sedation. Devices with simultaneous display of the white-light and fluorescence images are undergoing development and testing. These new devices will further shorten the procedure time and minimize re-imbursement issues that may be a barrier in some countries.

Current evidence supports the use of autofluorescence bronchoscopy in the following clinical situations:

1. Patients with severe atypia or malignant cells in their sputum cytology and a negative chest X-ray or CT scan;
2. As part of a diagnostic bronchoscopy in patients suspected to have lung cancer where a bronchoscopy is indicated; and
3. Patients with potentially curable carcinoma in-situ/micro-invasive cancer prior to therapy.

Patients who present with malignant cells in sputum cytology examination with a negative chest X-ray or CT scan – the so-called radiographically occult lung cancer represents a diagnostic challenge. When white-light bronchoscopy fails to localize the source of the malignant cells, repeat bronchoscopies with blind segmental bronchial brushings and multiple bronchial spur biopsies are required for diagnosis.[60–62] Although the procedure can be done under local anesthesia, it is more commonly done under general anesthesia. The examination generally takes 1–2 hours. There is also the problem of cross contamination from spilling of cells from one segment or lobe to another with coughing. With the introduction of autofluorescence bronchoscopy, these radiographically occult cancers can now be readily detected with one bronchoscopy as shown by the clinical experience reviewed above.

Severe atypia on sputum cytology examination has been reported in several studies to have a risk of developing lung cancer within 2 years of approximately 45%.[63–65] In the Johns Hopkins Early Lung Cancer Detection Project, moderate atypia was also found to have an increased risk of the subsequent development of lung cancer. Fourteen percent of the participants with moderate atypia developed lung cancer on long-term follow-up, compared to 3% of participants without atypia.[64] In the Colorado SPORE cohort of high-risk smokers and ex-smokers with airflow obstruction, there have been 83 incident lung cancers after more than 4469 years of observation. The relative risks of developing lung cancer, adjusted for age, gender, recruitment year, pack-years and smoking status, for increasing grades of cytologic atypia were 1.0 (normal), 1.10 (mild atypia), 1.68 (moderate atypia), 3.18 (moderate atypia or worse) and 31.4 (worse than moderate atypia).[65] Sputum cytologic atypia of severe dysplasia or worse clearly carries a risk of lung cancer that is high enough to warrant an aggressive diagnostic approach with combined white-light and fluorescence bronchoscopy. Two groups have reported results of bronchoscopy in subjects with moderate atypia sputum cytology and chest radiographs negative for carcinoma. Fujita reported, in abstract form only, a series of 25 subjects with moderate atypia sputum cytology and negative chest radiographs who underwent bronchoscopy. Two had carcinoma diagnosed.[66] Kennedy and colleagues have reported a series of 79 subjects with moderate atypia sputum cytology and chest radiographs negative for cancer.[67] Of the 79, lung cancer was found at bronchoscopy in five (6.3%; 95% CI = 0.7–11%). Two of the cancers were carcinoma in situ lesions and three were invasive. The rates of discovery of cancer at bronchoscopy reported in these studies exceed the rate of discovery of colon cancer when colonoscopy is performed for a positive fecal occult blood test. While moderate atypia in sputum cytology is not as compelling an indication for bronchoscopy as is severe dysplasia and the high rate of discovery of unexpected lung cancer in the reported studies may be partly due to chance, publication bias or a selection bias in which only subjects with moderate atypia and additional health problems were examined, consideration of bronchoscopy is certainly reasonable in a concerned patient with moderate atypia.

For patients with early lung cancer who are being assessed for curative surgical resection and those with carcinoma in-situ who are being evaluated for endobronchial therapies, autofluorescence bronchoscopy is useful in the delineation of tumor margins and to assess the presence of synchronous lesions in the bronchial tree.[46,47,68] Synchronous cancer can be found on autofluorescence bronchoscopy in up to 14% of these patients. Up to 27% of patients may also have other moderate/severe dysplastic lesions that will require bronchoscopic followup.[26,28,46,68]

Carcinoma in-situ is a potentially curable lesion with endobronchial therapy such as photodynamic therapy, electrocautery or cryotherapy if the lesion is ≤1 cm^2.[47,69] However, white light bronchoscopy is inadequate both for detection and for delineation of the margins of these lesions, whereas autofluorescence bronchoscopy improves staging of these occult cancers and has an impact on their management.[47,58] In addition, during endobronchial therapy with techniques such as electrocautery, autofluorescence can be used to ensure that the lesion is adequately treated.

The role of autofluorescence bronchoscopy for surveillance of second primary lung cancer in patients who have curative therapy for non-small-cell lung cancer or limited-stage small-cell lung cancer was examined in several studies.

This group of patients has a relatively high rate of development of metachronous tumors; 1–5% per year after non-small-cell lung cancer resection and 2–13% after small-cell lung cancer.[70–74] The number of patients in these studies was small. Lesions were identified in 3–6% of these patients who are thought to be disease-free.[37–39,75] Patients with prior squamous cell carcinoma appear to be a population that may warrant prospective study of postoperative fluorescence bronchoscopic surveillance.[39] Likewise, the prevalence of pre-invasive lesions in patients with cancer in the upper aerodigestive tract (head and neck cancer excluding nasopharyngeal cancer or esophageal cancer) may be sufficiently high due to the field cancerization effect of inhaled tobacco carcinogens to warrant a fluorescence bronchoscopy prior to curative therapy or for surveillance for second primary cancers. In patients with esophageal cancer up to 19% may have synchronous or metachronous cancers in other organs, and lung cancer contributed to approximately 10% of these second tumors.[76] In laryngeal cancer patients, up to 28% have been reported to have synchronous or metachronous tumors, and lung cancer was the most frequent second malignancy, contributing to 41% of second tumors.[28,77,78]

Currently, there are no established evidence-based guidelines to aid physicians in the ongoing surveillance of lung cancer patients following curative-intent therapy.[79] Although there has been stimulating research into lung cancer screening over the last decade with the emergence of techniques such as low-dose thoracic CT scans, autofluorescence bronchoscopy and new sputum biomarkers, we ultimately need the ability to both detect and reduce the development of metachronous pulmonary malignancies to impact lung cancer mortality. Evidence-based follow-up protocols need to be developed and their benefits need to be evaluated in larger prospective clinical trials.

RESEARCH APPLICATIONS

Autofluorescence bronchoscopy has a significant role in ongoing lung cancer research. The study of the natural history and genetic alterations in pre-neoplastic lesions accessible to the fiberoptic bronchoscope will lead to a better understanding of lung cancer pathogenesis and progression. It will in turn lead to the development of better biomarkers for early detection and novel molecular targets for intervention. Preliminary study suggests that fluorescence bronchoscopy plays an important role in an early lung cancer detection program in conjunction with spiral CT.[10] The ability to identify pre-neoplastic lesions and perform serial biopsies before and after treatment provides an intermediate endpoint to evaluate novel agents for chemoprevention of lung cancer.[80]

SUMMARY

Autofluorescence bronchoscopy is a sensitive technique for detection of intraepithelial neoplasia. In conjunction with white-light bronchoscopy, it has a definite clinical role in the localization of pre-invasive lung cancer in patients with abnormal sputum cytology and in determination of the extent of endobronchial spread in patients with early lung cancer prior to curative therapy. It may also play a role in patients with potentially curable esophageal and head and neck cancer in detection of second primary lung cancer, as well as in the postoperative surveillance of lung cancer patients, but further studies are required. Fluorescence bronchoscopy plays an important part in lung cancer

research particularly in the study of the natural history and the molecular biology of pre-neoplastic lesions, in lung cancer screening clinical trials as well as phase II trials of chemopreventive agents.

REFERENCES

1. Kaneko M, Eguchi K, Ohmatsu H, et al, Peripheral lung cancer: Screening and detection with low-dose spiral CT versus radiography. Radiology 1996; 210:798–802.
2. Henschke C, McCauley D, Yankelevitz D, et al, Early Lung Cancer Action Project: overall design and findings from baseline screening. Lancet 1999; 354:99–105.
3. Sone S, Li F, Yang Z-G, et al, Characteristics of small lung cancers invisible on conventional chest radiography and detected by population based screening using spiral CT. Br J Radiol 2000; 73:137–45.
4. Henschke C, Naidich D, Yankelevitz D, et al, Early Lung Cancer Action Project: Initial findings on repeat screening. Cancer 2001; 92(1): 153–9.
5. Sone S, Yang Z-G, Honda T, et al, Results of three-year mass screening program for lung cancer using mobile low-dose spiral computed tomography scanner. Br J Cancer 2001; 84(1): 25–32.
6. Sobue T, Moriyama N, Kaneko M, et al, Screening for lung cancer with low-dose helical computed tomography: Anti-lung cancer association project. J Clin Oncol 2002; 20(4):911–20.
7. Swensen SJ, Jett JR, Sloan JA, et al, Screening for lung cancer with low-dose spiral computed tomography. Am J Respir Crit Care Med 2002; 165:508–13.
8. Diederich S, Wormanns D, Semik M, et al, Screening for early lung cancer with low-dose spiral CT: prevalence in 817 asymptomatic smokers. Radiology 2002; 222(3):773–81.
9. Nawa T, Nakagawa T, Kusano S, et al, Lung cancer screening using low-dose spiral CT:

results of baseline and 1-year follow-up studies. Chest 2002; 122(1):15–20.

10. McWilliams A, Mayo J, MacDonald S, et al, Lung cancer screening; a different paradigm. Am J Respir Crit Care Med 2003; 168(10):1167–73.

11. Cortese DA, Pairolero PC, Bergstralh EJ, et al, Roentgenographically occult lung cancer. A ten-year experience. J Thorac Cardiovasc Surg 1983; 86:373–80.

12. Melamed MR, Flehinger BJ, Zaman MB, et al, Screening for early lung cancer. Results of the Memorial Sloan-Kettering study in New York. Chest 1984; 86(1):44–53.

13. Janssen-Heijnen ML, Coeburgh JW, Trends in incidence and prognosis of the histological subtypes of lung cancer in North America, Australia, New Zealand and Europe. Lung Cancer 2001; 31:123–37.

14. Wagnieres G, McWilliams A, Lam S, Lung cancer imaging with fluorescence endoscopy. In: Mycek M, Pogue B (eds) Handbook of Biomedical Fluorescence. Marcel Dekker, New York, 2003, pp. 361–96.

15. MacAulay C, Lane P, Richards-Kortum R, In-vivo pathology: Microendoscopy as a new endoscopic imaging modality. In: Gastrointestinal Endoscopy Clinics of North America – Optical Biopsy. Elsevier Science, 2004, 14:595–620.

16. Aguirre A, Hsiung P, Ko T, Hartl I, Fujimoto J, High-resolution optical coherence microscopy for high-speed, in vivo cellular imaging. Optics Lett 2003; 28(21):2064–6.

17. Hung J, Lam S, leRiche J, Palcic B, Autofluorescence of normal and malignant bronchial tissue. Laser Surg Med 1991; 11:99–105.

18. Qu J, MacAulay C, Lam S, Palcic B, Laser-induced fluorescence spectroscopy at endoscopy: tissue optics, Monte Carlo modeling, and in vivo measurements. Opt Eng 1995; 34: 3334–43.

19. Qu J, MacAulay C, Lam S, Palcic B, Optical properties of normal and carcinoma bronchial tissue. Appl Optics 1994; 33(31):7397–405.

20. Gardner C, Jacques S, Welch A, Fluorescence spectroscopy of tissue: recovery of intrinsic fluorescence from measured fluorescence. Appl Optics 1996; 35(10):1780–92.

21. Keith R, Miller Y, Gemmill R, et al, Angiogenic squamous dysplasia in bronchi of individuals at high risk for lung cancer. Clin Cancer Res 2000; 6:1616–25.

22. Wolfbeis O, Fluorescence of organic natural products. In: Schulman SG (ed.) Molecular Luminescence Spectroscopy, vol 1. J Wiley and Sons, New York, 1973, pp. 167–370.

23. Zellweger M, Grosjean P, Goujon D, et al, Autofluorescence spectroscopy to characterize the histopathological status of bronchial tissue in vivo. J Biomed Opt 2001; 6(1):41–52.

24. Woolner L, Pathology of cancer detected cytologically. In: Atlas Of Early Lung Cancer, National Institutes of Health, US Department of Health and Human Services. Igaku-Shoin, Tokyo, 1983, pp. 107–213.

25. Lam S, MacAulay C, leRiche J, Palcic B, Detection and localization of early lung cancer by fluorescence bronchoscopy. Cancer 2000; 89(11 Suppl):2468–73.

26. Lam S, MacAulay C, Hung J, et al, Detection of dysplasia and carcinoma in situ with a lung imaging fluorescence endoscope device. J Thorac Cardiovasc Surg 1993; 105:1035–40.

27. Häussinger K, Pichler J, Stanzel F, et al, Autofluorescence bronchoscopy: the D-light system. Interventional Bronchoscopy 2000; 30: 243–52.

28. Lam S, MacAulay C, leRiche J, Ikeda N, Palcic B, Early localization of bronchogenic carcinoma. Diag Therapeu Endo 1994; 1:75–8.

29. Lam S, Kennedy T, Unger M, et al, Localization of bronchial intraepithelial neoplastic lesions by fluorescence bronchoscopy. Chest 1998; 113: 696–702.

30. Lam S, LeRiche J, Zheng Y, et al, Sex-related differences in bronchial epithelial changes associated with tobacco smoking. J Natl Cancer Inst 1999; 91:691–6.

31. McWilliams A, Lam S, The utilization of autofluorescence in flexible bronchoscopy. In: Wang KP, Mehta AC, Turner JF Jr (eds) Flexible

Bronchoscopy, 2nd edn. Blackwell Science, Boston, 2004, pp. 138–45.

32. Goujon D, Zellweger M, Radu A, et al, In vivo autofluorescence imaging of early lung cancers in the human tracheobronchial tree with a spectrally optimized system. J Biomed Optics 2003; 8(1):17–25.

33. Beamis J, Ernst A, Mathur P, Yung R, Simoff M, A multi-center study comparing autofluorescence bronchoscopy to white light bronchoscopy. Lung Cancer 2003; 41(Suppl 2):S49.

34. Kakihana M, Okunaka T, Furukawa K, et al, Early detection of bronchial lesions using system of autofluorescence endoscopy (SAFE-1000). Diag Therapeu Endo 1999; 5:99–104.

35. Furukawa K, Kakihana M, Ikeda N, et al, Fluorescence bronchoscopy in the early detection of bronchial lesions. Lung Cancer 2000; 29(Suppl 2): 85.

36. Herth F, Becker H, Autofluorescence bronchoscopy – a comparison of two systems (LIFE and D-Light). Respiration 2003; 70(4): 395–8.

37. Weigel T, Kosco P, Dacic S, Yousem S, Luketich J, Fluorescence bronchoscopic surveillance in patients with a history of non-small cell lung cancer. Diag Therapeu Endo 1999; 6:1–7.

38. Weigel T, Yousem S, Dacic S, et al, Fluorescence bronchoscopic surveillance after curative surgical resection for non-small cell lung cancer. Ann Surg Onc 2000; 7(3):176–80.

39. Weigel T, Kosco P, Dacic S, et al, Post-operative fluorescence bronchoscopic surveillance in non-small cell lung cancer patients. Ann Thor Surg 2001; 71:967–70.

40. Kurie J, Lee J, Morice R, et al, Autofluorescence bronchoscopy in the detection of squamous metaplasia and dysplasia in current and former smokers. J Natl Cancer Inst 1998; 90(13): 991–5.

41. Kennedy T, Hirsch F, Miller Y, et al, A randomized study of fluorescence bronchoscopy versus white light bronchoscopy for early detection of lung cancer in high risk patients. Lung Cancer 2000; 29(1)(Suppl 1):244–5.

42. Hirsch F, Prindiville S, Miller Y, et al, Fluorescence versus white-light bronchoscopy for detection of preneoplastic lesions: A randomised study. J Natl Cancer Inst 2001; 93(18): 1385–91.

43. Venmans B, van der Linden H, Van Boxem T, et al, Early detection of preinvasive lesions in high-risk patients: a comparison of conventional flexible and fluorescence bronchoscopy. J Bronchology 1998; 5(4):280–3.

44. Venmans B, Van Boxem T, Smit E, Postmus P, Sutedja T, Results of two years experience with fluorescence bronchoscopy in detection of preinvasive bronchial neoplasia. Diag Therapeu Endo 1999; 5:77–84.

45. Vermylen P, Roufosse C, Pierard P, et al, Detection of preneoplastic lesions with fluorescence bronchoscopy. Eur Respir J 1997; 10:425S.

46. Van Rens M, Schramel F, Elbers J, Lammers J, The clinical value of lung imaging fluorescence endoscopy for detecting synchronous lung cancer. Lung Cancer 2001; 32:13–18.

47. Sutedja T, Codrington H, Risse E, et al, Autofluorescence bronchoscopy improves staging of radiographically occult lung cancer and has an impact on therapeutic strategy. Chest 2001; 120(4):1327–32.

48. Pasic A, Vonk-Noordegraaf, Risse E, Postmus P, Sutedja T, Multiple suspicious lesions detected by autofluorescence bronchoscopy predict malignant development in the bronchial mucosa in high risk patients. Lung Cancer 2003; 41: 295–301.

49. Venmans B, van Boxem A, Smit E, Postmus P, Sutedja T, Outcome of bronchial carcinoma in-situ. Chest 2000; 117; 1572–6.

50. Bota S, Auliac J-B, Paris C, et al, Follow-up of bronchial precancerous lesions and carcinoma in-situ using fluorescence endoscopy. Am J Respir Crit Care Med 2001; 164:1688–93.

51. Moro-Sibilot D, Jeanmart M, Lantuejoul S, et al, Cigarette smoking, preinvasive bronchial lesions, and autofluorescence bronchoscopy. Chest 2002; 122(6):1902–8.

52. Yokomise H, Yanagihara K, Fukuse T, et al,

Clinical experience with Lung-Imaging Fluorescence Endoscope (LIFE) in patients with lung cancer. J Bronchology 1997; 4(3):205–8.

53. Ikeda N, Honda H, Katsumi T, et al, Early detection of bronchial lesions using Lung Imaging Fluorescence Endoscope. Diag Therapeu Endos 1999; 5:85–90.

54. Ikeda N, Hiyoshi T, Kakihana M, et al, Histopathological evaluation of fluorescence bronchoscopy using resected lungs in cases of lung cancer. Lung Cancer 2003; 41(3):303–9.

55. Shibuya K, Fujisawa T, Hoshino H, et al, Fluorescence bronchoscopy in the detection of pre-invasive bronchial lesions in patients with sputum cytology suspicious or positive for malignancy. Lung Cancer 2001; 32:19–25.

56. Sato M, Sakurada A, Sagawa M, et al, Diagnostic results before and after introduction of autofluorescence bronchoscopy in patients suspected of having lung cancer detected by sputum cytology in lung cancer mass screening. Lung Cancer 2001; 32(3):247–53.

57. Lee F, Ng A, Weng Y, Early detection of lung cancer with the LIFE laser. Chest 1995; 108(Suppl):115.

58. Kusunoki Y, Imamura F, Uda H, Mano M, Horai T, Early detection of lung cancer with laser-induced fluorescence endoscopy and spectrofluorometry. Chest 2000; 118(6):1776–82.

59. Helfritszch H, Junker K, Bartel M, Scheele J, Differentiation of positive autofluorescence bronchoscopy findings by comparative genomic hybridization. Oncol Rep 2002; 9:697–701.

60. Sanderson DR, Fontana RS, Woolner LB, et al, Bronchoscopic localization of radiographically occult lung cancer. Chest 1974; 64:608–12.

61. Sato M, Saito Y, Nagamoto N, et al, Diagnostic value of differential brushings of all branches of the bronchi in patients with sputum-positive or suspected positive for lung cancer. Acta Cytol 1993; 37:879–83.

62. Sagawa M, Saito Y, Sato M, et al, Localization of double, roentgenographically occult lung cancer. Acta Cytol 1993; 38:392–7.

63. Risse EJK, Vooijs GP, van't Hof MA, Diagnostic significance of 'severe dysplasia' in sputum cytology. Acta Cytol 1988; 32:629–34.

64. Frost JK, Ball WC, Levin ML, et al, Sputum cytopathology: use and potential in monitoring the workplace environment by screening for biological effects of exposure. J Occup Med 1986; 22:692–703.

65. Prindville SA, Byers T, Hirsch FR, et al, Sputum cytological atypia as a predictor of incident lung cancer in a cohort of heavy smokers with airflow obstruction. Cancer Epidemiol Biomark Prev 2003; 12:987–93.

66. Fujita Y, Shimizu T, Sakai E, et al, Results of mass screening for early lung cancer detection and bronchoscopic approach for evaluation of moderate squamous cell atypia. Lung Cancer 1994; 11(suppl 1):70.

67. Kennedy TC, Franklin WA, Prindville SA, et al, High prevalence of endobronchial malignancy in high-risk patients with moderate dysplasia in sputum. Chest 2004; 125(suppl 1):109S.

68. Pierard P, Vermylen P, Bosschaerts T, et al, Synchronous roentgenographically occult lung cancer in patients with resectable primary lung cancer. Chest 2000; 117(3):779–85.

69. Fujimura S, Sakurada A, Sagawa M, et al, A therapeutic approach to roentgenographically occult squamous cell carcinoma of the lung. Cancer 2000; 8911(Suppl):2445–8.

70. Johnson B, Second lung cancers in patients after treatment for an initial lung cancer. J Natl Cancer Inst 1998; 90(18):1335–45.

71. Van Rens M, Zanen P, Riviere A, et al, Survival after resection of metachronous non-small cell lung cancer in 127 patients. Ann Thorac Surg 2001; 71:309–13.

72. Jeremic B, Shibamoto Y, Acimovic L, et al, Second lung cancers occurring in patients with early stage non-small lung cancer treated with chest radiation alone. J Clin Onc 2001; 19(4): 1056–63.

73. Nakamura H, Kawasaki N, Hagiwara M, et al, Early hilar lung cancer – risk for multiple lung cancers and clinical outcome. Lung Cancer 2001; 33:51–7.

74. Woolner L, Fontana R, Cortese D, et al, Roentgenographically occult lung cancer: Pathologic findings and frequency of multicentricity during a 10-year period. Mayo Clin Proc 1984; 59:453–66.

75. Means-Markwell M, Linnoila RI, Williams J, et al, Prospective study of the airways and pulmonary parenchyma of patients at risk for a second lung cancer. Clin Cancer Res 2003; 9:5915–21.

76. Kagei K, Hosokawa M, Shirato H, et al, Efficacy of intense screening and treatment for synchronous second primary cancers in patients with esophageal cancer. Jpn J Clin Oncol 2002; 32(4):120–7.

77. Holland J, Arsanjani A, Liem B, et al, Second malignancies in early stage laryngeal carcinoma patients treated with radiotherapy. J Laryngol & Otol 2002; 116:190–3.

78. Aydiner A, Karadinez A, Uygun K, et al, Multiple primary neoplasms at a single institution: Differences between synchronous and metachronous neoplasms. Am J Clin Oncol 2000; 23(4): 362–70.

79. Colice G, Rubins J, Unger M, Follow-up and surveillance of the lung cancer patient following curative intent therapy. Chest 2003; 123(1) (Suppl):272S–83S.

80. McWilliams A, Lam S, New approaches to lung cancer prevention. Curr Oncol Rep 2002; 4(6): 487–94.

10 The role of endobronchial ultrasound (EBUS) in diagnosis and treatment of centrally located early lung cancer

Heinrich D Becker

Contents   Introduction • Current imaging procedures • The development of endobronchial ultrasound (EBUS) • Technology of ultrasonography • Ultrasonic systems for endobronchial use • Clinical application • Sonographic anatomy • Studies on application of EBUS in diagnosis and staging of early lung cancer • Future developments • Conclusions and clinical implications

INTRODUCTION

For the majority of patients suffering from lung cancer despite all efforts during recent decades the prognosis has not been significantly changed. Neither refinement of surgical procedures nor improvement in chemotherapy and radiotherapy or combination thereof in a multimodality concept could improve the average 5-year survival of approximately 15%.[1] This is essentially due to the fact that lung cancer is mostly detected at advanced stages when therapeutic options are limited. As primary prevention by reduced smoking has only very limited effect so far, several attempts at early detection have been performed. Concerning the current knowledge of the natural history of lung cancer there should be a wide window for earlier diagnosis as the stepwise development from early premalignant precursor lesions such as metaplasia, mild and severe dysplasia are taking several years for development to carcinoma in situ and localized early lung cancer.[2] In turn these usually take another few years to progress to the advanced stages of lung cancer that we usually see now.

Large studies performed in the 1970s for early detection of lung cancer by screening, including conventional sputum cytology and chest X-ray examination versus symptom-related diagnosis proved insufficient for detecting lung cancer at earlier stages and were abandoned and screening was advised against.[1] With the introduction of new imaging technologies like high-resolution CT, low-dose spiral CT and autofluorescence bronchoscopy screening for early lung cancer has become of interest, again, especially as new minimally invasive treatment modalities for potential bronchoscopic curation of these lesions became widely available. These include high-frequency electrocautery (HF), Argon plasma coagulation (APC), Nd-YAG laser treatment and high-dose radiation by brachytherapy technique (HDR). Most data, however, are available for potentially curative treatment by photodynamic therapy (PDT) after sensitivization to laser light exposure by application of hematoporphyrin derivates and other photosensitizers.[3]

Although in up to 100% complete short time remission could be achieved by administering PDT, long-term recurrence rates of up to 50%

have been reported and were attributed to failure of treatment. How could it be, however, that treatment of early lesions of equal size should be successful in one patient and fail in another although by definition all lesions should be comparable by definition of election criteria. Those are limited local endoluminal extent by bronchoscopy and invisibility in conventional X-ray and in high-resolution CT, defined as radiological invisibility. Clinical observation also provided no data that successful treatment by PDT depended on histological differentiation. There obviously had to be another factor influencing treatment outcome.

Basically, the definite diagnosis of in situ cancer and so-called early lung cancer can only be established by pathoanatomical analysis of resected specimens. Carcinoma in situ is limited

to the mucosa and does not penetrate the basal membrane, whereas early lung cancer does not exceed beyond the submucosal layer towards the cartilage or the intercartilaginous connective tissue (Figure 10.1).[4] These structures cannot be differentiated by current radiological methods. Thus pathoanatomical analysis of resected so-called early lung cancers as defined by bronchoscopic aspect and radiological invisibility in a significant number of cases demonstrated that the tumors were much more advanced than anticipated. Some infiltrated the deeper layers of the bronchial wall or the surrounding mediastinal structures, some even were associated with lymph node metastases.[2] Thus failures probably were not so much failures of treatment but rather failures of local staging of the minute lesions by radiological and

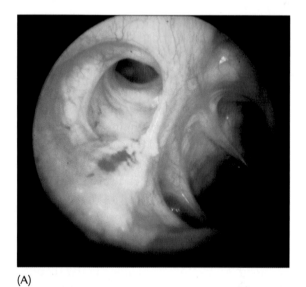

(A)

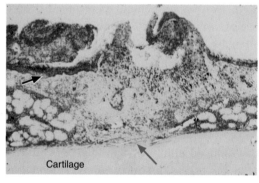

(B)

Figure 10.1
(A) This small cancer at the entrance of the middle lobe became apparent by blood traces in the sputum. The lesion appears as irregularity of the mucosa with whitish discoloration and small traces of blood. (B) The histological cross-section shows penetration of the basal membrane (lamina propria) by the tumor (black arrow). As the endochondrium is intact (red arrow), the tumor is an early cancer. (Histology courtesy of K.-M. Müller, Pathological Institute, University of Bochum, Germany.)

bronchoscopic imaging. This is why we felt it necessary to look for new imaging procedures so that we would be able to differentiate the layers of the bronchial wall. As the role for endobronchial ultrasound in early detection of small peripheral lesions currently is not clear yet, this chapter will deal with its role in early detection of central lesions only.

CURRENT IMAGING PROCEDURES

Improvement in white-light bronchoscopy (WLB)

By conventional white-light bronchoscopy with fiberoptics, detection of severe dysplasia and carcinoma in situ is difficult as these lesions are only a few cell layers thick and a few millimeters in surface diameter. However, there is a training effect once bronchoscopists are learning to recognize the subtle changes in early lesions as we experienced in a prospective study for evaluation of the Storz D-light system. Visualization with new video chip endoscopes is much superior and allows detailed analysis of the surface and intra- and supepithelial vascular structures which can be useful for differentiation of chronic bronchitis from dysplasia.[5]

Autofluorescence bronchoscopy (AF)

Since the development of autofluorescence bronchoscopy with illumination of the bronchial wall by blue light the detection rate of early lesions and precursors has been significantly increased.[6] AF is especially useful in diagnosing submucosal spread of pathological lesions and to improve exact diagnosis of their surface diameter. The details of the mechanisms are still under investigation, but besides metabolic alterations in early lesions a major contribution in alteration of fluorescence is epithelial thickening that results in drop of fluorescence

intensity, most of which comes from the submucosa and according to our observation especially from the connective tissue layer on the internal surface of the cartilages (endochondrium). Due to its origin pathological AF is unspecific and may be caused by metaplasia, dysplasia, in-situ cancer and early cancer, and also by benign lesions such as inflammation, scar formation and granulomas as well as by benign tumors. Thus biopsies are warranted in all cases for differential diagnosis. However, as the complete lesion can not usually be excised 'en block', pathoanatomical examination of endoscopic biopsy specimens is unable to diagnose the exact extent of the lesion, which can only be made on surgical resection specimens.

THE DEVELOPMENT OF ENDOBRONCHIAL ULTRASOUND (EBUS)

The view of the endoscopist is restricted to the lumen and the inner surface of the airways. Intramural processes or those adjacent to the airway, can only be assessed from indirect signs, such as discoloration and swelling of the mucosa, pathological vascularization, leveling of the cartilage relief and impression or distortion of the bronchial wall. Many pathologies of the airways also involve the parabronchial structures. Especially in malignant diseases exact diagnosis is decisive for the outcome of treatment. Therefore, the extension of the endoscopist's view beyond the tracheobronchial wall is essential as even recent radiological diagnostic procedures such as CT scan and MRI proved to be unreliable in staging of bronchial carcinoma with regard to these structures. Results of a prospective study for the validation of staging of bronchial carcinoma in our institution showed that clinical staging was congruent with

PTNM only in 60% of the cases. Especially diagnosis of involvement of mediastinal structures was very poor. Malignant involvement of lymph nodes is diagnosed correctly in only 50%; 25% were false positive, 25% false negative.[7] These results are in congruence with reports of other authors. As even invasive staging by mediastinoscopy proved to be negative in about 60%, 16% of which are false negative, some authors propose routine transbronchial needle biopsy (TBNA) of the hilar and mediastinal lymph nodes for staging in order to avoid futile thoratocomies in extensive tumor involvement of the mediastinum. For this reason it was necessary to improve diagnostic tools for exploration of the mediastinum. Endoluminal ultrasound proved superior to radiological exploration in other fields of medicine and has been established as a routine diagnostic procedure. This is especially true in gastro-intestinal endoscopy, where endoluminal ultrasound is firmly established in staging of esophageal carcinoma, carcinoma of the cardia and rectal cancer for diagnosis of primary tumor and lymph node metastasis as well as neighboring structures and has decisive influence on therapeutic procedures. In the investigation of mediastinal and parabronchial structures transthoracic ultrasound has been applied with some success in lesions of the anterior mediastinum and subcarinal region. The lower paratracheal structures and perihilar structures, however, are out of reach. Structures of the pretracheal region, the right hilum and most of the left hilum are out of reach for endoesophageal ultrasound (EUS) because of the interference of the central airways. Despite several attempts endoluminal ultrasound of the central airways has been established only recently as it took considerable time to solve the technical problems of application. From 1989 we started exploring endobronchial ultrasound at our institution. Besides developing new suitable instruments, we had to establish a sonographic anatomy of the airways and neighboring structures as well as investigation of its clinical use. Last but not least, the question of cost-effectiveness had to be addressed. Meantime EBUS use has spread widely and several prospective studies for validation of endobronchial ultrasound in comparison to established diagnostic procedures have been performed.[8]

TECHNOLOGY OF ULTRASONOGRAPHY

In contrast to radiological exploration of the chest where imaging depends mainly on the difference in absorption of the X-rays by water as compared to air or fat, imaging by ultrasound depends on differences in transmission, absorption, scattering and reflection of ultrasound waves by different tissues and tissue interfaces. The ultrasound waves are created by the inverse piezoelectric effect: when high-frequency alternating electric current is connected to a crystal, short mechanical vibrations of equal frequency are induced that are transmitted to the surrounding structures as sound waves. The sound waves are reflected by different tissues according to their specific resistance, called impedance, which in contrast to X-rays is only partially due to the water content. In the interval between emission of the short impulses the reflected sound waves induce mechanical vibrations in the crystal which result in electrical signals. These are transferred to an electronic ultrasound processor that transforms these signals into pixels on a gray-scale image. Generally speaking, the intensity of the reflected ultrasound waves is transformed to brightness (echogenicity) and the time elapsed from sending to receiving is shown as distance of the pixels from the ultrasonic probe. Water has very low resistance and ultrasound waves are traveling with high speed, whereas air is almost impenetrable and completely reflects ultrasonographic waves. Three major factors influence the ultrasonic image: (1) contact of the ultrasonic probe to the tissue; (2) depth of penetration of the ultrasonic wave and (3) spatial resolution of the different structures. In order to enhance contact of the ultrasonic probe to surfaces most of the probes are equipped with some kind of water cushion in front of the transducer. The lower the frequency of the ultrasonic wave, the higher the depth of penetration and vice versa. The higher the frequency, the higher is the resolution of structures.

ULTRASONIC SYSTEMS FOR ENDOBRONCHIAL USE

Currently two systems are applied for EBUS: ultrasonic endoscopes with linear electronic transducers at the tip of the instrument (Olympus XBF-UC160F-OL8; Processor EU-M60) and miniaturized probes with a mechanical rotating transducer at the tip, that can be inserted into the airways through flexible bronchoscopes with biopsy channels of at least 2.8 mm. As the former use frequencies of 7.5 MHz, the resolution is insufficient for analyzing the delicate layers of the bronchial wall. By 20 MHz the axial resolution is 0.12 mm and the lateral/radial resolution 0.23 mm, which should be sufficient for detailed imaging of these structures. The main problem of application inside the airways was coupling of the ultrasonic probe to the tracheobronchial wall. With the naked probe one gets only a very limited sectorial view. Whereas lobar bronchi can be filled with water it is impossible in the central airways. This is why we developed plastic introducer catheters for the Olympus

probes with a balloon attached at the tip. Once this balloon is filled with water the probe is gaining contact with the surrounding airway wall and provides a complete 360° view to the mediastinal structures. As the water filled balloon shifts the focus more to the periphery under favorable conditions the depth of penetration for the 20 MHz probes may be up to 5 cm while preserving the high resolution in the near field. Thus this system is now our preferred instrument for exploration of small bronchial lesions (probe UM-2R/3R, driving unit MH-240 and processor EU-M 20 and 30, Olympus Co, Tokyo, Japan) (Figure 10.2).

CLINICAL APPLICATION

Once the probe is placed inside the airways under visual control the balloon is filled until close contact to the wall is established. This can be achieved without any problems up to the main bronchi as long as both lungs are ventilated. If one bronchus is occluded by pathological structures, after contralateral pneumonectomy or during investigation of the trachea, complete occlusion of the airway under local anesthesia is tolerated up to 2 minutes after sufficient sedation and after thorough preoxygenation. In cases of impaired lung function the additional application of oxygen via a laryngeal mask or general anesthesia might be preferable, which allows up to 3 minutes of apnea for investigation, before it has to be deflated. This is sufficient for acquisition of images. If necessary the maneuver can be repeated after re-oxygenation.

SONOGRAPHIC ANATOMY

By in vitro studies of animal and human specimens as well as under clinical observation we

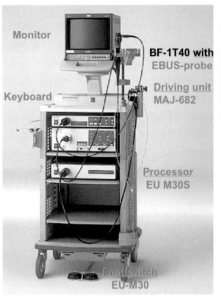

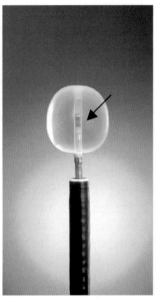

(A)   (B)

Figure 10.2
(A) Equipment for endobronchial ultrasound (EBUS) for miniaturprobe including probe, driving unit, processor with keyboard, footswitch and monitor. (B) Close-up view of the miniaturprobe, which is inserted via the biopsy channel of a flexible endoscope (Olympus BF-1T40) and the balloon is inflated. The arrow points towards the transducer inside the catheter.

could demonstrate a complex sonographic seven-layer structure of the central airway wall,[8] which is in contrast to other observations of only five layers.[9] The mucosa on the inner surface shows a very bright strong echo that is further enhanced by the adjacent balloon. The submucosa is comparatively echo-poor and clearly distinguishes the mucosa from the supporting structures of the tracheobronchial wall (first and second layers). The cartilages show a triple layer structure, consisting of a strong echo at the internal and external surface (endochondrium and perichondrium) whereas the spongiform internal structure is of low echogenity (third, fourth and fifth layers). The central airways are surrounded by a sheath of loose and dense connective tissue that appears as echo-poor and echo-dense layers respectively (sixth and seventh layers) (Figures 10.3 and 10.4). These structures have been confirmed by another experimental study and their analysis is essential in diagnosis and staging of lung cancer.[10]

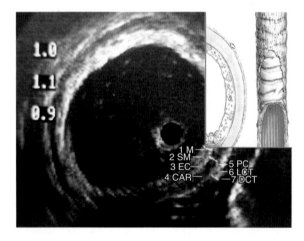

Figure 10.3
Echographic layers of the bronchial wall. Mucosa (M), submucosa (SM), internal surface of the cartilage (endochondrium, EC), internal spongiform structure of the cartilage (CAR), external surface of the cartilage (perichondrium PC), loose connective tissue sheath (LC) and dense connective tissue sheath (DC) surrounding the airways as adventitia. For comparison the illustration from Netter's atlas is inserted.

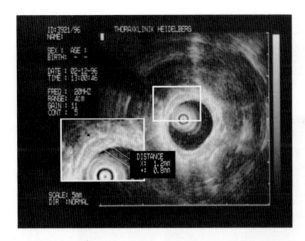

Figure 10.4
The seven-layer structure can be easily missed in low-power magnification and when the plane of the EBUS is not perpendicular to the wall. In higher magnification the seven layers can be clearly seen. The cartilage layer measures 1.2 mm, the mucosa/submucosa 0.8 mm.

STUDIES ON APPLICATION OF EBUS IN DIAGNOSIS AND STAGING OF EARLY LUNG CANCER

Already in our first experiences in several patients sent for endobronchial treatment of early bronchial carcinoma we could demonstrate deep infiltration of the bronchial wall and sometimes even regional lymph node metastasis which had escaped all other methods of diagnosis. In every case of macroscopic alteration of the mucosa we found concomitant alterations in the sonographic structure. The wall was more or less thickened and the delicate structures no longer visible. Usually the lesions are of low echogenity containing small black dots, that in our opinion represent the capillary blood vessels. They are extending sideways within the layers of the submucosa and in the case of deeper penetration into and beyond the cartilage. In many instances even if macroscopically the mucosa seemed to be intact we found sub-

mucosal tumor spread. In some instances it could be followed extending beyond the bronchial wall into the parabronchial structures (Figure 10.5). Meantime several crucial studies have been published to confirm these findings in the clinical setting and their impact on decision for treatment.

In 1999, Kurimoto and coinvestigators published a paper on endobronchial ultrasound for determination of depth of tracheobronchial tumor invasion.[9] They investigated the correlation of the anatomical structures of the tracheobronchial wall with the ultrasonic layer structure provided by the 20 MHz probe by sticking a fine needle into the different layers and comparing its appearance in the ultrasonic image. In addition they compared the ultrasonic determination of tumor invasion with the histopathologic findings on resected specimens. In vitro they described five layers of the bronchial wall: the first (hyperechoic) layer extended from the inner margin of the mucosal epithelium to the initial part of the submucosal tissue. The second (hypoechoic) layer is described as the deepest part of the submucosal tissue. The third (hyperechoic) layer was the internal surface of the cartilage, the fourth (hypoechoic) layer corresponded to the cartilage itself and the fifth (hyperechoic) sonographic layer comprised the external surface of the cartilage and the adventitia. At the dorsal membranaceous wall they found three layers. The first layer was the same as in the cartilaginous portion. The second (hypoechoic) layer corresponded to smooth muscle and the third (hyperechoic) layer again to the adventitia. Comparing the ultrasonic findings in small lesions with the histopathologic findings after resection they found exact correspondence in 23 of 24 lesions (95.8%). Only in one case did they mistake hypoechoic inflammatory lymphocytic infiltrates for tumor invasion to the deeper

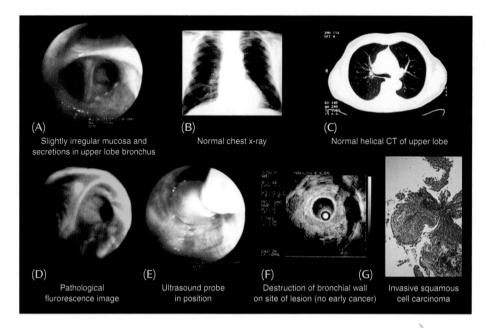

(A) Slightly irregular mucosa and secretions in upper lobe bronchus

(B) Normal chest x-ray

(C) Normal helical CT of upper lobe

(D) Pathological flurorescence image

(E) Ultrasound probe in position

(F) Destruction of bronchial wall on site of lesion (no early cancer)

(G) Invasive squamous cell carcinoma

Figure 10.5
Invading cancer in the right upper lobe bronchus. The patient was sent for endobronchial treatment of radiologically invisible cancer in the right upper lobe bronchus. (A) White light bronchoscopy shows a slight irregularity of the mucosa near the entrance of S1 of the right upper lobe with some mucus collection. (B) The chest X-ray and (C) the CT scan especially at the level of the right upper lobe are completely normal. (D) AF bronchoscopy (Life System, XILLIX Company, Vancouver, Canada) shows an extensive loss of normal fluorescence on the floor of the upper lobe bronchus. (E) The miniature probe is inserted into the upper lobe and the balloon is inflated. (F) The ultrasound image shows complete destruction of the bronchial wall (arrow) and (G) the histological section confirmed an invasive squamous cell cancer. (Histology courtesy of K-M Müller, Pathological Institute, University of Bochum, Germany.)

layers. From their results they concluded that endobronchial ultrasound was useful to determine the depth of tumor invasion and represented a major advance in bronchoscopic technology.

In another study by our group we investigated whether by EBUS we could improve classification of suspicious lesions detected by autofluorescence bronchoscopy.[11] In 74 of 332 patients examined by autofluorescence bronchoscopy we found suspicious lesions. In all patients the lesions were invisible to radiology. By combining ultrasonic analysis of the different layers we could improve diagnosis in malignant lesions to 97% as compared to AF diagnosis (69%), in benign lesions from 55% by AF to 92% in combination with EBUS. The correlation coefficient for AF/histology was 0.59 as compared to AF + EBUS/histology 0.91. Thus we proved that analyzing the structures of the bronchial wall by addition of EBUS to AF predicting the histology could be improved to 0.91 as compared to 0.59 by AF alone (Figure 10.6).

In 2000, Takahashi and coinvestigators published a prospective study on assessment of depth of invasion in early bronchogenic

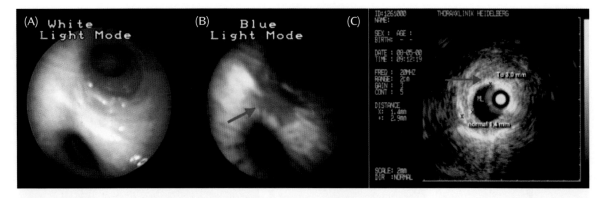

Figure 10.6
Early cancer on the middle lobe carina. (A) The lesion is hardly visible by white light bronchoscopy as whitish area on the carina. (B) By autofluorescence (AF, D-light system, Storz Company, Tuttlingen, Germany) the lesion becomes clearly visible (arrow). (C) Only by EBUS the true extent of the lesion becomes visible. The tumor measures 3 mm in depth as compared to the normal mucosa of 1.4 mm and is not invading the cartilage layer (arrow).

squamous cell carcinoma.[12] In 14 of 22 lesions they observed confinement of the lesion within the mucosal/submucosal layer and not invading the cartilage, of which they treated ten by PDT and achieved complete remission in nine. They analyzed the efficacy of pre-interventional evaluation by EBUS with respect to sensitivity and specificity according to the histopathological findings in case of surgery and to response after PDT, respectively. The sensitivity for evaluation of invasion by finding the lesion inside the bronchial cartilage was 85.7%, the specificity was 66% and the accuracy was 80.0%. The positive predictive value was 85.7%. However, the assumption that complete remission after PDT confirms accurate staging by EBUS is not proved. Thus when they restricted their analysis to the resected specimens sensitivity was 75% and specificity was 75%. The results must be taken with some caution as the numbers are very small.

In the fourth study, Miyazu and coworkers investigated the role of AF and EBUS in the choice of appropriate therapy for lung cancer, especially with regard to early stages.[13] In 54 patients they detected 29 lesions, 12 by addition of AF only. Six supposedly early lesions were evaluated by EBUS for the depth of tumor invasion. According to the ultrasonic appearance two patients were considered candidates for photodynamic therapy as the lesions were restricted to mucosa and submucosa, whereas the remaining four patients had invasive cancers, of whom three underwent surgery and one chemoradiotherapy. Despite the differences in definition of the layers the cartilage can be observed much more clearly than the other layers, and a lack of extension beyond the cartilage is essential for potentially curative bronchoscopic treatment of early lesions. Thus differentiating early lung cancer by EBUS according to its limitation to the structures inside the cartilage as compared to more advanced lesions involving the cartilage was considered much more reliable than radiology or the bronchoscopic appearance. In conclusion, the authors introduced EBUS in their routine work in making decisions regarding therapy, such as PDT, surgery or chemoradio-therapy.

In a subsequent paper the same authors report on a prospective study concerning EBUS in the assessment of early lung cancer before photodynamic therapy to confirm the results of the previous investigation.[14] In 12 of 93 patients that were explored by AF they found 18 biopsy-proven carcinomas considered to be early lesions by conventional definition of radiological invisibility and intraluminal tumor size of <2 cm. Ten by bronchoscopic appearance were superficial lesions (Figure 10.7), three nodular type and five polypoid. Five of 14 lesions less

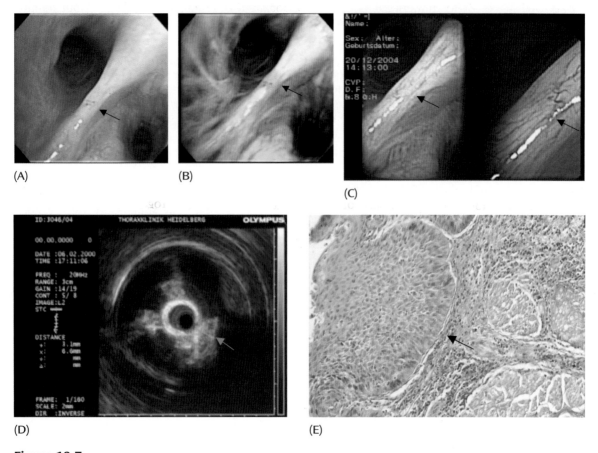

(A)   (B)

(C)

(D)   (E)

Figure 10.7
In-situ cancer on the middle lobe carina. (A) WLB by video bronchoscopy shows a slight vascular irregularity at the middle lobe carina. (B) AF bronchoscopy (AFI, Olympus Co., Tokyo) shows corresponding discoloration. (C) By magnification bronchoscopy, slight roughening of the mucosa and irregularity of vascularization can be seen, which is recognized by splintering and interruption of the light reflection. (D) EBUS shows a lesion 3.3 × 6.6 mm which is not extending beyond the connective tissue layer. As the lesion is located at the bronchial spur only tangential contact of the probe without inflation of the balloon is possible. (E) The histological specimen shows an in situ cancer, respecting the basal membrane of the mucosa. (Histology courtesy of K-M Müller, Pathological Institute, University of Bochum, Germany).

than 10 mm in diameter had already invaded the wall beyond the cartilage. Of all the 18 cancers only nine were confined to the intracartilaginous layers of the bronchial wall and thus considered to be candidates for endobronchial treatment by PDT. Six of the others were referred to surgery and three to chemotherapy or radiotherapy in combination with PDT. All patients staged by EBUS as early cancers and treated by PDT alone underwent long-term complete remission and no recurrence was observed in follow-up which extended up to more than 3 years. Interestingly, all three patients with more advanced cancers receiving additional PDT also had long-term complete remission. In all 18 patients there was no recurrence during the follow-up. The authors' conclusions are that complete remission by PDT depends on accurate patient selection based on an exact assessment of the tumor's dimensions. EBUS provides more accurate information than conventional bronchoscopy and HR-CT and currently is the only method to estimate the depth of tumor invasion.

FUTURE DEVELOPMENTS

Strategies in detection and treatment of early lung cancer

Improvements in detection and treatment of early lung cancer demand complex strategies, that will be based on three pillars. (1) Screening of large populations at risk for developing lung cancer, which comprises smokers and persons with occupational exposure to carcinogens by a non-invasive method, similar to conventional sputum cytology. (2) Localization of early lesions that are invisible by current radiological means. (3) Local staging of these lesions to decide for appropriate treatment, either by bronchoscopic means, surgery, radiotherapy or

chemotherapy and combination of different options.

Screening

Bronchoscopy as an invasive procedure will never be an instrument for screening of large numbers of candidates in a population at risk. Conventional sputum cytology, X-ray and HR-CT proved insufficient in detecting centrally localized early lung cancer. Thus in our opinion the most promising method for screening in the future might be molecular biomarkers in induced sputum, buccal mucosal swabs of the mouth or in blood samples. Molecular biomarkers recently attracted a lot of attention and several multicenter studies are currently under way to find candidates for a suitable testing system.[15] Some preliminary results have been published on automated sputum image cytometry[16] and molecular markers[17] but due to the complexity of cancerogenesis on a molecular base no such screening has been implemented routinely so far. A considerable number of early precursor lesions can undergo spontaneous regression. Thus for the bronchoscopist it would be desirable to obtain information from the pathologist as to which early lesion has developed to a 'point of no return' and has to be treated and which can be observed in follow up. As we are gaining more insight into the natural history of lung cancer in humans – as compared to experimental animal studies – by detecting those lesions with AF and EBUS, we hope that finally patterns of molecular biomarkers will emerge by which we will be able to make these decisions on a rational base.

Localization

There is no question that the introduction of AF increased the detection of early lesions significantly and has been the decisive technology to create new interest in early detection and chemoprevention, again. It has been the key technology for development of the additional technologies in screening, staging and minimally invasive therapy. The most important lesson by introduction of AF was to teach us to look for early lesions that were easily missed in routine white-light bronchoscopy. Thus during our prospective study in evaluation of the Storz D-light autofluorescence system we could observe an intra individual learning curve and improve our detection rate by WLB significantly. When comparing the results of Lam and coinvestigators' study to later publications there is a significant reduction in difference of detection rates between AF and WLB. With the recent introduction of videobronchoscopy resulting in a tremendous improvement in imaging the gap between WLB and AF is decreasing to such an extent, that according to our most recent experiences almost all CIS and early cancers can be recognized already by WLB and only detection of premalignant lesions by AF is superior. However, this is true for specialized centers with trained and well-experienced bronchoscopists and most recent technology available. With the advent of widespread screening programs referral of all persons with suspicious findings to expert centers for bronchoscopic evaluation is impossible. This is why AF will stay for much longer as an important instrument for the less-experienced bronchoscopist in localization of early cancer. Improvements in specificity by spectral analysis of the AF image supported by computerized processing might be a valuable adjunct in accuracy of early detection.

Imaging

With the introduction of AF and EBUS new imaging techniques have become of interest with regard to their ability in analyzing pathological lesions. The magnifying bronchoscopes have been mentioned before. Visualization of alterations in the capillary architecture have become possible by using their high-power magnification especially and computer-assisted analysis of the vascular pattern helped in differentiation of chronic bronchitis from dysplasia. Carrying magnification further by a rigid contact magnifying bronchoscope we were even able to observe the flow of the erythrocytes in the submucosal capillaries (Wolf, Co., Knittlingen, Germany). By analyzing the submucosal structures adjacent to the internal cartilage layer this instrument might be useful in future and support detection of lesions invading the cartilage. High-power magnification of the superficial layer with oblique illumination is able to visualize the cilia of the mucosa. In addition to diagnosis by alterations in structure such as loss of shining, fragmentation of light reflection and irregularity in the surface in WLB, local changes or loss of cilia might add to detection of these lesions. By micro confocal scanning microscopy (μCOSM) even individual cells become visible in vivo, and in vitro studies could demonstrate its capability to differentiate tumors from benign lesions. All these techniques could add considerably to the bronchoscopist's ability to recognize and classify early lesions within the bronchial mucosa. With recent communication technologies the pathologist could be easily connected to the bronchoscopy suite and actually participate in the procedure and help in directing diagnostic and therapeutic procedures to further improve accuracy.

Local staging

Twenty MHz EBUS currently is the only reliable method for staging of early bronchial cancer due to its ability to analyze the delicate layers of the tracheobronchial wall. As has been shown, decisions on local interventions based on staging by EBUS are very safe and therapy results in a high complete remission rate. Some problems, however, are remaining. (1) In rare instances differentiation of the submucosa from the internal cartilage layer may be difficult despite the high resolution (0.15 mm) of 20 MHz. The improved spatial resolution of 0.10 mm by 30 MHz probes might be useful to further differentiate the internal layers of the bronchial wall especially with regard to intramucosal in situ cancers. (2) The longitudinal extent of some lesions can be difficult to assess by current EBUS technology as the radial probe is providing only a limited cross-section (Figure 10.8). Thus the probe has to be advanced

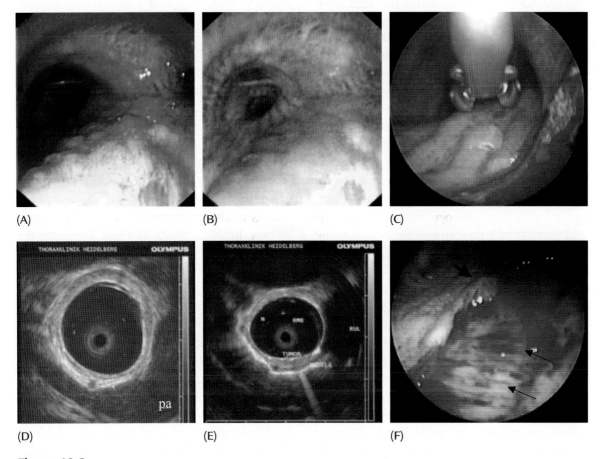

(A)   (B)   (C)

(D)   (E)   (F)

Figure 10.8
Extensive early cancer of the right main bronchus. (A) The dorsal wall of the right main bronchus shows an extensive irregularity of the mucosa extending towards the upper lobe spur. (B) AF bronchoscopy (AFI, Olympus Co., Tokyo) shows extensive corresponding pathological discoloration. (C) With rigid forceps biopsies can be performed including the deeper layers of the bronchial wall. (D) EBUS of the intermediate bronchus shows the normal structure including mucosa, submucosa, muscular layer and connective tissue. (E) At the site of the lesion the mucosa/submucosa are destroyed by the lesion, but the muscular layer and connective tissue are intact. (F) After rigid biopsy a large part of the lesion has been removed and the intact connective tissue layer can be seen (arrows). Histology confirmed an extensive in-situ carcinoma without invasion of the deeper layers.

stepwise along the lesion and images have to be reconstructed in a sequential way much like CT scans. By moving the probe automatically along the bronchial wall during image acquisition the spiral movement creates a continuous 3D ultrasound image that could be helpful in analyzing the longitudinal extent of early lesions. (3) At the site of bronchial spurs contact of the miniature probe can be difficult and depth of penetration is hard to assess, because the ultrasound wave is not directed frontally. In this situation theoretically a linear electronic transducer might be superior. However, with the current 7.5 MHz transducers on ultrasonic bronchoscopes resolution of the bronchial wall is too poor to detect early lesions. Thus electronic ultrasound bronchoscopes with transducers of higher frequencies would be desirable.

Currently, application of endoscopic optical coherence tomography (EOCT) is under investigation for its applicability within the airways. As by this method contact-free longitudinal application is possible, resulting in high-resolution images of the internal layers of the bronchial wall extending 2–3 mm in depth it might be another option for improved staging of localized early lesions. How it will compare to 20 MHz and 30 MHz EBUS remains to be seen. The definite advantage of 20 MHz EBUS is additional imaging of the deeper layers and of the adjacent structures including lymph nodes.

Current developments in conventional radiological imaging are too early in the stage of development to predict their usefulness in staging of early bronchial carcinoma. PET is not considered reliable in detecting lesions below 1 cm as yet and is useless in diagnosis of early bronchogenic carcinoma. The power in resolution of new 64-liner CT machines has yet to be awaited. High-resolution CT by these machines might be more apt to detect small intraluminal lesions and lesions extending outside the bronchial wall. However, intramural lesions might still be difficult, if not impossible, to detect and staged correctly. In contrast MRI by intraluminal application of miniaturized coils might be useful to stage early malignant lesions of the bronchial wall. If these new techniques are becoming available it still remains to be seen how they compare to the already well established technique of EBUS with regard to their applicability and cost effectiveness.

CONCLUSIONS AND CLINICAL IMPLICATIONS

The conclusion from current studies is that conventional staging of early lung cancer by WLB, X-ray and HR-CT is unreliable. Neither bronchoscopic diagnosis of endoluminal and intramural extent of the lesion below 10 mm nor intraluminal nodular protrusion of less than 5 mm exclude invasion of the cartilage layer and the parabronchial structures. In radiologically invisible lesions even lymph node metastasis can be observed. AF is useful to improve detection of early lung cancer and can show the true margins of tumors spreading in the submucosa but does not provide reliable information about the underlying histology nor especially about the depth of tumor invasion. In contrast EBUS can provide a reliable image of the delicate structures of the bronchial wall. It can improve prediction of the histological nature of the lesion with regard to malignancy or benign cause significantly as compared to AF. By accurately analyzing the depth of penetration of the lesion it currently is promising as a reliable method for local staging of early central lung cancer. As such it can provide the information needed to make a decision for appropriate treatment of these lesions, especially when potentially curative bronchoscopic treatment is taken into consideration. PDT based on local staging by EBUS resulted in an exceedingly high complete and long-lasting remission rate as compared to former studies based on conventional radiology and CT. Thus our assumptions and preliminary observations at the onset of development of EBUS with regard to local staging of early lung cancer have been widely confirmed and not only in this regard EBUS has been established as a routine instrument in a considerable number of institutions worldwide.

REFERENCES

1. Alberts WM, Colice GL, Diagnosis and management of lung cancer: ACCP evidence-based guidelines. 2003; Chest 123(suppl.):1S–337.
2. Lam S, Becker HD, Future diagnostic procedures. In: Feins RH (ed.) Thoracic Endoscopy; Chest Surgery Clinics of North America. W.B. Saunders, Philadelphia, 1996, pp. 366–80.
3. Edell ES, Future therapeutic procedures. In: Feins RH (ed.) Thoracic Endoscopy; Chest Surgery Clinics of North America. W.B. Saunders, Philadelphia, 1996, pp. 381–9.
4. Müller K-M, Early cancer of the lung. Rec Res Cancer 1988; 106:119–30.
5. Shibuya K, Hoshino S, Chiyo M, et al, Subepithelial vascular patterns in bronchial dysplasias using a high magnification bronchovideoscope. Thorax 2002; 57:902–7.
6. Lam S, Kennedy T, Unger M, et al, Localization of bronchial intraepithelial neoplastic lesions by fluorescence bronchoscopy. Chest 1998; 113:696–702.
7. Bülzebruck H, Bopp R, Drings P, et al, New aspects in the staging of lung cancer. Cancer 1992; 70(5):1102–10.
8. Becker HD, Herth F, Endobronchial ultrasound of the airways and the mediastinum. In: Bolliger CT, Mathur PN (eds) Progress in Respiratory Research, Vol. 30, Interventional Bronchoscopy. S. Karger, Basel-Freiburg, 1999, pp. 80–93.
9. Kurimoto N, Murayama M, Yoshioka S, et al, Assessment of usefulness of endobronchial ultrasonography in determination of depth of tracheobronchial tumor invasion. Chest 1999; 115:1500–6.
10. Shirakawa T, Tanaka F, Becker, HD, Layer structure of the central airways viewed using endobronchial ultrasonography (EBUS) In: Yoshimura H, Kida A, Arai T, Niimi S, Kaneko M, Kitahara S (eds) Bronchology and Bronchoesophagology: State of the Art. Elsevier, Amsterdam, 2001, pp. 921–3.
11. Herth FJF, Becker HD, LoCicero J, Ernst A, Endobronchial ultrasound improves classification of suspicious lesions detected by autofluorescence bronchoscopy. J Bronchol 2003; 10(4):249–52.
12. Takahashi H, Sagawa M, Sato M, et al, A prospective evaluation of transbronchial ultrasonography for assessment of depth of invasion in early bronchogenic squamous cell carcinoma. Lung Cancer 2003; 42:43–9.
13. Miyazu Y, Miyazawa T, Iwamoto Y, Kano K, Kurimoto N, The role of endoscopic techniques, laser-induced fluorescence endoscopy, and endobronchial ultrasonography in choice of appropriate therapy for bronchial cancer. J Bronchol 2001; 8:10–16.
14. Miyazu Y, Miyazawa T, Kurimoto N, et al, Endobronchial ultrasonography in the assessment of centrally located early-stage lung cancer before photodynamic therapy. Am J Respir Crit Care Med 2002; 165:832–7.
15. Available online at: www.EUELC.com.
16. Jaggi B, Deen MJ, Palcic B, Design of a solid state microscope. Optical Eng 1989; 28:675–82.
17. Mao L, Hruban RH, Boyle JO, Detection of oncogene mutations in sputum precedes diagnosis of lung cancer. Cancer Res 1994; 54:1634–7.

11 Bronchoscopic treatment of early lung cancer lesions

G Sutedja, Harubumi Kato, J Usuda

Contents Introduction • Clinical background • The criteria of early-stage lung cancer • Early-stage cancer lesions • Local treatment by bronchoscopy

INTRODUCTION

The awareness that early detection and treatment will be the way to improve the dismal survival rate of lung cancer patients has increased the interest to use minimal invasive techniques such as bronchoscopic treatment (BT) for the early management of this global epidemic.[1]

Many individuals at risk also suffer from smoking-related morbidities that hamper the application of conventional staging and treatment approaches.[2] Early intervention programs generally focus mainly on asymptomatic individuals in whom tiny early-stage lung cancer can be detected by high-resolution computed tomography (HRCT),[3] and on symptomatic individuals with cough, sputum and/or blood-tinged sputum. In centrally located early-stage lung cancer, more than 50% of individuals produce sputum, 80% have cough and more than 90% have some symptoms.[4] Therefore, the value of minimally invasive techniques to preserve quality of life is obvious, especially when treating patients considered marginally resectable or medically inoperable.[5–8]

Bronchoscopic treatment has established its potential for treating malignant airway obstruction.[9,10] Early detection, accurate staging in combination with local treatment with minimal morbidity are important to obtain an optimal cost-effective interventional strategy that pre-serves quality of life.[11] Based on sound onco-logical arguments for early treatment of cancer lesion at the N0M0 stage, one should consider the use of BT because surgery remains relatively morbid and wasteful.[8,12] Therefore, understanding the potentials and limits of BT are paramount in trying to implement a tailored strategy for each individual at risk.

CLINICAL BACKGROUND

The cure rate of patients with lung cancer has remained dismal at ~13%, because the majority is diagnosed with an advanced stage. The presence of either detected or unforeseen nodal and distant metastases will ultimately lead to cancer morbidity and death. Therefore, advanced-stage lung cancer poses a serious threat to quality of life. Central airway obstruction with imminent suffocation due to local tumor growth requires immediate action. Guidelines with regard to bronchoscopic treatment (BT) for palliation have been published.[9,13]

Patients referred to interventional broncho-scopists usually suffer from end-stage cancer recurrences failing previous chemo-radiotherapy regimens. The life-threatening situation provides little room for safe palliation. Diligent execution of bronchoscopic treatment (BT) by an experienced team is necessary to avoid disastrous complications. Against all odds, however, BT has established its cost-effectiveness for the palliative management of central airway lesions.[10] Refinements of various BT techniques have extended its potential for treating medically inoperable patients with centrally located early-stage cancer.[7,8,14,15]

Especially, based on histopathological study of centrally located early-stage squamous cancer, one can select more precisely candidates for minimal invasive local treatment such as BT.[16–18] Surgery with mediastinal lymph node dissection is considered the standard approach for resectable lung cancer. As screening involves asymptomatic individuals harboring N0 cancer, the integration of early diagnosis with minimally invasive treatment is a logical step.[2,3,19,20] This is important as the individuals at risk are susceptible to develop multiple subsequent cancer primaries and also suffer from non-lung-cancer-related morbidities.[21–23]

Newer staging and imaging procedures enable early detection and accurate staging to select the proper candidates for any treatment approach.[24–26] Accurate tumor staging is an absolute prerequisite before choosing the most appropriate strategy. The choice for a tailored approach in each individual, e.g. local treatment, should be based on data of accurate staging, i.e. tumor type, location, absence of both nodal and distant involvements and the functional status of each individual at risk.

Early detected lung cancers in a screening program are lesions in the order of 1 cm in size, either located in the lung parenchyma or in the central airways.[27] Bronchoscopic techniques have increasing potentials and we will primarily focus on the potential and limits of bronchoscopic treatment in this regard, especially as this is shown to be more cost-effective than standard surgical resection.[28]

THE CRITERIA OF EARLY-STAGE LUNG CANCER

Early-stage lung cancers can be divided into two categories, these are categories of the central or peripheral type, according to the developing sites. In Japan, the criteria of these categories of the disease have been strictly defined since 1975.[4] In the peripheral type, the tumor should be located in subsegmental or more peripheral bronchi, the lesion should be less than 2 cm in diameter without metastasis in an asymptomatic individual. In central-type early-stage lung cancer, most patients have symptoms such as cough, sputum production, e.g. blood-tinged sputum. The tumor must be located within the central area down to the segmental bronchi being carcinoma in situ or with only limited invasion into the bronchial wall. The histological type of superficial squamous cell cancer and the absence of metastasis should be confirmed. These criteria have been established based on extensive analyses of radiological, endoscopical and pathological data by the Ikeda Study Group of the Ministry of Health and Welfare in 1975.[4]

EARLY-STAGE CANCER LESIONS

Bronchoscopic procedures use miniaturized biopsy forceps and probes of ~2 mm cross-section which can be passed through the suction channel of the fiberoptic bronchoscope (Figure 11.1). Lesions beyond the visibility range of the bronchoscopists are anatomically off limits, such as in assessing tumor invasion into the airway wall and cancer locations or extension in the distal segmental bronchi or peripheral parenchyma.

New technical developments enable assessment beyond the visibility spectrum and microdynamic imaging techniques with bio-molecular

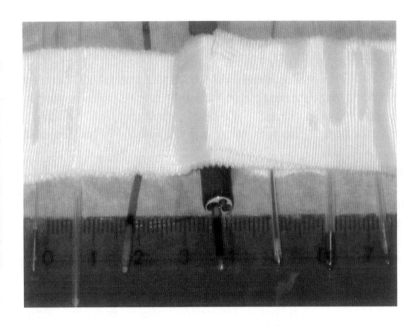

Figure 11.1
The various flexible applicators for local treatment using the fiberoptic bronchoscope, from left to right: photodynamic therapy (PDT) microlens fiber for surface illumination, PDT cylindrical-diffusor for intraluminal illumination, argon plasma catheter (blue) for non-contact mode diathermy coagulation, monopolar electrocautery probe for contact diathermy coagulation protruding out the working channel of the broncho-videoscope, high-dose-rate brachytherapy catheter for intraluminal irradiation, cryotherapy probe and Nd-YAG laser fiber.

data may help us understand carcinogenesis at the clonal level.[19,20,29] Examples of recent improvements are CT-based virtual bronchoscopy for navigational purposes and autofluorescence bronchoscopy, currently being applied for more accurate staging.[24,30–32]

Additional techniques for fiberoptic bronchoscopy widen the visibility spectrum using light and ultrasound analysis and enhance the image resolution down to the intracellular level, e.g. high-magnification endoscopy and confocal micro-endoscopy.[19,20,33,34] Additional use of CT-based navigational assistance and ultrasound pattern recognition of the fiberoptic bronchoscope widen our spectrum to lesions that were previously invisible and beyond reach.[30,35] This opens the opportunity to be increasingly accurate and precise in a less-invasive way for diagnostic and therapeutic interventions of early detected cancer lesions.

The recognition that accurate staging is the most important determinant for outcome also underscores the most important principles behind the logic of local treatment in N0M0 lung cancer.[16–18] Currently, >50% ground glass opacity (GGO) on high-resolution CT scan of small peripheral lesions <1 cm in size is shown to represent Noguchi type A/B adenocarcinoma, free of nodal involvement.[36] It can be expected that wedge resection without lymph node exploration may be replaced by non-invasive local treatment such as conformal stereotactic radiotherapy and radiofrequency ablation,[37,38] and transthoracic PDT.[39,40]

More data are available regarding central early-stage squamous cell cancers because sputum cytology programs have been detecting more individuals at risk.[16–18] Small lesions were detected and less-extensive surgical resection, such as surgical bronchoplasty for carefully selected individuals, has been adopted.[25,27,42] Minute lesions, being N0M0 cancers, frequently involve the bronchial spurs and therefore catalyze the interest to spare normal lung tissue as much as possible. Photodynamic therapy (PDT) prior to surgical exploration to enable less-extensive resection is based on the same perspective.[6]

The combined use of autofluorescence bronchoscopy (AFB), high-resolution CT scan, endobronchial ultrasound and PET scan have been reported to provide more accuracy for selecting candidates for BT.[25,43] AFB has recently been shown to be more accurate in assessing the extent of preneoplastic lesions and can predict malignant development in the individuals at risk.[32,44] Minimal invasive approaches for early diagnosis, accurate staging and curative local treatment for N0M0 lung cancer patients are comprehensive approaches to preserve quality of life.

Surgical data have shown central cancer lesions <1 cm with visible distal margin and no infiltration beyond the bronchial cartilage to be N0M0 cancer.[16–18] In many studies involving irresectable, marginally resectable and primarily resectable patients with central early-stage lung cancer, the high response rates after BT also in long-term survivors have shown its curative potential.[6–8,14] Some early recurrences had been successfully retreated,[14,45] which indicates ample lead time before nodal disease involvement.

Provided accurate staging can exclude nodal and distal disease,[11,12,25,26,43] one should therefore carefully consider to exploit this lead time opportunity in choosing a tailored approach for each particular individual.[23,27]

Thus, selection of the proper candidates with superficial early-stage cancer at the N0M0 stage has to be combined with the choice for local treatment based on staging consideration rather than treatment technique per se,[11,12,46] be it surgery or otherwise. Also the preservation of quality of life due to the persistent risk for subsequent primaries in the population at risk has to be taken into account.[21–23,27]

LOCAL TREATMENT BY BRONCHOSCOPY

Bronchoscopic treatment modalities include tumor removal by biopsy, photodynamic therapy (PDT), brachytherapy, cryotherapy, electrocautery, argon plasma coagulation and the vaporization by various lasers such as Nd-YAG laser.[9–12] These therapies have been used for early-stage lung cancers.

Photodynamic therapy (PDT)

Photodynamic therapy (PDT) destroys cancer cells through the use of a fixed-frequency laser light in combination with a photosensitizing agent, the photosensitizer. PDT was first applied in Japan for endoscopically early-stage lung cancer using argon dye laser combined with a photosensitizer, hematoporphyrin derivative (HpD) in March 1980.[47] A phase II multicentric clinical study on PDT with Photofrin for centrally located early-stage lung cancer was conducted using excimer dye laser and demonstrated excellent PDT efficacy (CR rate: 84.8%).[7] The US National Cancer Institute therefore recommends PDT as one of the standard treatment options for centrally located early-stage lung cancer, i.e. for stage 0 (TisN0M0) and stage IA (T1N0M0).

In such cases where the incidence of second primary cancers is high, PDT is an alternative, as many individuals at risk are considered marginally resectable because of limited pulmonary function.[48] PDT is potentially tissue sparing, thus can preserve lung function and can be repeated if subsequent cancers develop or local recurrence reappears, without precluding additional surgical intervention when deemed necessary.

The new diode laser system is developed to improve PDT applications using second-generation photosensitizer, mono-L-aspartyl chlorine e6 (NPe6) which has excellent anti-tumor activity with rapid clearance from the skin.[49] NPe6-PDT has recently been shown in humans to be safe and has excellent anti-tumor effects with negligible skin phototoxicity.[49]

The efficacy of PDT for treating centrally located early-stage cancer has been reviewed (Table 11.1).[12] PDT as an alternative for surgical resection for early-stage cancer has been

reported to spare 43% of the patients from surgical resection.[8]

From recent studies on second-generation photosensitizers such as NPe6, tetra (m-hydroxyphenyl) chlorine (m-THPC) and 5-amino laevulinic acid (5ALA) for treating early-stage cancers,[14,50,51] one can see the important correlation between response rate and tumor size

Table 11.1 Centrally located early-stage cancers treated with intraluminal bronchoscopic treatment modalities: photodynamic therapy, brachytherapy, electrocautery

Study group	Number of lesions/patients	Treatment	CR	Remarks
Furuse[7]	49 patients 59 lesions	PDT	85%	*duration CR 2–32 months (median 14) *long-term response 76%
Cortese[8]	21 patients 23 lesions	PDT as alternative for surgery	70%	*CR >12 months in 52% of patients *follow-up 24–116 (mean 68)
Hayata[14]	75 patients 95 lesions	PDT	83%	*duration CR 3–176 months *long-term response 75%
Kato[49]	35 patients 39 lesions	PDT with NPe-6	83%	*85% <2 weeks skin photosensitive
Marsiglia[52]	34 patients	Brachytherapy	94%	*85% response at 2 years; 73% at 3 years *78% survival at 2 years *median follow-up 29 months (5–50)
Perol[53]	19 patients	Brachytherapy	83%	*75% response at 1 year *78% survival at 1 year; 58% at 2 years *mean follow-up 28 months (7–49)
Vonk[45]	32 patients	PDT (5) Nd-YAG (1) Electrocautery (24) Argon (2)	97%	*50% survival at 5 years *28% lung cancer deaths (previous advanced-stage cancer related) *follow-up: 5 years (2–10)
Deygas[55]	35 patients	Cryotherapy	91%	*20% local failure >4 years

*CR: endoscopically and histologically proven complete responses.

based on better staging methods. For PDT to be successful, it is necessary that tumor growth is limited to the mucosa and submucosa. The depth of tumor invasion is an important factor for response as well as tumor location, size and the absence of nodal involvement.[16–18] It has been reported that the depth of tumor invasion as estimated by surface diameter was not always accurate when histopathologic specimens were examined, and that some tumors <1.0 cm may show extracartilaginous invasion on endobronchial ultrasonography (EBUS) imaging that was later confirmed histopathologically.[26] We now can clearly determine the tumor margin using light-induced autofluorescence endoscopy while it remains difficult to evaluate this using conventional bronchoscopy.[32] Improving the assessment of tumor margin and depth invasion into the bronchial wall will greatly improve the quality and efficacy of PDT.

Local treatment by other bronchoscopic methods

Brachytherapy uses catheter positioning by fiberoptic bronchoscopy in the region where cancer is located.[52,53] The catheter is connected to a remote afterloading device, which transports small radioactive Iridium-192 seed into several fixed positions according to the dosimetric calculation of the target volume. Brachytherapy is an expensive facility and several fractions are required to minimize normal tissue damage.[10] Accurate dosimetry remains difficult as breathing and cough lead to constant catheter movement inside the bronchial tube while early cancer lesions are neither perfectly symmetrical nor circumferential. There is potential damage for bronchial mucosa as well.

Tumor coagulation by using heat or cold has been widely applied by many surgical disciplines prior to the BT era.[11,12,15] Lasers such as Nd-YAG and argon, together with electrocautery

and argon plasma coagulation are causing heat leading to coagulation necrosis. Nd-YAG laser is popular as 1064 nm wavelength light photons scatter deeply in tissue.[9,13] Extensive necrosis can be obtained due to the enormous heat sink effect inside a small target volume. Electrocautery and argon plasma coagulation are widely used surgical techniques and can be applied for early cancer treatment.[15,45] A visible superficial tissue effect of only several millimeters deep can be achieved in a matter of seconds, because electrons easily disperse into deeper tissue layers and do not scatter.[15,54] Cryotherapy is repetitive cooling and thawing of the target tissue using liquid gas and specially designed flexible applicators to crystallize cellular contents of the target tissue causing late necrosis.[55]

For palliation, techniques that obtain late or secondary necrosis such as PDT, brachytherapy and cryotherapy are not suitable for immediate palliation, while coagulation techniques – Nd-YAG laser, electrocautery and argon plasma coagulation – combined with mechanical tumor debulking are straightforward.[9,10,13] For treatment with curative intent, however, there is no such limitation due to the limited volume of the targeted tumor tissue within reach of the bronchoscopic instruments. All techniques can then be performed under local anesthesia with minimal treatment related morbidity and without any record of treatment-related mortality.

Arguments have been frequently raised that the limited number of patients with occult cancer treated in several BT series so far reported, does not justify its role. Understanding carcinogenesis and the importance of accurate staging, the extended use of the fiberoptic bronchoscope under local anesthesia is obviously an attractive approach.[14,15,21,23,24,27] So far, marginally resectable patients with early-stage cancer have been the main candidates for BT. However, there is no reasonable argument against the use of any BT modality being potentially curative for early superficial intraluminally located N0M0 lesions while surgical bronchotomy as a less-extensive resection technique is well accepted (Table 11.1).[18,23,27]

If the consideration for quality of life is similarly important for those considered marginally operable or being high-risk surgical candidates, there is no reason why BT modalities being superiorly cost-effective should be excluded as an alternative approach.[28,56]

Tumor invasion in the deeper layers of the bronchial wall >3 mm may already have tumor spread to regional lymph nodes.[16–18,21] Therefore, only superficial lesions such as carcinoma in situ and microinvasive cancer fulfilling the criteria of <1 cm in size with distinct border is suitable for BT, being a valid alternative for surgical bronchoplasty.[11,12] New diagnostic imaging and staging facilities have become more practical and accurate to properly select the best candidates for BT by exploiting the lead time of early detection. Initial BT treatment may also enable less-extensive surgical resection. BT is therefore a cost-effective alternative modality – unfortunately too frequently not considered – in the era of early detection that can greatly reduce screening-related morbidities and mortalities which are important issues influencing the controversies about overdiagnosis and treatment of pseudo diseases.[6,7,57]

REFERENCES

1. Parkin DM, Pisani P, Ferlay J, Global cancer statistics. Ca Cancer J Clin 1999; 49:33–64.
2. Petty TL, Screening strategies for early detection of lung cancer: the time is now. JAMA 2000; 284:1977–80.
3. van Klaveren RJ, de Koning HJ, Mulshine J, Hirsch FR, Lung cancer screening by spiral CT. What is the optimal target population for screening trials? Lung Cancer 2002; 38: 243–52.
4. Ikeda S, Atlas of early cancer of major bronchi. Tokyo, Igakushoin, 1976.
5. Endo C, Sagawa M, Sato M, et al, What kind of hilar lung cancer can be a candidate for segmentectomy with curative intent? Retrospective clinicopathological study of completely resected roentgenographically occult bronchogenic squamous cell carcinoma. Lung Cancer 1998; 21: 93–9.
6. Kato H, Konaka C, Ono J, Preoperative laser photodynamic therapy in combination with operation in lung cancer. J Thorac Cardiovasc Surg 1985; 90:420–9.
7. Furuse K, Fukuoka M, Kato H, et al, A prospective phase II study on photodynamic therapy with photofrin II for centrally located early-stage lung cancer. J Clin Oncol 1993; 11: 1852–7.
8. Cortese DA, Edell ES, Kinsey JH, Photodynamic therapy for early stage squamous cell carcinoma of the lung. Mayo Clin Proc 1997; 72:595–602.
9. Bolliger CT, Mathur PN, Beamis JF, et al, European Respiratory Society/American Thoracic Society. ERS/ATS statement on interventional pulmonology. Eur Respir J 2002; 19:356–73.
10. Sutedja G, Postmus PE, Bronchoscopic treatment of lung tumors. Lung Cancer 1994; 11: 1–17.
11. Mathur PN, Edell E, Sutedja G, Vergnon JM, Treatment of early stage non-small cell lung cancer. American College of Chest Physicians. Chest 2003; 123(1 Suppl):176S–80S.
12. van Boxem TJ, Venmans BJ, Postmus PE, Sutedja G, Curative endobronchial therapy in early-stage non-small cell lung cancer. Review. J Bronchology 1999; 6:198–206.
13. Dumon JF, Shapshay S, Bourcereau J, et al, Principles for safety in application of neodymium-YAG laser in bronchology. Chest 1984; 86: 163–8.

14. Hayata Y, Kato H, Furuse K, et al, Photodynamic therapy of 169 early stage cancers of the lung and oesophagus: a Japanese multi-centre study. Laser Med Sci 1996; 11:255–9.

15. van Boxem TJ, Venmans BJ, Schramel FM, et al, Radiographically occult lung cancer treated with fibreoptic bronchoscopic electrocautery: a pilot study of a simple and inexpensive technique. Eur Respir J 1998; 11:169–72.

16. Usuda K, Saito Y, Nagamoto N, et al, Relation between bronchoscopic findings and tumor size of roentgenographically occult bronchogenic squamous cell carcinoma. J Thorac Cardiovasc Surg 1993; 106:1098–103.

17. Konaka C, Hirano T, Kato H, et al, Comparison of endoscopic features of early-stage squamous cell lung cancer and histological findings. Br J Cancer 1999; 80:1435–9.

18. Nagamoto N, Saito Y, Ohta S, et al, Relationship of lymph node metastasis to primary tumor size and microscopic appearance of roentgenographically occult lung cancer. Am J Surg Pathol 1989; 13:1009–13.

19. McWilliams A, MacAulay C, Gazdar AF, Lam S, Innovative molecular and imaging approaches for the detection of lung cancer and its precursor lesions. Oncogene 2002; 21:6949–59.

20. Sutedja G, New techniques for early detection of lung cancer. Eur Resp J Suppl 2003; 39: 57s–66s.

21. Woolner LB, Fontana RS, Cortese DA, Roentgenographically occult lung cancer: Pathologic findings and frequency of multicentricity during a 10-year period. Mayo Clin Proc 1984; 59:453–66.

22. Marcus PM, Bergstrahl EJ, Fagerstrom RM, et al, Lung cancer mortality in the Mayo Lung Project: impact of extended follow-up. J Natl Cancer Inst 2000; 92:1308–16.

23. Nakamura H, Kawasaki N, Hagiwara M, et al, Early hilar lung cancer risk for multiple lung cancers and clinical outcome. Lung Cancer 2001; 33:51–7.

24. Lam S, MacAulay C, Hung J, et al, Detection of dysplasia and carcinoma in situ with a lung imaging fluorescence endoscope device. J Thorac Cardiovasc Surg 1993; 105:1035–40.

25. Sutedja G, Codrington H, Risse EK, et al, Autofluorescence bronchoscopy improves staging of radiographically occult lung cancer and has an impact on therapeutic strategy. Chest 2001; 120:1327–32.

26. Miyazu Y, Miyazawa T, Kurimoto N, et al, Endobronchial ultrasonography in the assessment of centrally located early-stage lung cancer before photodynamic therapy. Am J Respir Crit Care Med 2002; 165:832–7.

27. Fujimura S, Sakurada A, Sagawa M, et al, A therapeutic approach to roentgenographically occult squamous cell carcinoma of the lung. Cancer 2000; 89:2445–8.

28. Kato H, Okunaka T, Tsuchida T, et al, Analysis of the cost-effectiveness of photodynamic therapy in early stage lung cancer. Diagnostic Therapeutic Endoscopy 1999; 6:9–16.

29. Brambilla C, Fievet F, Jeanmart M, et al, Early detection of lung cancer: role of biomarkers. Eur Respir J Suppl 2003; 39:36s–44s.

30. Shinagawa N, Yamazaki K, Onodera Y, et al, CT-guided transbronchial biopsy using an ultrathin bronchoscope with virtual bronchoscopic navigation. Chest 2004; 125:1138–43.

31. Sutedja TG, Venmans BJ, Smit EF, Postmus PE, Fluorescence bronchoscopy for early detection of lung cancer: a clinical perspective. Lung Cancer 2001; 34:157–68.

32. Ikeda N, Hiyoshi T, Kakihana M, et al, Histopathological evaluation of fluorescence bronchoscopy using resected lungs in cases of lung cancer. Lung Cancer 2003; 41:303–9.

33. Shibuya K, Hoshino H, Chiyo M, et al, Subepithelial vascular patterns in bronchial dysplasias using a high magnification bronchovideoscope. Thorax 2002; 57:902–7.

34. MacAulay C, Lane P, Richards-Kortum R, In vivo pathology: microendoscopy as a new endoscopic imaging modality. Gastrointest Endosc Clin N Am 2004; 14:595–620.

35. Kurimoto N, Murayama M, Yoshioka S, Nishisaka T, Analysis of the internal structure of peripheral

pulmonary lesions using endobronchial ultrasonography. Chest 2002; 122:1887–94.

36. Nakata M, Sawada S, Saeki H, et al, Prospective study of thoracoscopic limited resection for ground-glass opacity selected by computed tomography. Ann Thorac Surg 2003; 75: 1601–5.

37. Uematsu M, Shioda A, Suda A, et al, Computed tomography-guided frameless stereotactic radiotherapy for stage I non-small cell lung cancer: a 5-year experience. Int J Radiat Oncol Biol Phys 2001; 51:666–70.

38. Schaefer O, Lohrmann C, Langer M, CT-guided radiofrequency ablation of a bronchogenic carcinoma. Br J Radiol 2003; 76:268–70.

39. Kato H, Tsuchida T, Usuda J, et al, The new trial of PDT and PDD in the peripheral lung tumors. 30th Annual Meeting American Society for Photobiology, Quebec City, Canada, 2002.

40. Okunaka T, Kato H, Photodynamic therapy for lung cancer: state of the art and expanded indications. IPA 9th World Congress of Photodynamic Medicine, Miyazaki, Japan, 2003.

41. Saito Y, Nagamoto N, Ota S, et al, Results of surgical treatment for roentgenographically occult bronchogenic squamous cell carcinoma. J Thorac Cardiovasc Surg 1992; 104:401–7.

42. Saito M, Furukawa K, Miura T, Kato H, Evaluation of T factor, surgical method, and prognostic factors in central type lung cancer. Jpn J Thorac Cardiovasc Surg 2002; 50:413–17.

43. Herder GJ, Breuer RH, Comans EF, et al, Positron emission tomography scans can detect radiographically occult lung cancer in the central airways. J Clin Oncol 2001; 19: 4271–2.

44. Pasic A, Vonk-Noordegraaf A, Risse EK, Postmus PE, Sutedja G, Multiple suspicious lesions detected by autofluorescence bronchoscopy predict malignant development in the bronchial mucosa in high risk patients. Lung Cancer 2003; 41:295–301.

45. Vonk Noordegraaf A, Postmus PE, Sutedja G, Bronchoscopic treatment of patients with intraluminal microinvasive radiographically occult lung cancer not eligible for surgical resection: a follow-up study. Lung Cancer 2003; 39: 49–53.

46. Boxem TJ van, Westerga J, Venmans BJ, Postmus PE, Sutedja G, Photodynamic therapy, Nd-YAG laser and electrocautery for treating early stage intraluminal cancer: Which to choose? Lung Cancer 2001; 31:31–6.

47. Hayata Y, Kato H, Konaka C, et al, Fiberoptic bronchoscopic laser photoradiation for tumor localization in lung cancer. Chest 1982; 82: 10–14.

48. Usuda J, Okunaka T, Furukawa K, et al, Photodynamic therapy for bronchogenic carcinoma. Lasers Surg Med 2001; suppl 13: 40.

49. Kato H, Furukawa K, Sato M, et al, Phase II clinical study of photodynamic therapy using mono-L-aspartyl cholorin e6 and diode laser for early superficial squamous cell carcinoma of the lung. Lung Cancer 2003; 42:103–11.

50. Braichotte D, Savary JF, Glanzmann T, et al, Optimizing light dosimetry in photodynamic therapy of the bronchi by fluorescence spectroscopy. Laser Med Sci 1996; 11:247–54.

51. Awadh N, MacAulay C, Lam S, Detection and treatment of superficial lung cancer by using δ-aminolevulinic acid: a preliminary report. J Bronchology 1997; 4:13–17.

52. Marsiglia H, Baldeyrou P, Lartigau E, et al, High-dose-rate brachytherapy as sole modality for early-stage endobronchial carcinoma. Int J Radiat Oncol Biol Phys 2000; 47:665–72.

53. Perol M, Caliandro R, Pommier P, et al, Curative irradiation of limited endobronchial carcinomas with high-dose rate brachytherapy. Results of a pilot study. Chest 1997; 111:1417–23.

54. van Boxem TJ, Westerga J, Venmans BJ, Postmus PE, Sutedja G, Tissue effects of bronchoscopic electrocautery: bronchoscopic appearance and histologic changes of bronchial wall after electrocautery. Chest 2000; 117: 887–91.

55. Deygas N, Froudarakis M, Ozenne G, Vergnon JM, Cryotherapy in early superficial bronchogenic carcinoma. Chest 2001; 120:26–31.

56. Pasic A, Brokx HA, Vonk Noordegraaf A, et al, Cost-effectiveness of early intervention: comparison between intraluminal bronchoscopic treatment and surgical resection for T1N0 lung cancer patients. Respiration 2004; 71:391–6.

57. Black WC, Overdiagnosis: An underrecognized cause of confusion and harm in cancer screening. J Natl Cancer Inst 2000; 92:1280–2.

12 CT screening for lung cancer

Claudia I Henschke, Anthony P Reeves, Dorith Shaham,
Rowena Yip, David F Yankelevitz, Christian Brambilla,
Shusuke Sone

Contents   Introduction • Background • Screening for lung cancer: its essence
• Diagnostic-prognostic trials • Current knowledge about the benefit of CT
screening • Randomized trials • Summary

INTRODUCTION

In this chapter, we review the research and practice initiatives on CT screening for lung cancer and the information currently available. This includes a discussion of the two alternative approaches currently being used in the research to assess the usefulness of CT screening; (1) the traditional 'randomized control trial' comparing screening with either 'no screening' or 'screening with another modality' and (2) the 'diagnostic-prognostic trial' which assesses the diagnostic component separately from that of the subsequent interventive component. A full understanding of the differences between these two approaches is important as there is much at stake for the individuals at high risk for lung cancer.

BACKGROUND

Helical CT was introduced in the early 1990s and for the first time images of the entire thorax could be obtained in a single breath. Previously each cross-sectional image was obtained in a single breath which meant that the imaging was time consuming and resulted in misregistration due to different inspiratory effort for each image so that potentially significant areas of the lungs could be missed. The use of helical CT led to many small pulmonary nodules being identified on CT[1] and it was recognized that the management of these small nodules was problematic as there was little understanding about the frequency of lung cancer among them on which to base follow-up recommendations or of how to measure growth.

In weekly thoracic oncology conferences at Cornell University Medical College, now Weill Medical College of Cornell University, cases were regularly encountered in which incidental nodules were identified on CT scans and these discussions led to multi-disciplinary research meetings starting in 1991 to which an epidemiologist, OS Miettinen and a statistician, BJ Flehinger were also invited. BJ Flehinger had been responsible for the analysis of the NIH-funded Memorial Sloan-Kettering Lung Project that was initiated in the 1970s,[2] and was also involved in the analysis of the two other NIH-funded randomized screening trials concerning lung cancer screening, the Mayo Lung Project[3] and the Johns Hopkins Lung Project[4] being performed at the same time. Later, Dr Flehinger and her co-workers developed a mathematical model of lung cancer based on this screening experience.[5] The Cornell group asked her to use it to predict the potential benefit of CT screening and the results showed that helical CT imaging held promise for early diagnosis of lung cancer and, thereby, for enhanced curability of this highly fatal disease.[6]

In light of an analysis of the controversy surrounding the prior screening studies on lung cancer[2–4] and the difficulties encountered due to their study design, the Cornell group was decided to develop a different approach, called a 'diagnostic-prognostic trial' to evaluate CT screening for lung cancer[7] as it distinguishes between the evaluation of the diagnostic and interventive components. Using this approach, the Early Lung Cancer Action Project (ELCAP) screened 1000 high-risk people and provided results for baseline[8] and annual repeat[9] screening. These two publications showed CT-based imaging's great superiority over traditional chest radiography in leading to diagnoses of small lung cancers, and that workup of positive results, while common in baseline, are much less common in repeat screening. Thus, CT screening could be managed with no notable excess of biopsies or thoracotomies when following the ELCAP protocol.

In Japan starting in 1993, CT was added to an already long-existing practice of screening for lung cancer using chest radiography,[10] presumably for similar reasons which led to the initiation of ELCAP and CT was superior to chest radiography in detection of small, early-stage lung cancer. In another study in Nagano Prefecture,[11,12] screening using CT and chest radiography using a mobile van was started in 1996. In 1996, baseline screenings on 5483 men and women were performed followed by a total of 8303 annual repeat screenings. At baseline, 279 (5%) of the 5483 had a suspicious finding which required further work-up and among them 23 had lung cancer. Among the 8303 repeat screening, 309 (4%) required further workup and 37 had cancers. Among the 60 screen-diagnosed lung cancers, 55 (88%) of

them were stage I. These two studies in Japan, like ELCAP, demonstrated the marked superiority of CT over chest radiography. These two studies enrolled smokers and non-smokers so that the prevalence of cancer was much lower than in ELCAP.

The ELCAP report led to considerable public[13] and professional interest in the practice of CT-based screening for lung cancer. Suddenly, screening for lung cancer became a hot topic with researchers initiating projects to study it, the public demanding it, and medical institutions offering it. The nihilistic North American public policies on lung-cancer screening[14] were suddenly being reconsidered and the American Cancer Society started to update its recommendations. The demand for information on screening led to the International Conferences on Screening for Lung Cancer to which all those already performing screening or wishing to start it were invited.[15] This initiative was an outgrowth of the already extensive role of ELCAP in helping other investigator groups at the University of Muenster in Germany,[16] Hadassah Medical Center in Israel,[17] University of South Florida in the United States, the Mayo Clinic in the United States,[18] the University of Navarra[19] and Hirslanden Lung Centre in Switzerland[20] to initiate their research projects patterned after the original ELCAP.

The First International Conference on Screening for Lung Cancer in October 1999[15] identified the urgent need for further research as to the benefit of CT screening and how best to determine its magnitude in preventing death from lung cancer. It was recognized that this area of medical technology was advancing rapidly as single-slice scanners were being replaced by ever-increasing multidetector-row scanners so that instead of 10 mm images of the lungs, sub-millimeter images could be obtained in a single breath. Other advances included the use of computer monitors for the reading of the images (instead of printing them on film) allowing for easier identification of small nodules. Image analytic techniques were being developed to characterize and classify pulmonary nodules on CT[21] and in the future these advances will be integrated in the reading and management process.[22] Thus, this first Conference led to the general recognition that the rate of refinement of CT imaging is so rapid that 1999 state-of-the-art CT will be obsolete within several years.

By the Second International Conference in February 2000,[15] it was generally agreed that CT screening presented a breakthrough opportunity in preventing death from lung cancer and thus there was an urgency for rapid assessment of the magnitude of its benefit so that it could then be made available to the community at large. Critical diagnostic and interventive issues were identified including the need for quality control and documentation of the entire screening process starting with the initial CT and ending with the diagnosis of lung cancer, including long-term follow-up of all diagnosed cases. The Third International Conference in October 2000[15] presented the new research initiatives being developed throughout the world and acknowledged the marked increase in the practice of screening. The desirability of an international consortium with a focus on pooling of data for rapid accumulation of policy-relevant information on screening for lung cancer was raised. In response to this call for an international consortium, the International (I)-ELCAP was formed, drawing its members from participants in the conferences.[23] Integral to the I-ELCAP collaboration is a shared set of principles and the use of a common protocol and management system which would allow for pooling of the data from participating institutions. Its first task was to define an optimal

regimen for 'CT screening' for lung cancer which was presented at the Fourth International Conference on Screening for Lung Cancer in April 2001[15] and unanimously adopted with the recommendation to quickly publish it.[24] Since then it has been updated every 6 months and the latest version is available on the web.[23] Any given conference focuses on issues that are particularly topical at the time. The subsequent conferences[15] have provided an update on the relevant interim meetings, publications and new trials, updates of I-ELCAP screening and pathology protocols, and focused on the relevant diagnostics which might impact the screening regimen or early interventions which might impact the curability of lung cancer and have sought to develop consensus on these topics. As of the 10th Conference in April 2004, over 25 000 screenees had been enrolled.

In 2001, the Director of the National Cancer Institute organized the Lung Cancer Progress Review Group (PRG) to identify high-priority areas of research in lung cancer.[25] This process led to the following major recommendations: to create and foster scientifically integrated, multi-disciplinary, multi-institutional research consortia organized around lung cancer; develop and expand new approaches to the biology and treatment of nicotine addiction; evaluation of population-based tobacco control efforts; to facilitate and hasten the evaluation of CT to detect lung cancer at an early stage; to reverse the current stage distribution at presentation, and reduce mortality from lung cancer; to elucidate the contributions of injury, inflammation and infection to the genesis of lung cancer; design, implement and study 'best practices' in lung cancer management; facilitate and encourage training programs that emphasize multi-disciplinary science and clinical care. The PRG also recognized that no single approach or trial will answer all of the questions which needed to be answered about lung cancer screening.

In March 2001, the National Cancer Institute and the American Cancer Society jointly sponsored the Early Lung Cancer Screening Workshop[26] with the aim of bringing together experts to address issues of study design. The workshop concluded that both traditional randomized trials and non-randomized studies were necessary to answer key questions about early lung cancer detection. Since then, it has been recognized that both randomized and non-randomized studies are desirable and that subsequent pooling of data from all these studies would be a worthwhile investment for the future, as it would allow clearer interpretation of the body of evidence from all studies.

In Europe, research efforts in lung cancer had culminated in a European Union research grant being awarded to the European Union Early Lung Cancer Detection Group in 2001.[27] Stimulated by the success of this collaborative effort and the International Conferences on Screening for Lung Cancer, different trial designs were developed in Europe. Under the auspices of the EU Early Lung Cancer Detection Group, the American Cancer Society and the National Cancer Institute multiple meetings were held which expressed support for the two different study designs and had as the goal to harmonize the core elements of the radiology, pathology and biomarker protocols for the future trials with a view to pooling of the data rather than later meta-analysis.

SCREENING FOR LUNG CANCER: ITS ESSENCE

The ultimate aim of screening is the pursuit of early diagnosis which provides the opportunity for early intervention and thus the prevention of the cancer's fatal outcome. The death which is prevented is due to the early intervention that is made possible by early diagnosis CT screening. Two approaches to address this question have been developed.

In the traditional approach, screening for a cancer is viewed as the application of a single diagnostic test to an asymptomatic person and the thought is that this testing is supposed to reduce mortality from the cancer. According to this traditional viewpoint, the diagnostic test is viewed as the 'intervention', and it is supposed to have 'effectiveness' in that it should prevent the cancer's fatal outcome. To test the hypothesis that the diagnostic test reduces mortality, a randomized trial is performed in which one cohort receives the test and the other cohort does not. After several rounds of screening and further follow-up of both cohorts, the cumulative mortality rates in each cohort are compared. If the cumulative mortality rate in the cohort which received the diagnostic test is significantly reduced when compared to that of the cohort which did not receive the test, then the 'intervention' is deemed effective. This approach to the evaluation of the effectiveness of screening has been called a hybrid approach even by its strongest proponents[28] as it applies the methodology developed for evaluating competing *interventions* to analyze the benefit of a *diagnostic* test. In these randomized trials, the diagnostic test, the 'intervention', is typically specified in detail while the entire process of further work-up leading to diagnosis of lung cancer is left to the usual care and not specified by the protocol.

At variance with this traditional viewpoint is that a sharp distinction is to be made between diagnostic testing and intervening. The useful property of a diagnostic test is its informativeness; the test in itself has no effect on the course of health.[29] An intervention, by contrast, is intended to change the course of health, hopefully, for the better, that is, to have effectiveness. For example, the use of chest radiography to diagnose pulmonary tuberculosis did not change its course; rather, the intervention with streptomycin did.[30,31] This alternative viewpoint considers screening as the pursuit of early diagnosis which starts with an initial test and proceeds along a well-defined path to diagnose lung cancer (i.e., a clearly defined regimen of screening), as exemplified by ELCAP.[24,32,33] Early intervention follows the early diagnosis and, typically, in the evaluation of screening the intervention to be used is the usual standard of care and is not itself being evaluated. The diagnostic-prognostic trial, however, allows for evaluation of alternative interventions using either a randomized or non-randomized approach. For this reason, this design is called a 'diagnostic-prognostic' trial as it is not simply a 'cohort', 'observational' or 'single-armed' study. The usefulness of the screening regimen is assessed by evaluating the diagnostic performance of the regimen and then by determining how many deaths are prevented by the early diagnosis and early intervention. The latter information is provided by the reduction in the case-fatality rate of lung cancer among those who have the intervention as compared to those who do not.[32–36]

DIAGNOSTIC-PROGNOSTIC TRIALS

The results of ELCAP led to the planning of the New York (NY)-ELCAP in the fall of 1999[37] with the intention to perform baseline and a single annual repeat screening in high-risk people using the same design and entry criteria as ELCAP in institutions throughout NY State. Twelve institutions decided to participate and screening started in 2001. A total of 6295 high-

risk people were enrolled using the same entry criteria as ELCAP. The study was completed in 2004 and the results confirm those of the ELCAP.[38] During the same time, the international consortium called International (I)-ELCAP was being formed and includes institutions throughout the world and by 2005 it has enrolled more than 28 000 screenees.[23] Other studies have also started in Japan.

It needs to be stressed that the 'diagnostic-prognostic' trial studies the two component issues of screening – the diagnostic regimen and its prognostic implications. Evaluation of the screening regimen, the diagnostic component, requires no control group as the information about the performance of the regimen can only be obtained from those receiving it. Assessment of early intervention following early diagnosis may include the use of randomized control trials to compare different interventions. The deaths prevented by obtaining early diagnosis and early intervention are determined from the case-fatality rates of the cases that had early diagnosis with and without early intervention.[32–36]

The diagnostic-prognostic approach asserts that the ultimate usefulness of screening cannot be determined without specifying the particular way in which the early diagnosis might be pursued. This requires specification of a particular regimen of screening for diagnosing lung cancer, and more particularly one that is, at the time, potentially optimal for the purpose. For this reason, the I-ELCAP protocol focuses on the most-promising regimen of early (pre-symptomatic) diagnosis of lung cancer at any particular time and is continually updated.[23,24] The regimen of screening starts with the initial low-dose CT, and if the result is positive, other testing follows along a well-thought-out algorithm which eventually leads to a (rule-in) diagnosis of lung cancer. The particulars of the regimen have been evolving over the years, but its fundamental nature has remained stable. A particularly notable feature of the screening regimen for lung cancer is the difference between the baseline and repeat screenings in the definition of a positive result and the algorithm for further work-up. In the repeat screenings, the focus is on growing nodules in comparison with previous screening. At baseline, by contrast, multiple non-calcified nodules are commonly visible in the CT images and the definition of a positive result poses a considerable challenge given the lack of prior information, particularly as the decreasing slice thickness of the CT images permits for identification of smaller nodules. Thus, this definition has been frequently updated in light of new information.[39–41] Assessment of growth is an integral part of the regimen.[42–46] Ultimately, the diagnosis of lung cancer derives from a biopsy of the suspicious nodule followed by the specimen's cytologic reading and interpretation. Given the critical role of pathology, a separate protocol was developed to assure the quality and consistency of the diagnoses and all cases were reviewed by an expert pathology panel.[47,48]

CT screening for lung cancer leads to exceptional types of diagnosis as for the nature of the lesion – 'nodule' – in CT imaging. The lesion can be extraordinarily small; and it can be only part-solid in appearance or even completely non-solid. These diagnoses of cancer raise some legitimate questions about their significance. The principal question concerns the frequency with which a lesion actually has a benign rather than malignant behavior; and insofar as it is malignant, the question is about its typical degree of aggressiveness. Thus, for the prognostic component, the aim is to determine the significance of these screen-diagnoses which is a matter of determining the case-fatality rates without and with intervention (in the absence of

competing causes of death), together with the respective timings of fatal outcomes.[32–36]

These questions of significance will be answerable in quite definitive terms once adequate numbers of such cases have been followed long enough, unresected cases in particular. Early on, the significance or genuineness of the screen-diagnosed cases can be addressed by pathologic review by the expert pathology panel and by assessment of the growth rates.[49,50] Later in the follow-up of unresected lesions, the genuine cancers express themselves in spread to lymph nodes and other organs. In this later follow-up experience, the rate of curability is manifest in the extent to which the frequency of spread is lower in the early-resected cases relative to the unresected ones, given control of confounders. Finally, the answer is provided by following the deaths of the unresected and resected cases as previously done by Flehinger et al[51] and Sobue et al[52] for chest radiographic screening and as has already been demonstrated for small lung cancers using the SEER registry data.[36]

The diagnostic-prognostic approach has been criticized as it is not a traditional randomized trial, but the estimate of deaths prevented by the early diagnosis and early intervention is determined so that there is no lead-time and overdiagnosis bias.[32–36] The approach also allows for distinguishing between overdiagnosis and competing causes of death, quite different from the randomized trial approach which uses mortality rates to avoid biases due to these two components, but cannot distinguish between them nor produce any estimate of them.

In the diagnostic-prognostic approach, overdiagnosis is not a bias but an important parameter to be estimated by the case-fatality rate of those cases of lung cancer not being treated.[34–36] Furthermore, it is not enough to obtain an overall estimate of overdiagnosis, but it also needs to be assessed for each relevant subtype of cancer. Curability is obtained from the case-fatality rates, both without and with intervention (in the absence of competing causes of death), together with the respective timings of fatal outcomes. Again, curability needs to be assessed for each relevant subtype of cancer. Knowledge of the risk of competing causes of death, on the other hand, is needed in determining who should be screened.

Obtaining estimates of overdiagnosis and curability requires long-term follow-up of a reasonably large number of cases. Prior to the availability of such cases, an estimate can be determined from prior studies and registries. Based on analysis of chest radiographic screening, the case-fatality rate of untreated lung cancers was over 90% and of resected ones was below 30%. This implies that some 10% might be overdiagnosed cases and the overall curability of lung cancer is thus $(90\% - 30\%)/90\% = 67\%$.[35] As screening using chest radiography produced stage I diagnoses in only about 30% of the diagnosed cases of lung cancer despite the high frequency (every 4 months) of screening,[3] the overall cure rate was some 20% ($30\% \times 67\%$).

It is important to understand that in light of advancing technology and knowledge, the diagnostic regimen and treatment are continually being updated. Thus, for example, more limited treatment is already being performed in those institutions with more experience with screening, even without the benefit of scientific assessment. The diagnostic-prognostic approach allows for separate assessment of each component and thus provides the capability of performing randomized treatment trials to provide scientific evidence for such treatment decisions.

An ancillary aim of the 'diagnostic-interventive' approach is to assess the indications for screening and the resulting frequency – prevalence – of cases that are diagnosable by the regimen. This ancillary aim provides the additional information needed to determine appropriate screening policies and the cost-effectiveness of these policies and should also consider the risk of competing causes of death.[53] Analyses have shown that CT screening for lung cancer is very cost-effective[54–57] with the exception of one theoretical study.[58] These analyses look at the overall cost per life-year saved, but ideally a cost-effectiveness assessment would be done on an individualized basis. Such an individualized assessment would determine the life expectancy of the person (in light of the personal risk indicators) and the risk of competing causes of death in order to determine how many years of life might be saved by the screening round that is being contemplated.

An important advantage of the diagnostic-prognostic approach is that information can be pooled across studies with varying indications for screening so long as the same regimen of screening is being followed.[59]

CURRENT KNOWLEDGE ABOUT THE BENEFIT OF CT SCREENING

Assessment of the diagnostic performance of any regimen of screening is provided by estimates of (1) how frequently a positive result of the initial CT occurs, (2) how frequently screen-diagnoses are made in comparison to all diagnoses (including interim-diagnoses), separately for baseline and repeat screening, and (3) how early the screen-diagnoses are achieved. This is a matter of determining the distribution of the diagnosed cases by prognostic indicators, foremost by stage and within stage, by size. The diagnostic subclassification is further refined by other prognostic indicators, notably cell type and, for the earliest diagnoses, CT-based measures of the tumor's rate of growth.

Frequency of positive result of the initial test

Screening in the original ELCAP was done using 10 mm CT slice thickness and on baseline 23% had 1–6 non-calcified nodules.[8] Using the same definition but obtaining thinner section CT images, Diederich et al[16] and Swensen et al[18] both had higher rates (43% and 53%, respectively), however, they found that most of the nodules were small (50% of the nodules <5 mm and 89% <7 mm, respectively). In terms of the work-up of these nodules on baseline, Diederich et al ignored all nodules <10 mm and Swensen et al ignored all nodules ≤4 mm, effectively changing the definition of a positive result. Pasterino et al[60] had already defined a positive result on baseline as any person having a nodule greater than 5 mm and found that only 6% had a positive result. Recall that in Sone's study, the rate was 5%.[12]

Review of screening results also yielded new insights that nodules are not all solid, that is completely obscuring the entire parenchyma in it. This is a topic peculiar to CT imaging of the chest, and the significance of other types of nodule in CT-based screening for lung cancer was not fully appreciated at the beginning.[39,40] Such nodules had been called 'ground-glass opacities', but this descriptor is non-specific and in no way describes the underlying pathology.[40] Thus, a better descriptor was needed and to this end the nodules were described as being solid, part-solid or non-solid; a solid nodule is one which completely obscures the entire lung parenchyma in it, part-solid (Figure 12.1) as having parts that are solid in this sense, and non-solid (Figure 12.2) as not having any solid parts. A review of the ELCAP results showed that the frequency of these part-solid and non-

solid nodules in relation to that of solid ones in CT-based lung cancer screening at baseline is appreciable (circa 20%)[40] and that about half of the cancers are diagnosed in these part-solid and non-solid nodules.[59,61] On the other hand, on annual repeat screening, few malignancies were seen in part-solid or non-solid nodules.[40] With thinner CT slices due to advancing technology, the relative frequency of part-solid and especially non-solid nodule detection presumably will be even higher.

More striking was that the malignancy rate was significantly higher for part-solid nodules than for either solid or non-solid ones. The distribution by malignancy type also was strikingly different in the part-solid and non-solid nodules as compared with the solid ones as

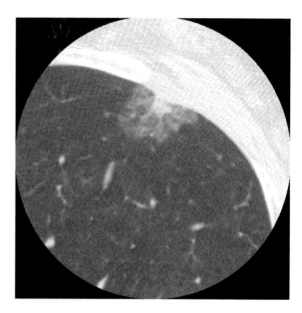

Figure 12.1
High resolution CT image of a 58 year-old woman shows a part-solid 18 mm right upper lobe nodule abutting the pleura. The diagnosis was adenocarcinoma, mixed subtype, Noguchi C.

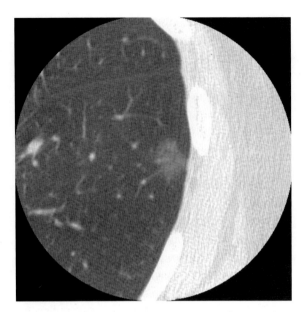

Figure 12.2
High resolution CT image of a 75 year-old woman shows a non-solid 10 mm right lower lobe nodule abutting the pleura. The diagnosis was adenocarcinoma, mixed subtype, Noguchi C.

the malignancies in part-solid and non-solid nodules were either adenocarcinoma with bronchioloalveolar features or adenocarcinoma-mixed subtype, while malignancy in solid nodules included the entire spectrum of small-cell and non-small-cell lung cancer except adenocarcinoma with bronchioloalveolar features.[59]

Similar results were seen by Yang et al.[39] They identified four patterns on high-resolution CT: pure ground-glass opacity (ggo) (non-solid), hetergeneous (part-solid), solid with ggo in the periphery (part-solid, but with a large solid component), and solid. They showed that the malignancies typically found non-solid nodules were classified as Noguchi type A and part-solid were typically Noguchi type B (both types A and

B are non-invasive and classified according to WHO as adenocarcinoma with bronchioloalveolar features) and that the malignancies with a larger solid component were classified as type C (WHO classification as invasive, adenocarcinoma-mixed subtype). All of their solid cases were adenocarcinoma, Noguchi type D. The Noguchi classification of types A–F[62] was developed for adenocarcinomas and the WHO classification is given above.

With the advances in multidetector-row CT, the slice thickness has decreased from 10 mm to 1.25 mm or less, leading to identification of an increasing number of small nodules and thus the definition of a positive result needed updating. It was shown that the work-up of non-calcified nodules less than 5 mm in diameter found in the initial baseline CT was not productive in diagnosing malignancy[41] and consequently, the definition of a positive result of the initial CT on baseline screening in the I-ELCAP changed. It is currently: identification of at least one solid or part-solid nodule 5 mm or more in diameter, and/or at least one non-solid nodule 8 mm or more in diameter and this result calls for immediate further diagnostic work-up.[23] When non-calcified nodules are identified but all of them were too small to imply a positive result, the result is called 'semi-positive' in the sense of calling for repeat CT 1 year later. Using this definition, a positive result of the initial CT was 12% (95% CI: 11–14%) in ELCAP[59] and 14% (95% CI: 14–15%) in NY-ELCAP.[38] With advancing knowledge and technology, the definition of a positive result will continue to be updated so that even the smaller malignancies can be identified in the baseline cycle.

For repeat screening, the definition of a positive result of the initial CT has remained the same throughout: any non-calcified nodule that evidently had grown in the interim, regardless of size. Growth was defined as either enlargement, identified visually by the radiologist, of the entire nodule or of the solid component of a part-solid nodule, or the development of a solid component in a previously non-solid nodule. Using this definition, a positive result on annual repeat was found in 6% (95% CI: 5–6%) in ELCAP[59] and 6% (95% CI: 5–16%) in NY-ELCAP.[38]

In summary, by judicious definition of a positive result on baseline, unnecessary work-up can be markedly reduced. All subjects having a 'semi-positive' finding being referred to the first annual repeat screening. On repeat screening, the proportion having a growing nodule has always remained low. The definition of a positive result, however, should continue to be updated as further advances in knowledge and technology are made.

Frequency of screen-diagnoses

The frequency of screen-diagnoses (prompted by a positive result) as compared with all diagnoses (including interim-diagnoses prompted by symptoms in between screenings) is an important performance measure. To completely identify interim diagnoses, each subject must be contacted 1 year after the last screening. A diagnosis of lung cancer was classified as a baseline interim-diagnosis in the baseline cycle, if the result of the initial CT at baseline was negative and the diagnostic work-up was prompted by suspicion-raising symptoms (or an incidental finding) before the scheduled first annual repeat. A screen-diagnosis is one which results from work-up prompted by findings on the initial CT, regardless of when the diagnosis is achieved. For baseline screening, the diagnosis was classified in this way even when the result is 'semi-positive' in the sense of calling for a repeat CT 1 year later. Analogous attribution is applied in the context of repeat-screening cycles.

Interim diagnoses for ELCAP have been few, 3% (2/79) in the baseline cycle and 4% (1/29) in the annual repeat cycles (Table 12.1). Other than Pasterino et al,[60] who reported no cases of interim-diagnosis, the other studies have reported on the frequency of interim-diagnosis. In summary, annual CT screening produces very few interim-diagnoses.

Diagnostic distribution by prognostic indicators

How early the diagnoses are made depends on the frequency of stage I screen-diagnoses, first and foremost (Table 12.1), and then by size. The distribution of diagnosed cases by stage of studies reported by Sone of 88%[12] and by Sobue et al[63] and Nawa et al[64] were essentially the same or higher than ELCAP. The frequency of stage I cancers in the studies by Pasterino et al,[60] Diederich et al[16] and Swensen et al[18] were slightly lower, perhaps in part as all of the baseline cases as defined in this section were not included in the initial publications, some of the included cases may have been symptomatic, because the diagnostic work-up of the smallest nodules on baseline was delayed by 1 year, or simply because of the statistical variation expected for such small samples of cases.

The diagnostic distribution by cell-type is given for the baseline and annual repeat cycles in Table 12.2. Adenocarcinoma represents a higher proportion of the diagnoses in the baseline than in annual repeat cycles of screening (82% vs. 59%). Only diagnoses of adenocarcinoma are made in sub-solid nodules, while all cell-types are diagnosed in solid nodules.

Significance of screen-diagnoses

As illustrated in the preceding section, preliminary estimates of the extent of overdiagnosis and curability can be obtained from the currently available data. Annual CT screening

Table 12.1 Diagnosis in the baseline cycle and annual repeat cycles of screening in ELCAP: frequency of screen-diagnosis subclassified by presurgical tumor size and stage

		Baseline (N = 79)	Annual repeat (N = 29)
Interim-diagnosis:	n	2	1
	%	3	3
	CI (%)[1]	0–9	0–18
Screen-diagnosis: tumor diameter (mm)			
<10	n	9	15
	%	11	52
10–19	n	50	11
	%	63	38
20–29	n	11	0
	%	14	0
30+	n	7	2
	%	9	7
Any	n	77	28
	%	97	97
Stage I	n	75	27
	%	95	93
	CI (%)[1]	88–99	77–99

[1] 95% exact confidence interval for the percentage.

produces stage I diagnoses in a very high proportion, in at least eight out of ten cases, as shown by the already extensive evidence. Thus, even if the curability of these stage I cases is no higher than the 67% associated with radiographic screening or 71% as shown using SEER data for cancers less than 15 mm in diameter,[35] the overall cure rate would already be higher than 50% (8/10 × 67%). Preliminary reports[63,64] suggest an even higher curability rate of some 80–90% which would yield an even higher overall cure rate of more than 64% (8/10 × 80%).

As to the question of overdiagnosis of CT screen-diagnosed lung cancers, review of some 300 baseline and annual repeat screen-diagnosed cancers by the Expert Pathology Panel has confirmed all the original diagnoses of cancer to be genuine, meeting the WHO criteria of malignancy.

Review of the growth rates of the earliest screen-diagnosed malignancies, those with no evidence of invasion or lymph node metastases at baseline, suggested that about 10% of the cases diagnosed under baseline screening might be overdiagnosed ones,[50] similar to that found

Table 12.2 Diagnosis in baseline and annual repeat cycles in ELCAP: frequency distributions by cell-type (interim-diagnosed cases included)

Cell-type	Baseline		Annual repeat
	Solid	Sub-solid	All solid
	n	n	n
Adeno	18	47	17
Non-small	0	0	3
Squamous	4*	0	3*
Large/neuroendocrine	6	0	3
Small	4**	0	2
Other	0	0	1
Total	32	47	29

*One interim diagnosis.

by Flehinger et al[51] and Sobue et al[52] Further follow-up of the unresected cases will provide the even better estimates by subtype of nodule. Similarly, Wang et al[44] reviewed 12 cancers (in solid, part-solid and non-solid nodules) in the Nagano Project for which doubling times could be calculated and found that they varied between 54–132 days and thus were rapidly growing cancers.

Overdiagnosis on annual repeat screening is highly unlikely for the following reason. The definition of a screen-diagnosis on annual repeat requires that it was not seen on the initial, baseline CT screening, thus, the cancer was below the visibility threshold (approximately 2 mm) and it now becomes visible 1 year later when it reaches a size of at least 3 mm. The slowest possible doubling time for such a cancer would be 300 days, which represents the doubling time of a typical cancer. All repeat cancers larger than 3 mm would have a more rapid doubling time.

Indications for screening

An ancillary aim of the 'diagnostic-interventive' approach is to assess the frequency – prevalence – of cases diagnosable by the regimen which depends on the indications for screening as defined by risk indicators, such as age, smoking history, occupational exposure and gender, together with the risk of competing causes of death. Such knowledge is important as it directly impacts the cost-effectiveness of the screening.

Comparison of the existing CT screening studies shows that the older the person and the higher the pack-years of smoking, the higher the malignancy rate[16,61] as is already well-known in lung cancer epidemiology. Further, Henschke and Miettinen[66] found that women were at higher risk for lung cancer than equally smoking and aged men and Li et al[61] found a higher frequency of cancer in non-smoking women than in non-smoking men.

The only data about CT screening of non-smokers comes from Japan.[61,64] Li et al[61] compared 4251 non-smokers with 3596 smokers and, surprisingly, found that the malignancy rate was the same for both (44/4251 vs. 35/3596), although adjusted rates for potential confounders (age, smoking history, occupational exposure, gender) are needed to better understand these results. For example, most of the non-smokers were women (3310/4251 = 78%) while most of the smokers were men (3347/3596 = 93%).

Although it seems reasonable for high-risk people to have annual screening based on the current information on the prognostic distributions of cancers found on annual repeat, it might not be needed so frequently for lower-risk people. Nawa et al,[64] for example, suggested that non-smokers have a single baseline scan. Further research is needed to determine the optimal frequency of screening for various risk groups.

RANDOMIZED TRIALS

The promising results of ELCAP led to the funding of several large national randomized trials. In the United States, starting in late 2002, the National Lung Screening Trial (NLST) started recruitment of 50 000 participants and completed its enrollment in early 2004.[67] The trial specifies two cohorts, one to receive the CT test and the other a chest radiograph. There will only be three rounds of screening with follow-up to 5 years so that its designers envision that it will provide an answer about the benefit of CT screening, or lack thereof, about 10 years after its start. These trials are very costly. The NLST will cost well over $200 million.

In France, a pilot randomized trial, the DepiScan (Depistage par scanner) started in 2002 in which 1000 men and women were randomized into one of two cohorts, one receiving low-dose CT screening and the other a chest radiograph.[68] This pilot study will be expanded to the GranDepiScan trial of 40 000 individuals in 2004 in which a total of five screening rounds and 5 years of follow-up will be performed. The results are anticipated on a yearly basis through a sequential design with the final results becoming available about 12 years after its start.

In the Netherlands and Belgium, the Nelson trial (NEderlands Leuvens Longkanker Screenings ONderzoek) trial was started in 2004. It is a randomized trial of 10 000 men and women, each randomized to one of two cohorts. One cohort will receive CT screening and the other cohort will not be screened; both will be receiving smoking cessation advice. A total of three screening rounds will be performed in years 1, 2 and 4 (second interval being 2 years) with 6 years of follow-up. The first results from baseline screening are anticipated by the end of 2005 and the final results about 10 years after the start.

In Italy, the ITALUNG_CT (Italy Lung CT) project starting in 2004 will randomize 3000 men and women who are living in the cities where the screening centers are located (Firenze, Pisa and Pistoia in Tuscany) and in 2005, another 1500 men and women will be enrolled at screening centers of the Emilia Romagna Region. One cohort will have CT screening and the other the usual care and all current smokers in both cohorts will have a smoking cessation visit. Starting in 2001, a total of four screening rounds performed and the subsequent follow-up will be for 6 years. Results on indicators of screening performance are anticipated at the end of each round of screening. Blood and sputum of participants who signed the specific informed consent will also be collected and stored for evaluation of biomarkers. The investigators of the European randomized trials recognized that the screening regimen needs to be specified in detail starting with the initial test and proceeding to diagnosis and they have all coordinated their approach to essentially follow the I-ELCAP protocol. It was also agreed that the screening regimen will be updated as needed, there will be interim reports, and regular meetings of the leaders of the trials so as to enhance the feasibility of pooling of the data at the end of the trials.[27] The Coordinating Centers of randomized controlled trials (RCTs) contrasting CT screening with either no screening or some other type of screening are also working together with the I-ELCAP consortium.

The final results from these randomized trials on CT screening, other than the interim reports, are probably at least a decade away. Following the traditional approach, the benefit of CT screening in these trials will be determined by a test of hypothesis which compares the cumulative mortality rates of the two cohorts over the entire period of screening and follow-up at the completion of the trial, typically several years after the last round of screening. Typically, these trials must enroll a large number of people (e.g., 50 000 in NLST) so several years may be required for the enrollment process. The number of years of screening and follow-up must also be sufficiently long, particularly in view of the lead-time afforded by CT (i.e., 4–5 years), and thus, these trials are costly in terms of time and money.

The long duration of randomized trials for assessment of the benefit of screening is problematic as technology is changing rapidly and as a consequence so is the optimal management protocols. Thus, the screening practice at the beginning of the trial is likely quite outdated by the time the trial is completed. Protocol compliance is difficult to maintain during the long period that screening must be performed, particularly in the cohort not receiving the diagnostic test, and this may vary between countries

depending on the existing medical system. To decrease the cost and duration of these trials, the screening rounds are typically decreased, but this affects the validity of the outcome. Even when the screening rounds are shortened considerably, as in the NLST to 3 years, and the number of participants is restricted, NLST will require at least 10–12 years to provide results. The power of the test of hypothesis is critical when designing a randomized trial and thus realistic assumptions must be made in planning these trials.[70] Although randomized trials are still considered the 'gold standard' for formulation of public health policy, previous trials for lung cancer[2–4] ended with much controversy,[5,69–75] in particular as to the extent of over-diagnosis,[71] while screening continued to be practiced in the United States.[76] Today, there is increasing recognition of the limitations of these trials[77] as has also been recognized in the mammography trials for breast cancer.[78–81]

SUMMARY

Currently available results on CT screening are all based on diagnostic-prognostic trials and show that (1) by appropriate definition of a positive result the work-up on baseline screening was confined to less than 15% and on annual repeat less than 6%, (2) that screen-diagnoses represented more than 95% of all diagnoses and (3) that over 80% of all the diagnoses were of stage I. As to the preliminary results (4) of the significance of the screen-diagnoses, all diagnoses of malignancy were confirmed by the expert pathology review. Estimates based on growth rates suggest that about 10% of the baseline-diagnosed cancers and essentially none of those diagnosed on repeat screening. The preliminary results of (5) the overall cure rate of screen-diagnosed lung cancer suggest that it may be raised to 50–60% as compared with that of usual care of 10% and that of chest radiographic screening of 20%.

It is hoped that continued reporting of the long-term follow-up of 'diagnostic-prognostic' trials which started in 1993 in the United States and Japan together with preliminary results of the ongoing randomized trials will allow for progressive updating of the national policies for screening for lung cancer. Progress was made in this direction, as in 2004, the US Preventive Services Task Force changed its recommendation for screening for lung cancer from D (recommend against) to I (neither for or against) and suggested that individuals task to their physicians about whether they should be screened.[82] Previously, the American Cancer Society had made a similar recommendation.[83] Other physicians are now suggesting this as well.[84] It is also hoped that further analysis of the results of these trials will allow for the development of methodologies of evaluation which provide information on new diagnostic tests and their benefit in reducing death from cancer in a more reasonable time frame.

REFERENCES

1. Remy-Jardin M, Remy J, Giraud F, Marquette CH, Pulmonary nodules: detection with thick-section spiral CT versus conventional CT. Radiology 1993; 187:513–20.
2. Melamed MR, Flehinger BJ, et al, Screening for early lung cancer. Results of the Memorial Sloan-Kettering study in New York. Chest 1984; 86: 44–53.
3. Fontana RS, Sanderson DR, Woolner LB, et al, Lung cancer screening: the Mayo program. J Occup Med 1986; 28:746–50.
4. Tockman MS, Survival and mortality from lung cancer in a screened population. The John Hopkins Study. Chest 1986; 89:324s–5s.
5. Flehinger BJ, Kimmel M, The natural history of lung cancer in a periodically screened population. Biometrics 1987; 43:127–44.
6. Flehinger BJ, Kimmel M, Polyak T, Melamed MR, Screening for lung cancer. The Mayo Lung Project revisited. Cancer 1993; 2:1573–80.
7. Henschke CI, Miettinen OS, Yankelevitz DF, Libby D, Smith JP, Radiographic screening for cancer: New paradigm for its scientific basis. Clin Imag 1994; 18:16–20.
8. Henschke CI, McCauley DI, Yankelevitz DF, et al, Early Lung Cancer Action Project: overall design and findings from baseline screening. Lancet 1999; 354:99–105.
9. Henschke CI, Naidich DP, Yankelevitz DF, et al, Early Lung Cancer Action Project: preliminary findings on annual repeat screening. Cancer 2001; 92:153–9.
10. Kaneko M, Eguchi K, Ohmatsu H, et al, Peripheral lung cancer: Screening and detection with low-dose spiral CT versus radiography. Radiology 1996; 201:798–802.
11. Sone S, Takahima S, Li F, et al, Mass screening for lung cancer with mobile spiral computed tomography scanner. Lancet 1998; 351:1242–5.
12. Sone S, Li F, Yang Z-G, et al, Results of three-year mass screening programme for lung cancer using mobile low-dose spiral computed tomography scanner. Br J Cancer 2001; 84:25–32.
13. Grady D, CAT scan process could cut deaths from lung cancer. Small tumors detected. New York Times, July 9,1999, p. 1.
14. Eddy DM, Screening for lung cancer. Ann Intern Med 1989; 11:232–7.
15. Consensus Statements of the International Conferences on Screening for Lung Cancer. http://www.IELCAP.org.
16. Diederich S, Wormanns D, Semik M, et al, Screening for early lung cancer with low-dose spiral CT: Prevalence in 817 asymptomatic smokers. Radiology 2002; 222:773–81.
17. Shaham D, Breuer R, Coppel L, et al, Hadassah Early Lung Cancer Action Project. Findings on baseline and annual repeat screening of an I-ELCAP study. Submitted.

18. Swensen SJ, Jett JR, Sloan JA, et al, Screening for lung cancer with low-dose spiral computed tomography. Am J Respir Crit Care Med 2002; 165:508–13.

19. Bastarrika G, Garcia Velloso MJ, Lozano MD, et al, Early lung cancer detection using spiral CT and positron emission tomography (FDG:PET). Am J Respir Crit Care Med 2005 Mar 24 (Epub).

20. Klinger K, Scherer T, Inderbitzi R, et al, Early detection of lung cancer by CT screening. International St. Gallen Oncology Conference: controversies and Prevention and Genetics 2004.

21. Henschke CI, Yankelevitz DF, Mateescu I, et al, Neural networks for the analysis of small pulmonary nodules. Clin Imag 1997; 21:390–9.

22. Reeves AP, Kostis WJ, Yankelevitz DF, Henschke CI, A web-based database system for multi-institutional research studies on lung cancer. Radiologic Society of North America Scientific Session, November 27, 2001, Chicago, IL.

23. International Early Lung Cancer Action Program and Protocol. website: www.IELCAP.org.

24. Henschke CI, Yankelevitz DF, Smith JP, Miettinen OS, Screening for lung cancer: the early lung cancer action approach. Lung Cancer 2002; 35:143–8.

25. Report of the Lung Cancer Progress Review Group. National Cancer Institute. Chantilly, Virginia, August 2001 (website: http://prg.nci.cih.gov/lung/default.html).

26. Early Lung Cancer Screening Workshop, National Cancer Institute, Washington, DC, 2001 (website: http://www3.cancer.gov/bip/dipsponsored.htm).

27. First, Second, and Third Early Lung Cancer Detection Workshop. A European strategy for developing lung cancer imaging and molecular diagnosis in high risk populations. Liverpool, England. November, 1999, 2001, 2003.

28. Welch HG, Black WC, Evaluating randomized trials of screening. JGIM 1997; 12118–24.

29. Miettinen OS, The modern scientific physician. 6. The useful property of a screening regimen. CMAJ 2001; 165:1219–20.

30. Hill AB, Suspended judgment. Memories of the British Streptomycin Trial in Tuberculosis. The first randomized clinical trial. Control Clin Trials 1990; 11:77–9.

31. Medical Research Council, Streptomycin treatment of pulmonary tuberculosis. British Medical Journal 1948; 2:769–82.

32. Henschke CI, Yankelevitz DF, Smith JP, Miettinen OS, The use of spiral CT in lung cancer screening. In: DeVita VT, Hellman S, Rosenberg SA (eds) Progress in Oncology 2002. Jones and Barlett, Sudbury, MA, 2002.

33. Henschke CI, Yankelevitz DF, Wisnivesky UP, et al, CT screening for lung cancer. In: Pass HI, Carbone DP, Johnson DH, Minna JD, Turrisi AT (eds) Lung Cancer: Principles and Practice, 3rd edn. Lippincott, Williams and Wilkins, 2004.

34. Henschke CI, Yankelevitz DF, Kostis WJ, CT screening for lung cancer: bias, shift and controversies. In: Schoepf UJ (ed.) Multidetector-Row CT of the Thorax. Springer Verlag, Berlin, Germany, 2003.

35. Henschke CI, Wisnivesky JP, Yankelevitz DF, Miettinen OS, Screen-diagnosed small stage I cancers of the lung: genuineness and curability. Lung Cancer 2003; 39:327–30.

36. Wisnivesky JP, Yankelevitz DF, Henschke CI, The effect of tumor size on curability of stage I non-small-cell lung cancers. Chest 2004; 126: 761–765.

37. New York Early Lung Cancer Action Project. website: www.IELCAP.org.

38. Henschke CI, Rifkin M, Kopel S, et al, NY Early Lung Cancer Action Project: A multi-institutional study of CT screening for lung cancer. Radiological Society of North America Scientific Abstract. Chicago, IL, December 2, 2003.

39. Yang Z-G, Sone S, Takashima S, et al, High-resolution CT analysis of small peripheral lung adenocarcinomas revealed on screening helical CT. AJR 2001; 176:1399–407.

40. Henschke CI, Yankelevitz DF, Mirtcheva R, et al, CT screening for lung cancer: Frequency and significance of part-solid and nonsolid nodules. AJR 2002; 178:1053–7.

41. Henschke CI, Yankelevitz DF, Naidich D, et al,

CT screening for lung cancer: Suspiciousness of nodules at baseline according to size. Radiology 2004; 231:164–8.

42. Yankelevitz DF, Gupta R, Zhao B, Henschke CI, Repeat CT scanning for evaluation of small pulmonary nodules: preliminary results. Radiology 1999; 212:561–6.

43. Yankelevitz DF, Reeves A, Kostis W, Zhao B, Henschke CI, Determination of malignancy in small pulmonary nodules based on volumetrically determined growth rates: Preliminary results. Radiology. Radiology 2000; 217:251–6.

44. Wang J-C, Sone S, Feng L, et al, Rapidly growing small peripheral lung cancers detected by screening CT: correlation between radiological appearance and pathological features. Br J Radiology 2000; 72:930–7.

45. Kostis WJ, Reeves AP, Yankelevitz DF, Henschke CI, Three-dimensional segmentation and growth-rate estimation of small pulmonary nodules in helical CT images. IEEE Transaction on Medical Imaging 2003; 22:1259–74.

46. Kostis WJ, Yankelevitz DF, Reeves AP, Fluture SC, Henschke CI, Small pulmonary nodules: reproducibility of three-dimensional volumetric measurement and estimation of time to follow-up CT. Radiology 2004; 231:446–52.

47. Vazquez M, Flieder D, Travis W, et al, Early Lung Cancer Action Project Pathology Protocol. Lung Cancer 2003; 39:231–2.

48. Vazquez M, Flieder D, Travis W, et al, Early Lung Cancer Action Project Pathology Protocol. Website: http://ICScreen.med.cornell.edu.

49. Yankelevitz DF, Kostis WF, Henschke CI, et al, Overdiagnosis in traditional radiographic screening for lung cancer: Frequency. Cancer 2003; 97:1271–5.

50. Henschke CI, Shaham D, Yankelevitz DF, et al, CT screening for lung cancer: significance of diagnoses in the baseline cycle of screening. Submitted.

51. Flehinger BJ, Kimmel M, Melamed MR, The effect of surgical treatment on survival from early lung cancer. Chest 1992; 101:1013–18.

52. Sobue T, Suzuki T, Matsuda M, et al, Survival for clinical stage I lung cancer not surgically treated. Comparison between screen-detected and symptom-detected cases. Cancer 1992; 69: 685–92.

53. Miettinen OS, Screening for lung cancer: Can it be cost-effective? Can Med Assoc J 2000; 162: 1431–6.

54. Wisnivesky JP, Mushlin AI, Sicherman N, et al, The cost-effectiveness of low-dose CT screening for lung cancer: preliminary results of baseline screening. Chest 2003; 124:614–21.

55. Marshall D, Simpson KN, Earle CC, et al, Potential cost-effectiveness of one-time screening for lung cancer (LC) in a high risk cohort. Lung Cancer 2001; 32:227–36.

56. Marshall D, Simpson KN, Earle CC, et al, Economic decision analysis model of screening for lung cancer. Eur J Cancer 2001; 37:1759–67.

57. Chirikos TN, Hazelton T, Tockman M, et al, Screening for lung cancer with CT: a preliminary cost-effectiveness analysis. Chest 2002; 121: 1507–14.

58. Mahadevia PJ, Fleisher LA, Frick KD, et al, Lung cancer screening with helical computed tomography in older adult smokers: a decision and cost-effectiveness analysis. JAMA 2003; 289: 313–22.

59. Henschke CI, Yankelevitz DF, Smith JP, et al, CT screening for lung cancer: assessing a regimen's diagnostic performance. Clinical Imaging 2004; 28:317–21.

60. Pasterino U, Bellomi M, Landoni C, et al, Early lung-cancer detection with spiral CT and positron emission tomography in heavy smokers: 2-year results. Lancet 2003; 362:593–7.

61. Li F, Sone S, Abe H, MacMahon H, Doi K, Low-dose computed tomography screening for lung cancer in a general population: characteristics of cancer in non-smokers versus smokers. Acad Radiol 2003; 10:1013–20.

62. Noguchi M, Moricawa A, Kawasaki M, et al, Small adenocarcinoma of the lung. Histologic characterisation and prognosis. Cancer 1995; 75: 2844–52.

63. Sobue T, Moriyama N, Kaneko M, et al,

Screening for lung cancer with low-dose helical computed tomography: anti-lung cancer association project. J Clin Oncol 2002; 20:911–20.

64. Nawa T, Nakagawa T, Kusano S, et al, Lung cancer screening using low-dose spiral CT. Chest 2002; 122:15–20.

65. Henschke CI, Yankelivitz MD, Faroogi MBBS, et al, Lung cancers diagnosed under annual repeat CT screening in the ELCAP. Radiological Society of North America Scientific Abstract. Chicago, IL, December 2, 2003.

66. Henschke CI, Miettinen OS, Women's susceptibility to tobacco carcinogens. Lung Cancer 2004; 43:1–5.

67. National Lung Screening Trial. Website: http://cancer.gov/nlst and http://acrin.org.

68. Frija G, Flahault A, Lemarie E, Spiral CT: is it time for lung cancer screening? Bull Acad Natl Med 2003; 187(1):153–60. Website: http//www.u444.jussieu.fr/depiscan.

69. Fontana RS, Sanderson DR, Woolner LB, et al, Screening for lung cancer: A critique of the Mayo Lung Project. Cancer 1991; 67:1155–64.

70. Kimmel M, Gorlova OY, Henschke CI, Modeling lung cancer screening. In: Edler L, Kitsos C (eds) Quantitative Methods for Cancer and Human Health Risk Assessment. Wiley and Sons, New York, 2005.

71. Black WC, Overdiagnosis: An underrecognized cause of confusion and harm in cancer screening (Editorial). J Natl Cancer Inst 2000; 92:1–6.

72. Marcus PM, Bergstralh EJ, Fagerstrom RM, et al, Lung cancer mortality in the Mayo Lung Project: Impact of extended follow-up. J Natl Cancer Inst 2000; 92:1308–16.

73. Sobue T, Nakayama T, Re: Lung cancer mortality in the Mayo Lung Project: impact of extended follow-up. UNCI 2001; 93:320–1.

74. Gorlova OY, Kimmel M, Henschke C, Modeling of long-term screening for lung cancer. Cancer 2001; 92:1531–40.

75. Dominioni L, Imperatori A, Rovera F. Paolucci M, Paddeu A, The fairy-tale of overdiagnosis of lung cancer. Website: http://www.predica.it/forum_02.pdf.

76. Epler GR, Screening for lung cancer. Is it worthwhile? Postgrad Med 1990; 87:181–6.

77. Dominioni L, Strauss GM, Consensus statement. International Conference on Prevention and Early Diagnosis of Lung Cancer, Varese, Italy. Cancer 2000; 89:2329–30.

78. Jackson VP, Screening mammography: controversies and headlines. Radiology 2002; 225:323–6.

79. Miettinen OS, Henschke CI, Pasmantier MW, et al, Mammographic screening: No reliable supporting evidence? Lancet 2002; 359:404–5.

80. Miettinen OS, Henschke CI, Pasmantier MW, et al, Mammographic screening: No reliable supporting evidence? www.Lancet.com Feb 2, 2002.

81. Miettinen OS, Yankelevitz DF, Henschke CI, Evaluation of screening for a cancer: annotated catechism of the Gold Standard creed. J Evaluation Clin Pract 2003; 9:145–50.

82. Smith RA, von Eschenback AD, Wender R, et al, American Cancer Society guidelines for the early detection of cancer: update of early detection guidelines for prostate, colorectal, and endometrial cancer; also update 2001 – testing for early lung cancer detection. CA Cancer J Clin 2001; 51:38–75.

83. Humphrey LL, Johnson M, Teutsch S, Lung cancer screening with sputum cytologic examination, chest radiography, and computed tomography: an update of the U.S. Preventive Services Task Force. Ann Intern Med 2004; 140:738-53. Also on http://ahrg.gov/clinic/cps3dix.htm.

84. Strauss GM, Dominioni L, Jett JR, et al, Como International Conference Position Statement. Chest 2005; 127:1146–51.

13 New directions in spiral CT image processing and computer-aided diagnosis

Anthony P Reeves, Andinet A Enquobahrie

Contents Introduction • Visualization • Detection • Characterization • Documentation and health evaluation • Discussion • Conclusion

INTRODUCTION

Recent developments in computer image analysis methods and the ongoing technical development in CT scanners will significantly impact diagnostic radiology. The methods in which computer analysis may assist the physician in the context of CT images of the lung are discussed with a particular focus on lung cancer. Future directions that may be anticipated once these computer methods mature are also discussed.

Domains of computer methods for image analysis

From the initial realization of CT scanners, and other electronic imaging modalities, the computer has been an integral part of the imaging system. The fundamental images that the physician reviews are the result of applying computer algorithms to the raw CT data; the raw data by themself are not suitable for viewing the organs of the body or diagnosing disease. Modern computer methods offer several additional capabilities as follows:

1. Image visualization: by providing different viewing options the computer may present images to the radiologist in a more convenient form for diagnosis in such a way that anatomic relationships may be more easily recognized and that abnormalities and disease may be more readily perceived and identified.

2. Detection: the computer may be used to automatically detect lung nodules, especially in typical situations where whole-lung scans consist of many (hundreds) images and the nodule is small and may only be visible on one image.

3. Characterization: the computer may make measurements on a nodule to determine its malignancy status. Currently the most accurate non-invasive method for predicting malignancy in small nodules is based on determining growth rate from the change in nodule volume in two time-separated scans.

4. Abnormality documentation and treatment evaluation: When there are many nodules present, the computer is ideal for the tedious task of cataloging and documentation. Furthermore, for treatment evaluation, the computer may be used to quantitatively measure the overall treatment response in the entire lung.

CT images of the lung

The lung is a particularly receptive organ for CT image analysis because of the inherent natural contrast between the abnormalities, that typically show up as brighter image regions on the 'dark' lung parenchyma background; this is in contrast to other organs in which the contrast is much less and the delineation of abnormal tissue is typically more difficult. On the other hand, the lung presents unique challenges due to its compressible nature. Image analysis is complicated, for example, by change in patient position, degree of inspiration, heart motion image artifacts and body movement image artifacts.

CT technology has made considerable advances over the last decade providing both better information and new challenges for the radiologist. Modern, multi-slice scanners can obtain many more images in a single breath hold. Consequently, the radiologist is confronted with the task of examining several hundred images for a single whole-lung scan rather than the tens of images characteristic of older scanners. Furthermore, these images are now performed with a view towards using low-dose protocols, particularly in the domain of lung cancer screening, which means that there is more image noise, making the reading more difficult. However, for computer analysis, the thinner slices provide a tremendous opportunity for considering the CT scan as a single three-dimensional (3D) image rather than the traditional viewpoint of a set of individual two-dimensional images. Computer methods can use true three-dimensional geometric analysis, which is more powerful, simpler and more direct than the two-dimensional counterpart.

For three-dimensional geometrical techniques to be used, the 3D image must have close to isotropic voxel size. That is, the resolution in the axial direction (slice thickness) must be similar to the in-plane resolution (pixel size). For example, a typical whole-lung image has a pixel size of about 0.6×0.6 mm. If the slice-thickness is 10 mm then there is an anisotropic mismatch of 10 mm to 0.6 mm or about 18 to 1.

For a 1 mm slice thickness the ratio is 1 to 0.6 or about 1.8 to 1. The most recent multi-slice scanners are offering 0.5 mm slice thickness in which the ideal 1 to 1 ratio is achievable.

Benefits of computer-aided diagnosis

The main benefits of computer-aided image analysis will be realized when quantitative methods are used for measuring and classifying image characteristics. Image visualization, where the computer provides a more convenient presentation of the image data, has been the more traditional use of computer assistance; however, such a qualitative approach leaves the image analysis and decision making entirely up to the radiologist. In contrast, quantitative data analysis can provide four major benefits to the radiologist.

1. More accurate and repeatable measurements: The computer does not suffer from fatigue and will consistently use the same measurement algorithm with the same parameters every time it is applied. In contrast, the human uses a number of subjective judgments in making measurements and there are many sources of measurement variation. However, the computer occasionally makes errors in locating the correct boundary for a region of interest. Therefore, a good strategy is to have the human observe the decisions made by computer and to manually override the measurement process when any incorrect computer decisions are observed.

2. Large database for diagnosis: Diagnosis by computer involves comparing the quantitative information from an image with knowledge of all previous examples that the computer has information in its database. There are many ways that this 'knowledge' may be recorded in the computer, from a set of actual images to a

set of derived measurement parameters. However the data are organized, the general result is that the larger the knowledge database (in terms of number of cases) the better the quality of the computer diagnosis. Given that memory to store these cases is no longer a major consideration for modern computer technology, we may anticipate that performance of computer diagnosis methods will continue to improve with time. Compare this to the physician, who must typically make a judgment based on their own personal experience, with a tendency to give greater weight to those cases that may have had unanticipated outcomes.

3. Management of large data sets: The computer is an excellent data manager, ideally suited to the tedious task of documenting all the abnormalities that may be present in a single whole-lung scan. Furthermore, it is equally well suited to matching two time-separated whole-lung scans and documenting the changes that have occurred in the period between them. For the radiologists this is an arduous time-consuming task that is difficult to perform consistently over long periods of time.

4. Evaluation of all the image data: Modern imaging technology can now provide far more data than the radiologist can examine in a reasonable amount of time. Computers are ideal for examining every region of the image data in the greatest possible detail without suffering any loss of performance due to fatigue.

In the following we first consider recent advances in the 'qualitative' image visualization. We then consider the advantages of using quantitative methods for detection, characterization and general documentation.

VISUALIZATION

Unlike chest radiographs, the original standard for chest radiography, the visualization of CT images has always required computer assistance in the form of digital reconstruction algorithms, even when the images are presented to the radiologist on film. In order to acquire the CT image data, several parameters including the dose and slice thickness need to be pre-established. However, to view a CT image, a radiologist must specify a number of post hoc parameters once the raw CT image data have been acquired. These parameters include brightness and contrast (level and window), spatial enhancement and the field of view (magnification). The use of film fixes these parameters while the use of a soft copy computer display device permits the radiologist to modify these parameters in real time while viewing the image data.

The standard radiology soft-copy viewing station is designed to accommodate a range of imaging modalities. Constraints on projection images such as chest radiographs and mammograms require high resolution and a well-controlled viewing environment; hence most soft-copy systems are very costly and involve a special high-resolution grayscale monitor.

The viewing requirements for the high-contrast lung CT scans are, in general, less stringent than for projection images. Many standard PCs offer adequate quality for viewing CT image data especially for the characterization of previously identified nodules. Furthermore, they offer color as one means of drawing attention to regions of interest such as lung abnormalities. Standard computer graphics methods coupled with simple computer analysis offer alternative modes for viewing CT image data. Vendors are introducing such methods. Acceptance of these methods by radiologists has been rather slow;

possibly one factor here is the difficulty in incorporating such techniques on the traditional high-resolution, grayscale, soft-copy workstations.

To illustrate some of the visualization options, we can consider the visualization of a single lung nodule. In Figure 13.1, a conventional axial CT image of the lung is shown with a 6 mm nodule outlined in the left lung. This is the conventional visualization supported by all scanners and soft-copy workstations. In Figure 13.2, we show all the image slices through that nodule at the same time in a montage display. Figure 13.3 shows an alternative method of viewing these data using standard computer-graphics techniques. A visualization is generated to resemble how the nodule might look if it were perfectly extracted from the lung, if it had a perfect reflecting matt surface, and if it was illuminated by a single simple light source with

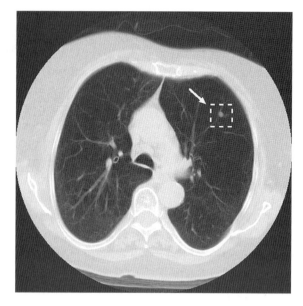

Figure 13.1
Axial CT image with a small pulmonary nodule outlined. (Courtesy of the Early Lung Cancer Action Program, Cornell University, New York.)

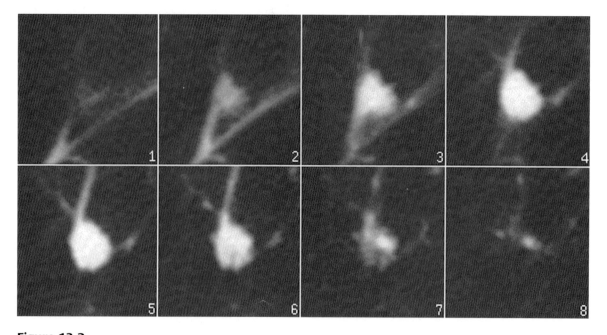

Figure 13.2
Consecutive 1 mm image slices through the nodule shown in Figure 13.1. (Courtesy of the Early Lung Cancer Action Program, Cornell University, New York.)

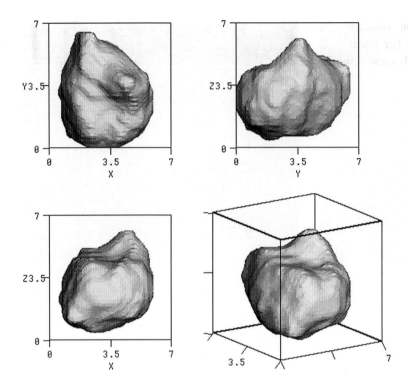

Figure 13.3
3D reconstructions of the nodule shown in Figure 13.2 rendered from three orthogonal viewing directions: axial (top left), sagittal (top right) and coronal (lower left) and one oblique (lower right) viewing direction. (Courtesy of the Early Lung Cancer Action Program, Cornell University, New York.)

some uniform background illumination. Since this method involves creating a three-dimensional model of the nodule (which is made possible by the isotropic property of the thin slice scan), the nodule may be viewed from different viewpoints, rather than just the conventional axial direction. On a viewing workstation the nodule may be rotated and viewed from any arbitrary direction. In Figure 13.3, visualizations from the three canonical viewpoints: axial, sagittal, and coronal and an additional oblique view are provided.

A targeted reconstruction of the nodule in Figure 13.1 is shown in Figure 13.4. The visualization of that nodule using standard solid-modeling techniques is shown in Figure 13.5, where computer algorithms to identify the nodule region itself have colorized the other dense image objects in the lung according to their

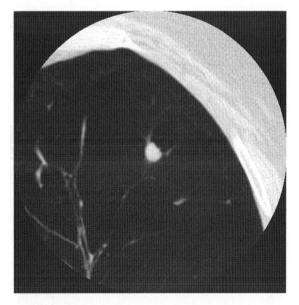

Figure 13.4
Conventional targeted study image of a small solid pulmonary nodule. (Courtesy of the Early Lung Cancer Action Program, Cornell University, New York.)

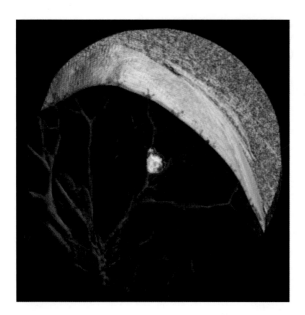

Figure 13.5
Color-coded ray-traced rendering of the nodule shown in Figure 13.4. (Courtesy of the Early Lung Cancer Action Program, Cornell University, New York.)

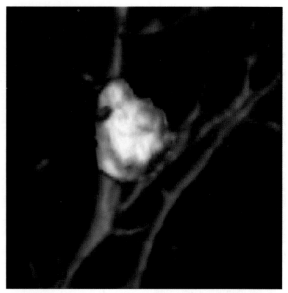

Figure 13.6
Magnified view of nodule shown in Figure 13.5. (Courtesy of the Early Lung Cancer Action Program, Cornell University, New York.)

geometric form, hence using color to highlight the region of prime interest to the radiologist. A magnified image of the nodule is shown in Figure 13.6.

In Figure 13.7A a CT image of a non-solid nodule or GGO (ground-glass opacity) is shown. For this important nodule type, there is a distinctive difference in density between the non-solid material and other solid tissue (e.g. vessels and chest wall). In order to visualize the non-solid tissue we use a translucent rendering method as shown in Figure 13.7B. The inter-action between the vessels and the nodule can now be seen. Further, we can remove the vessels from consideration as shown in Figure 13.7C in order to have an unobstructed view of the whole nodule's shape.

While visualization is important, especially for the correct interpretation of image data by radiologists, the real power of the computer is in the *quantitative* analysis of the data to directly determine clinically relevant information. The visualizations in Figure 13.3 show renderings of a geometrical model of a nodule, derived from the nodule size measurements extracted by the computer segmentation process. That is, these renderings are derived from the quantitative analysis while the other (ray-tracing and direct image viewing) renderings are computed without explicit segmentation and from which measurements cannot be made.

DETECTION

A computer assistant for detection will examine a whole-lung CT scan for any evidence of pulmonary nodules and will report the location of

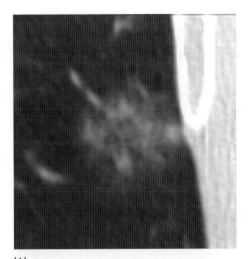

(A)

Figure 13.7
Visualization of a non-solid nodule: CT image (A), Rendered as a translucent blue region with vessels marked in red (B), and with vessels removed (C). (Courtesy of the Early Lung Cancer Action Program, Cornell University, New York.)

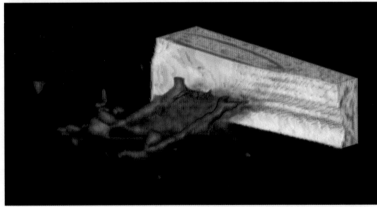

(B)

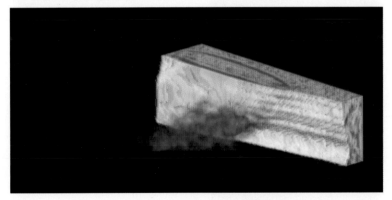

(C)

suspected nodules to the radiologist. One method of presentation is to highlight regions of the scan as the radiologist sequentially views the scan images. An alternative more-focused method of presentation is illustrated in Figure 13.8. The locations of nodule candidates as identified by the CAD detection system are superimposed on a simulated coronal projection image. The radiologist can then move directly to the image view (as illustrated in Figure 13.1) by clicking the mouse on each nodule candidate in turn. The radiologist then determines whether to discount the candidate from further consideration or to view additional 'characterization' analysis as described in the following section.

Following the lead from mammography CAD, R2 has FDA approval to use the computer detection results as a 'second read'. That is, once the radiologist has performed a conventional sequential reading of the scan the computer will highlight possible nodule candidates that have not been documented by the radiologist. The radiologist will then examine these locations with a view to modifying his or her report. Future systems are likely to integrate the CAD process with the primary radiology reading; however, methodology to assess the usefulness of this approach is a topic of active research.

The critical issue for a detection system is that it must be sensitive enough to detect essentially all the nodules without indicating too many false alarms (false positives). To achieve this performance the detection algorithm must have both a high sensitivity and specificity; furthermore, a 'sensitivity' parameter will need to be set to fix the sensitivity/specificity tradeoff to the optimal value for a given clinical reading task.

Of importance to a detection system is the definition of a nodule or a reportable event. In general, large nodules are easier to identify for both the radiologist and the machine. The task of nodule identification becomes increasingly more difficult as the nodule size approaches the voxel size of the scanner. Furthermore, as nodules of a smaller size are being detected and

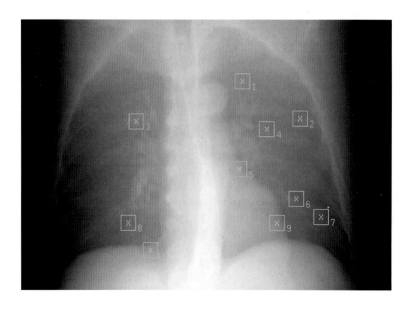

Figure 13.8
Nodule candidate locations on a coronal projection image of the lungs.

characterized, there is a higher probability of benign nodules for the smaller sizes. In the context of lung cancer screening, clinically relevant nodules are currently considered to be in the 3 mm to 3 cm size range. In addition other lung abnormalities may be of interest to the radiologist, and the issue of reporting these abnormalities should be addressed.

A number of commercial products are now available for nodule detection, nevertheless, this remains an active area of research and new methods continue to be developed. The basic algorithms currently available for nodule detection[1-8] need to be optimized before they will be useful in the general clinical setting. For example, the specification of exactly what abnormalities are to be reported, and the appropriate size and sensitivity settings commenserate with acceptable rates of false positives for clinical use must be determined.

A current barrier to the development of detection CAD systems is the need for large documented databases of whole-lung CT scans for system training and evaluation. Establishing these databases requires a large amount of resources, as do any clinical trials that are needed to evaluate the performance of a radiologist–CAD system combination. Most of the work in this field suffers from this limitation. This was the driving motivation behind the NCI's Lung Imaging Database Consortium (LIDC); a consortium of institutions whose mission is to make a publicly accessible database of well documented nodules available to the imaging community. As technology improves and more experience is gained, it is anticipated that future methods will achieve a significant improvement with respect to sensitivity and specificity.

CHARACTERIZATION

The computer may aid the physician in a number of different ways for characterizing the detected nodule; beyond a variety of special visualizations, it may provide quantitative measurements on that nodule for the physician to interpret or it may perform a classification on these measurements (based on a large number of previously diagnosed nodules) to directly determine the probability of malignancy.

The basic procedure for nodule characterization is:

(a) Segmentation: Determining which voxels belong to the nodule and which do not.
(b) Feature extraction: Making quantitative measurement on the nodule voxels.
(c) Diagnosis/classification: Determining the probability of malignancy from a statistical analysis of the extracted features.

Two basic methods have been explored to determine the malignancy status of a nodule by computer evaluation: (a) shape features and (b) size change. In the shape feature method a number of measurements are made on the nodule voxels from a CT scan and these features are used to predict malignancy via a classifier that has been trained on a database consisting of documented malignant and benign nodules. This method has been explored in research settings and while the initial results are quite promising,[9-13] more research is needed. The second method is to measure growth rate from the nodule volume change in two time-separated CT scans. In preliminary studies[14-16] a rapid growth rate has been found to be an excellent predictor of malignancy. However, this approach has the drawbacks of requiring a second CT scan and the delay in diagnosis caused by the required time period between scans.

CT manufacturers and other vendors are now providing 3D nodule growth estimation tools. Issues with this approach are (a) the two scans must be of a high quality and recorded with the same CT scan parameters, and (b) the time delay between scans must be long enough to obtain a sufficiently accurate measurement to predict malignancy but this delay needs to be minimized to reduce patient anxiety. For current CT scanner technology this optimal time period may be several months for small nodules reducing to perhaps less than a month for larger (1 cm) nodules.

DOCUMENTATION AND HEALTH EVALUATION

Beyond detecting and measuring nodules, the computer system should also be capable of facilitating other operations such as whole-lung health monitoring and automated nodule cataloging. This is especially important for repeat scans either in a screening or treatment scenario. This operation, in itself, does not require any new technological developments; rather it requires the development of a patient management system that goes beyond conventional Radiology Information Systems (RIS). For example, we have built into our data management system a whole-lung volume and emphysema analysis capability. The computer automatically delineates the

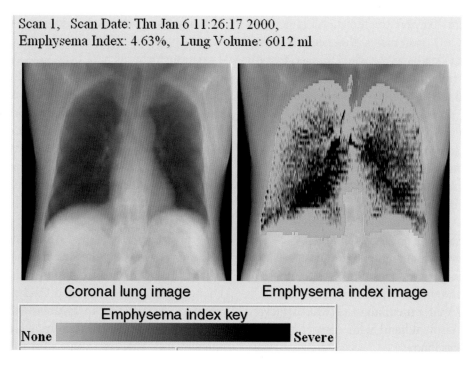

Figure 13.9
Emphysema visualization on a coronal projection of the lungs. (Courtesy of the Early Lung Cancer Action Program, Cornell University, New York.)

whole-lung parenchyma region from the CT images and computes the lung volume. In addition, an analysis of the density distribution of the lung parenchyma is computed to allow visualization of the spatial distribution of emphysema. The outcome of this analysis presented in the coronal plane is shown in Figure 13.9. Whole-lung analysis of this type may be automatically applied to all CT scans prior to physician evaluation on a routine basis.

DISCUSSION

Recently developed computer methods have been used to enhance the visualization of CT images for diagnostic purposes and to provide quantitative measurements on these images. It is in the latter respect that computer methods are most powerful as a diagnostic tool.

There are many improvements, both quantitative and qualitative, to be anticipated from an anatomical analysis of the chest CT. Algorithms have been developed for the automatic segmentation of major anatomical regions from chest CT scans; however, we anticipate that future algorithm development will result in the automatic segmentation of all major bone and soft tissue regions in the thorax. The lung regions themselves are easily extracted, as are the trachea, major bronchi and major blood vessels.

CAD methodology

To anticipate the way the future may evolve, it is instructive to consider how CAD systems are developed. Solving problems using conventional artificial intelligence methods requires knowledge about the problem at hand and a specific method of applying that knowledge to an instance of the problem. For most CAD systems the 'knowledge' is defined by a set of example cases that are documented by the best information available. For

example, for lung cancer characterization, lung scans with lesions identified that have been proven to be cancer and lung scans with lesions that have proven to be benign would be the knowledge examples. The knowledge engineer takes these samples, plus any other information from an expert on the problem (e.g., a chest radiologist in this case) and develops a suitable set of features to be extracted from the data and the best method to classify these features into a decision (probability of cancer).

Most classification algorithms provide a numerical output that relates to the probability of a positive classification. A sensitivity parameter is set to indicate a 'yes' or 'no' decision. Increasing the sensitivity usually diminishes the specificity of the decision (as sensitivity is increased more lesions are correctly identified as cancer but also more benign lesions are labeled as cancer). An optimal operating point needs to be set to match the competing risks for any given clinical situation.

CAD system performance evaluation

To evaluate the performance of a CAD system, a dataset of documented test images is typically used. The actual performance *sensitivity* (fraction of cancers correctly labeled as cancer) and *specificity* (fraction of benign lesions labeled as benign) achieved for a given sensitivity parameter setting is known as an operating point. The performance for different operating points is typically plotted on a graph called a receiver operating characteristic (ROC) curve, where the axes are the normalized sensitivity (range 0–1) vs 1 – normalized specificity (range 0–1). A typical curve is shown in Figure 13.10A. Consider a characterization task in which, given a nodule, the problem is to indicate cancer or not cancer. The ROC curves for two different CAD systems are shown for a test set of nodules with known outcomes. Curves start at (0,0)

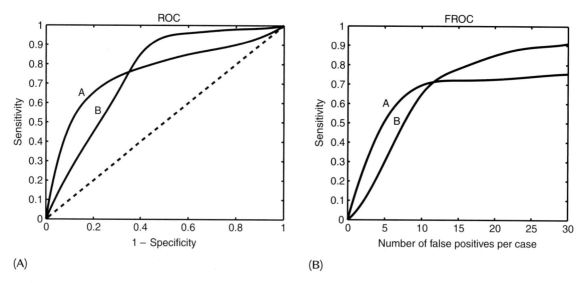

Figure 13.10
(A) ROC curves for two characterization systems and (B) FROC curves for two detection systems.

(no cancers identified) and end at (1,1) all nodules identified as cancer. In general, the closer that the curve approaches the (1,0) corner of the graph (all nodules correctly identified) the better the performance of the system. As a lower bound on performance, the diagonal (0,0 to 1,1) indicates the performance that would be expected by chance (i.e. using no problem knowledge such as flipping a coin to make a diagnosis). For the two CAD systems shown, we see that algorithm A is better than algorithm B when a low sensitivity operating point is selected while algorithm B has a better performance than algorithm A when a high-sensitivity operating point is selected.

The task of detecting cancer is different to the task of characterizing a nodule, since the number of locations that might be incorrectly identified as containing a nodule is essentially unbounded; hence, specificity cannot be simply normalized. The usual approach in this case is to plot sensitivity (fraction of known nodules detected) vs. number of false positives (loca-

tions identified as nodules that do not contain a nodule) as shown in Figure 13.10B; this curve is known as a free-response receiver operating characteristic or FROC curve. Usually this curve is plotted until the number of false positives exceeds a reasonable number for practical use (if the sensitivity has not reached 1.0).

The ROC and FROC curves are good ways of showing the performance options (locus of operating points) for a given validation dataset. There has been considerable research on estimating the relative performance of different CAD systems by derived measurements from the ROC curves such as computing the area under the curve (AUC), such methods for CAD should be used with care. For example, the AUCs for the two systems shown in Figure 13.10A are very similar; however the performances of the systems are significantly different for different clinical situations (selections of the sensitivity parameter).

In using ROC analysis it is very important to realize that the ROC curve is highly dependent on both the dataset being used for evaluation and the task of the system. As an example, Figure 13.11 shows a set of ROC curves for one of our experimental detection algorithms. Each curve corresponds to a different nodule size range. We see that for nodules 5 mm and above we achieve very high sensitivity at less than five false positives per case. If we try to detect smaller nodules, close in size to the slice thickness of the scans (2.5 mm in this case), then there are many more false positives; on the order of 30 per case for very high sensitivity. The dataset we used was taken sequentially from a cancer screening study of asymptomatic cases in which small nodules dominate. We would expect that the ROC curve for this same system would look very different if the database was taken from a general clinical practice, with different underlying clinical risk factors. Also the curves would be significantly different if the scans had been reconstructed with a different slice thickness.

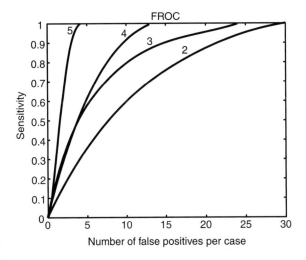

Figure 13.11
Detection FROC curves for different nodule size ranges.

Generalization

The key property of a CAD method is known as generalization; that is, how well does the system perform on a case that it has not seen before? This is a critical feature since there exist simple methods that will guarantee correct identification of all of the training cases, but may not do well on a different set of cases. The only way to correctly measure the useful performance of a CAD system is, therefore, to only evaluate it on cases that it has not seen before (i.e., cases that are not in the training dataset). In practice, great care is needed to maintain this separation; once a case has been used for training it cannot be used for evaluation.

In summary, the development of a CAD system involves an appropriate set of example data (documented cases) plus appropriate computer algorithms. The evaluation of CAD system requires a very well documented validation dataset that does not contain any cases that are in the training dataset.

How good can the CAD system be expected to perform compared to an expert physician with many years of experience? Much work is first needed to identify the most useful computer algorithms and to acquire the needed database of knowledge; however, as knowledge of the problem and its solution is acquired, the performance of the computer system continues to improve. An illustrative example of the development of a knowledge-based methodology is the academic exercise of computer chess. The computer chess problem was inspired by a presentation and paper by Claude Shannon in 1950[17] where the basic algorithm for solving the problem was presented. The first attempts at making computers play chess were very slow and naïve and, initially, computers would more often just play other computers. However, as more attention was given to the task, both the knowledge base and the computer technology (speed) improved dramatically over ensuing years. By 1983 a computer had reached national master level and in 1997, by careful engineering, an IBM supercomputer (Deep Blue) bested the world champion Grandmaster (Gary Kasparov).[18] More recently, a much more modest computer (Deep Junior) built on off-the-shelf parts has also proved to be a match for Kasparov. In time and with due attention, it is reasonable to assume that computers may match or surpass the world experts in many endeavors. Further, that once this capability has been achieved, it may be provided at a low cost to all who need it. Today, CAD systems are still at the very start of their development. The computer resources currently used for CAD are very small (typically, in the order of 0.001 of the cost of a CT scanner) and the large databases are yet to be developed.

What should the CAD datasets contain?

The validation dataset must be very carefully selected; a critical issue is how many cases should the dataset contain and, just as important, what types of cases should it contain. This is of prime interest to the FDA, as they are responsible for certifying that vendor's claims concerning a CAD system are valid. A further complication is the nature of the claim that vendors currently make and that, for now, the FDA finds acceptable. Usually the claim is that the product enhances the performance of the radiologist compared to using standard methods. To establish this claim a proactive clinical trial must be conducted in which the radiologist without CAD is compared to the radiologist using the CAD. There has been considerable interest in this area[19–23] and one vendor, R2, has obtained FDA approval for a nodule detection system based on 152 cases. In addition the selection of cases for the validation set is critically important. For example, if a CAD system is designed to detect nodules for a screening task then a test set consisting of nodules larger than 15 mm would not be appropriate. Addressing the question what would be the best distribution of nodule types would require understanding the frequency of the different nodules that would be anticipated in clinical practice for the target application. Finally, we note that any validation for a dataset only applies to that dataset. It does not apply directly to a dataset that has a different subtype distribution or even different scanner parameters.

For the training dataset we can pose the question how much training is enough? To which the intuitive answer would be: the more training the better. And this is the case for CAD. Then the question becomes how much data can be used for training within a reasonable amount of time and effort. As training sets become large, the documentation costs and the computation resources required for training also becomes large. However, consider that when you make a web data search on Google you are in fact addressing a database that has over two billion documents indexed. Consequently, it is not unreasonable with current technology to consider a training set of millions of cases providing a significant number of examples for all subtypes of the target.

Currently CAD vendors sponsor the collection of training data and conduct a clinical trial to validate the trained CAD system; data collection and documentation is a very expensive part of product development, consequently, competing vendors are reluctant to share their data. There are two problems with this approach. First, the very expensive cost of product development limits the number of products that are developed. Second, since the dataset used by each vendor is different, the results cannot be directly compared with each other. ROC and FROC curves may be very different for different datasets.

The best way to move CAD forward would be to create a vast documented dataset available to all vendors for developing CAD systems, and maintaining a separate validation dataset that would have no overlap with the training dataset. Subsets of these datasets would be defined for different diseases and disease sub-types. These datasets would need to be continually updated to keep track with new technology (and disease) developments. Securing the necessary resources to establish these datasets requires a significant paradigm shift from current research funding practices. There have been some initial demonstration projects to promote this paradigm. The ELCAP group has provided web-access to a small set of documented lung scans so that for the first time, CAD research groups can report the performance of their systems with reference to a common standard dataset (http://www.via. cornell.edu/lungdb.html). As described earlier, the NIH funded Lung Image Database Consortium (LIDC) is a 5-year project involving five institutions to provide a pilot database of lung CT scans with careful documentation. The LIDC group has developed a process involving multiple radiologist reads for data documentation and plans to release its first documented scans through the NCI in the near future.[24] There are ongoing activities involving both the NIH and vendors focused on developing such datasets.

CONCLUSION

The computer may be used in a number of ways to aid the physician to interpret CT lung images. New visualization tools are being introduced to assist the radiologist in viewing the increasing amount of information resulting from evolving CT technology. At this time commercial CAD tools are becoming available to assist the radiologist in the detection of nodules and in growth-rate determination and hence cancer diagnosis. When used correctly, these tools can improve the performance of the radiologist and provide superior quantitative analysis of the data leading to a more timely and accurate diagnosis for lung cancer. A further advantage is the workflow management component of these tools. The management of a large number of small nodules and the matching of these nodules from scan to scan, which is essential for lung cancer evaluation, can be highly automated; this is one of the major benefits of these tools. In the near future the release of additional tools that permit evaluation of other aspects of lung health may be anticipated.

Current systems are only a preview of systems that will ultimately be developed. Like the pioneering flights by the Wright brothers at Kitty Hawk, these prototype systems give insight as to what may be ahead including much needed further development. These systems may also be very useful in clinical practice when used with due care. What are needed are resources for the development of computer methods and for the creation of shared datasets; a new medical research paradigm. What are not needed are extensive clinical trials on the efficacy of current CAD systems since, at this stage of CAD technology any such system should be significantly improved before the results of the trial are known.

For the future we can anticipate that CT scanners will provide far more data than current systems such that the concept of the radiologist carefully reviewing every image is simply impractical (in fact this is already the case with many multislice scanners, wherein images are reconstructed with lower resolution than they are acquired). Rather, computer analysis will be more integrated into the reading process than it already is and the physician may be presented with just a summary of the CAD results plus selected image visualizations. The task of the radiologist for lung cancer then returns back to diagnosing disease rather than identifying and measuring tiny nodules. One example of how a CAD device may reduce the physician's workload is the AutoPap system[25] which in 1998 received FDA approval to be used as an automated primary screening device for Pap smear samples. With this device the pathologist only has to evaluate samples that the device identifies as potentially problematic; this frees the pathologist from evaluating samples that the device determines are not potentially problematic.

Computer assistance has been more readily embraced in arenas other than medicine such as manufacturing industry and the military. Experience gained from these other areas would indicate that at some point we can anticipate that the performance of the CAD system will exceed the performance of the typical human physician (as computer systems have already done, for example, in the playing of chess, and in many other human endeavors), and ultimately it will match and perhaps exceed the performance of the most experienced physicians. At that time, the concept of providing the best possible care for all patients becomes much closer to a reality.

REFERENCES

1. Lee Y, Hara T, Fujita H, Itoh S, Ishigaki T, Automated detection of pulmonary nodules in helical CT images based on an improved template-matching technique. IEEE Trans Med Imaging 2001; 20(7):595–604.

2. Fan L, Qian J, Ordy B, et al, Automatic segmentation of pulmonary nodules by using dynamic 3D cross-correlation for interactive CAD systems. Proceedings of the SPIE 2002; 4648: 1362–9.

3. Taguchi H, Kawata Y, Niki N, et al, Lung cancer detection based on helical CT images using curved surface morphology analysis. SPIE Conference on Image Processing 1999; 3661: 1307–14.

4. McCulloch CC, Kaucic RA, Mendonca PRS, Walter DJ, Avila RS, Model-based detection of lung nodules in computed tomography exams. Acad Radiology 2004; 11:258–66.

5. Wiemker R, Rogalla P, Zwartkruis A, Blaffert T, Computer aided lung nodule detection on high resolution CT data. Proceedings of the SPIE 2002; 4684:677–88.

6. Arimura H, Katsuragawa S, Suzuki K, et al, Computerized scheme for automated detection of lung nodules in low-dose computed tomography images for lung cancer screening. Acad Radiology 2004; 11:617–29.

7. Lu X, Wei G, Qian J, Jain AK, Learning-based pulmonary nodule detection from multislice CT data. 18th International Congress of CARS 2004.

8. Enquobahrie AA, Reeves AP, Yankelevitz DF, Henschke CI, Automated detection of pulmonary nodules from whole lung CT scans: Performance comparison for isolated and attached nodules. Proceedings of the SPIE 2004; 5370:791–800.

9. Reeves AP, Kostis WJ, Yankelevitz DF, Henschke CI, Three-dimensional shape characterization of solitary pulmonary nodules from helical CT scans. In: Lemke HU, Vannier MW, Inamura K, Farman AG (eds) Proceedings of Computer Assisted Radiology and Surgery (CARS '99). Elsevier Science, June, 1999, 83–7.

10. Sluimer IC, Van Waes PF, Viergever MA, Van Ginneken B, Computer-aided diagnosis in high resolution CT of the lungs. Medical Physics 2003; 30(12):3081–90.

11. McNitt-Gray MF, Wyckoff N, Goldin JG, Sayre JW, Aberle DR, Computer-aided diagnosis of the solitary pulmonary nodule imaged on CT: 2D, 3D and contrast enhancement features. Proceedings of SPIE 2001; 4322:1845–52.

12. Ichikawa W, Kawata Y, Niki N, et al, Classification experiments of pulmonary nodules using

high resolution CT images. Proceedings of SPIE 2002; 4684:1280–91.

13. Armato SG, Altman MB, Wilkie J, et al, Automated lung nodule classification following automated nodule detection on CT: A serial approach. Medical Physics 2003; 30(6):1188–97.

14. Yankelevitz DF, Reeves AP, Kostis WJ, Zhao B, Henschke CI, CT evaluation of small pulmonary nodules based on volumetrically determined growth rates. Radiology 2000; 217:251–6.

15. Kostis WJ, Reeves AP, Yankelevitz DF, Henschke CI, Three-dimensional segmentation and growth-rate estimation of small pulmonary nodules in helical CT images. IEEE Trans Med Imaging 2003; 22(10):1259–74.

16. Kostis WJ, Yankelevitz DF, Reeves AP, Fluture SC, Henschke CI, Small pulmonary nodules: Reproducibility of three-dimensional volumetric, measurement and estimation of time to follow-up CT. Radiology 2004; 231:446–52.

17. Shannon CE, Programming computer for playing chess. Philosophical Magazine 1950; 41:256–75.

18. Hsu F-H, Computer chess, then and now: The Deep Blue Saga. Proceedings of International Symposium for VLSI Technology, Systems and Applications, 1997, 153–6.

19. Wagner RF, Beiden SV, Campbell G, Metz CE, Sacks WM, Assessment of medical imaging and computer-assist system. Acad Radiology 2002; 9:1264–77.

20. Beiden SV, Wagner RF, Doi K, et al, Independent versus sequential reading in ROC studies of computer-assist modalities, Acad Radiology 2002; 9:1036–43.

21. Dodd LE, Wagner RF, Armato SG, et al, Assessment methodologies and statistical issues for computer-aided diagnosis of lung nodules in computed tomography. Acad Radiology 2004; 11:462–75.

22. Beiden SV, Maloof MA, Wagner RF, A general model for finite-sample effects in training and testing of competing classifiers. IEEE Transactions on Pattern Analysis and Machine Intelligence 2003; 1(1):1–9.

23. Wagner RF, Beiden SV, Campbell G, Metz CE, Sacks WM, Contemporary issues for experimental design in assessment of medical imaging and computer-assist systems. Proceedings of the SPIE 2003; 5034:213–24.

24. Armato SG, McLennan G, McNitt-Gray MF, et al, Lung Image Database Consortium: developing a resource for the medical imaging research community. Radiology 2004; 232(3):739–48.

25. Wilbur DC, Prey MU, Miller WM, Pawlick GF, Colgan TJ, The AutoPap system for primary screening in cervical cytology. Comparing the results of a prospective, intended-use study with routine manual practice. Acta Cytol 1998; 42(1):214–20.

14 Diagnostic workup of screen-detected lesions

David E Midthun, Stephen J Swensen, James R Jett

Contents   Introduction • Nodule detection • False-positive findings • Baseline versus new nodule • Age • Smoking • Nodule characteristics • Ground-glass opacities • What to do? • Observation • Further imaging • Positron emission tomography • Magnetic resonance (MR) • Biopsy • Surgical resection • Future directions

INTRODUCTION

The goal of computed tomography (CT) screening is to detect lung cancer at an earlier stage when intervention may be more likely to lead to cure. Toward achieving this goal, the desire is to identify cancers when they are small and before they have developed nodal or distant metastases. CT is inherently limited in detection of early, centrally located airway cancers. Consequently, nearly all screen-detected early-stage cancers will be identified nodular opacities in the parenchyma. As cancer growth requires time, and assuming similar growth rates, a smaller nodular cancer implies it is earlier in development than a larger one. The desire to detect small cancers is made problematic by the potential number of small benign lesions from which the malignant ones require identification. Herein lies the crux of the problem presented to the clinician or researcher evaluating the patient or participant who has been screened. Optimal evaluation of screen-detected lesions identifies cancer with haste and avoids resection of benign lesions.

The results of prospective single-arm studies in various countries show rates of nodule detection at baseline screening ranges from 5–60% in participants at high risk for lung cancer.[1–9] In contrast, annual repeat scanning lowers the rate of non-calcified nodule detection to 3–18%.[5,6,8,10,11] Whether at base line or subsequent annual scanning, CT screening frequently results in the need for decisions regarding nodule management. Optimal management of nodules of various sizes and character is in evolution. This chapter seeks to examine the current literature of relevance to the diagnostic workup of lesions detected by CT screening and to identify the issues required to further our understanding.

NODULE DETECTION

Critical to decision making in management of screen-detected nodules is the assessment of likelihood of malignancy. As long as radiology is the means of screening, to be detected a nodule has to be seen. An important aspect of likelihood of malignancy is specifically how the nodule was detected. A nodule detected on chest X-ray screening would be of higher concern for malignancy than a nodule detected on CT screening. In reporting the results of chest X-ray screening in the Johns Hopkins study, Frost et al reported that of 10 387 baseline chest roentgenograms, 82% were negative for cancer, 1518 (15%) were indeterminate, and 57 (0.5%) were suspicious for cancer.[12] Of the 57 participants with chest roentgenograms suspicious for cancer, 34 (60%) did demonstrate cancer; whereas, only 35 (2%) of the 1518 radiographs described as indeterminate were later confirmed to be a cancer. In contrast, CT screening studies have shown much lower rates of malignancy among detected nodules, ranging from 1% to 12%.[3–9]

Although CT is less specific, it is much more sensitive than CXR in detecting lung cancer (Figure 14.1). The initial report of CT screening by Kaneko showed that 11 of the 15 cases of lung cancer detected by CT were missed by simultaneous chest X-ray.[2] Similarly, the study by Sone et al found 19 peripheral lung cancers detected by CT at baseline and only four of these were visible on chest X-ray.[1] CT obviously increases the detection of cancer over chest X-ray but also increases the detection of benign nodules, thereby reducing the likelihood of malignancy among nodules detected. An understanding of the algorithm used to screen with CT is important in assessing subsequent likelihood of malignancy.

Sensitivity and specificity of low-dose spiral CT and conventional-dose CT for detecting lung nodules are comparable.[13] The nodule detection rates vary among prospective studies of low-dose CT and can be explained by differences in slice thickness or collimation (Table 14.1) and the number of detectors used. Both the Kaneko and Sone studies used 10 mm collimation as well; Kaneko reported that 17% had abnormal shadows, and Sone reported 5% had CT findings described as suspicious or indeterminate.[1,2] Baseline scanning in the Early Lung Cancer Action Project (ELCAP) revealed presence of non-calcified nodules of various sizes in 23% of the 1000 participants studied.[3] The ELCAP algorithm used 10-mm collimation and single detector scanning and radiologists viewed images on films. Cine viewing of images on workstations results in detection of 30% more nodules than viewing the same images on film.[14,15] Nawa et al reported finding one or more baseline nodules detected in 26% of nearly 8000 participants screened and also used 10-mm collimation.[5] Higher rates of nodule detection have been reported using 5 mm collimation. The Mayo Clinic study found that 51%

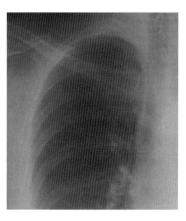

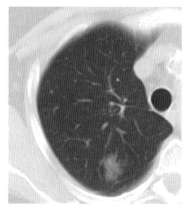

Figure 14.1
Nodule detection with CT is much more sensitive than chest radiography. (A) Normal coned view of the right upper lobe (RUL). (B) CT done within a day of the radiograph shows a ground-glass nodule in the RUL that was an adenocarcinoma with bronchoalveolar features at resection.

(A)   (B)

Table 14.1 Nodule detection: effect of slice thickness

Study	# Participants	# Non-calcified nodules at baseline	Participants with nodules	CT collimation
Kaneko[2]	1369	588*	17%	10 mm
Sone[1]	3967	217**	5%	10 mm
ELCAP[3,10]	1000	233	23%	10 mm
Nawa[5]	7956	2099	26%	10 mm
Diederich[7]	817	350	43%	5 mm
Mayo[4]	1520	782	51%	5 mm
McWilliams[9]	561	431	36%	7 mm
			60%	1.25 mm

*CT findings described as abnormal shadows.
**CT findings described as suspicious or indeterminate.

of the 1520 participants had one or more non-calcified nodules at baseline and used 5-mm collimation at 3.5-mm overlap intervals as well as a 4-detector scanner.[4] Similarly, Diederich et al reported that 43% of 817 participants had one or more non-calcified nodules when scanned using 5-mm collimation.[7] Pastorino reported a lower rate of 19% non-calcified nodule detection using 5-mm collimation.[8] McWilliams et al reported that use of 1.25-mm collimation resulted in nodule detection in 60% of participants.[9] Studies using thinner slice thickness and soft copy viewing generally show more nodules and smaller nodules and, consequently, have a lower overall percentage of malignant nodules than do the studies using algorithms with larger slice thickness. The high rate of benign nodules on CT in high-risk patients does not appear to be due to granulomatous disease given high rates of detection in diverse geographic regions.

FALSE-POSITIVE FINDINGS

The desire to find earlier lung cancer as a small, parenchymal opacity puts sensitivity in direct conflict with specificity. Studies using 5-mm collimation for a screening algorithm report twice the nodule detection rate as 10-mm studies and it is unclear if this has resulted in even greater sensitivity for cancer detection. A discussion of the proposed efficacy of CT screening is not appropriate for this chapter; however, the potential high false-positive rate of CT screening has been one of the criticisms levied against the enthusiasm for the technique. Ideally, CT would identify every cancer present at the time of screening. The similarity of characteristics of benign and malignant nodules of small size does not allow malignant detection in isolation from detection of benign lesions. If the evolving technologic advances of CT lead to the detection of smaller and smaller malignancies at greater benefit to the patient, then it would appear that an increasing number of false-positives might be the good news rather than the bad news. Concern over high false-positive rates has led some investigators to propose changing the definition of a positive scan. By considering non-calcified nodules that are 3 mm or less as negative, the rate of false-positive scans can be reduced.[16] Unfortunately, some of these small nodules are malignant and considering all nodules of this size as 'negative' will increase the rate of false-negative scans. A false-negative scan would seem to be a much greater problem in the pursuit of early lung cancer than would be the false-positive scan. The impact of false-positive scans from small nodules can be mitigated with 1-year interval follow-up for nodules <4 mm.

In the baseline reporting of the ELCAP study, one of the 27 CT-detected cancers was 2–5 mm in size at detection, and upon annual repeat scanning, three of the seven CT-detected cancers were 5 mm at detection.[3] Within the baseline and repeat scanning results of the Mayo study, Swensen et al have reported that five of 40 lung cancers identified were less than 5 mm in diameter at initial detection.[17] As mentioned, the ideal screening study would have a zero false-negative rate. If we, by convention, decide that nodules of a few millimeters in size are to be considered negative, we will increase the number of false-negative scans. This concern is borne out in the results reported by Pastorino et al, wherein they considered non-calcified nodules of 5 mm or less in maximal diameter as negative.[8] Annual repeat scanning identified 11 cancers, and six of these were classified as benign or negative at baseline scanning because of their small size or inflammatory character. False-positives will occur with CT screening and false-positive rates may be high, but lowering these rates at the consequence of increasing the false-negative studies may not be appropriate.

The evaluation of screen-detected nodules needs to take into account the high prevalence of benign nodules. In the National Lung Screening Study (NLST) the very small nodule is considered as a 'micronodule'.[18] Perhaps it is semantics, but calling a 4 mm nodule a micronodule appears to be the more appropriate way to indicate the high likelihood of benignancy in nodules of this size rather than to consider it as negative. Perhaps CT follow-up at 1 year is all that is needed for the vast majority of nodules detected at CT screening, but this should be considered recommended follow-up. Calling a scan containing micronodules negative and starting anew at 12 months as though the nodules never existed risks missing the chance to see growth on the subsequent film.

BASELINE VERSUS NEW NODULE

Whether or not a nodule is detected on an initial, baseline scan or is detected on a subsequent scan may affect its likelihood of malignancy. Although studies to date have varied results, most show a significant increase in the likelihood of malignancy if a nodule is new (and not present in retrospect) at annual scanning compared to a nodule present at baseline (Table 14.2). In the ELCAP study, there were 233 baseline nodules in 1000 participants.[3] Twenty-seven nodules or 11.5% were proven malignant. On repeat annual scanning, there were 63 new nodules identified, and 23 of these were identified on baseline scanning in retrospect.[10] Of the nodules remaining, seven were proven malignant or 17.5% of the new nodules. In the Mayo study, there were 2053 nodules present at baseline with 22 subsequently proven malignant for a rate of 1.07%.[4] At repeat first and second annual scans, there were 336 new nodules identified and 11 of these were proven malignant for a rate of 3.3% – nearly three times the rate of malignancy among the baseline nodules (Figure

Study	# Participants	# Nodules at baseline	Malignancy	%	# Nodules at repeat scanning	Malignancy	%
Sobue[6]	1611	192	14	7.3	721	11	1.5
ELCAP[3,10]	1000	233	27	11.5	40	7	17.5
Swensen[4,11]	1520	2053	22	1.07	336	11	3.3
Nawa[5]	7956	541	36	6.7	148*	4	2.7
Pastorini[8]	1035	284	11	3.9	127	11	8.6

Table 14.2 Likelihood of malignancy baseline vs new nodule

*Number of nodules further evaluated with thin-section CT.

14.2).[11] Also favoring a higher rate of malignancy among new nodules detected was the study by Pastorini.[8] There were 284 nodules identified at baseline of which 11 were malignant (3.9%). On first annual scan, there were 127 new non-calcified nodules, and 11 of these were malignant for a rate of 8.6%.

A significant increase in the rate of malignancy among nodules detected at repeat scanning was not seen in Japanese studies. In the study reported by Sobue there were 192 nodules identified at baseline with 14 (7.3%) proven malignant.[6] On annual repeat scanning, 721 new non-calcified nodules were identified and 11 of these were malignant for a lower rate of 1.5%. Similarly, Nawa reported that 36 of 541 (6.7%) of nodules further evaluated with thin-section CT were proved malignant.[5] On

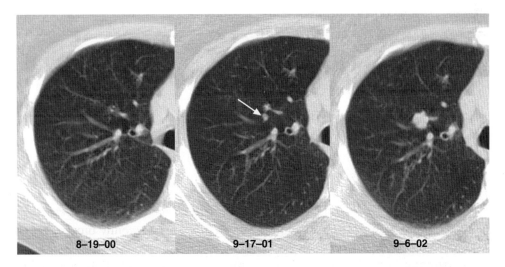

Figure 14.2
New nodule. The screening CT from 9–17–01 shows a new 3-mm nodule in the RUL not present on the scan of 8–19–00. Follow-up scan at 1-year shows obvious growth. Resection showed a 1.4-cm, stage IA, adenocarcinoma.

repeat annual scanning, there were 148 nodules that were recommended to have further evaluation with thin-section CT and four of these were malignant (2.7%). The likely difference between these studies relates to what constituted a positive scan, and to the threshold for calling smaller nodules as intermediate or suspicious. The differences in screening methodology as well as threshold for defining a scan abnormal make comparison between studies difficult. However, results from the majority of the studies support a higher index of suspicion for malignancy for a new nodule detected at an annual scan versus one detected at baseline.

AGE

Age is a recognized risk factor for lung cancer. According to the surveillance epidemiology and end results (SEER data), the incidence rates for lung cancer in those less than age 50 is less than 50 per 100000, and this rate peaks (dependent on race and sex) to between 300–700 cases per 100000 by age 75.[19] The age-related increase is reflected in the design of current screening studies in which participants were required to be 50–60 years or older at entry.[3,4] Sobue reported increased likelihood of a positive screening CT with advancing age, but this was only statistically significant on the repeat scan and not on baseline.[6] Nawa reported increased rate of nodule detection among men 65 years or older when compared to those in their early 50s but no difference in nodule detection by age for women.[5] In the Mayo study, 28 of 735 (3.8%) of the participants aged 55–64 years had prevalence or incidence cancers, whereas 34 of 309 (11%) of the participants aged 65–74 years had cancer.[20] Nodule detection has significance in determining when screening should begin, but beyond

that, participant age does not appear to greatly assist nodule evaluation.

SMOKING

A history of smoking has been a participant requirement for nearly every study trial to date. The ELCAP study[3] required a ten or more pack-year history, and the Mayo Clinic study[4] required a 20-pack-year history or more and, if they had quit smoking, it had to be within 10 years of enrollment. Quantitative data regarding risk based on number of pack years is not available. The only information available regarding never smokers is from Japan. Sobue reported that among 1611 participants screened, 225 were never smokers and one cancer was detected; a rate of 0.44%.[6] This was less than half the rate among former or current smokers at baseline. On repeat annual screening, there were two cancers identified in never smokers for a rate of 0.27% – similar to that of current smokers (0.33%) and higher than that of former smokers (0.17%). Never smokers made up 23% of the population in the study reported by Nawa.[5] At baseline screening, the prevalence rate for cancer detection was 0.44% of all participants, and surprisingly, 22 of 36 cancers were detected in never smokers. There were only four lung cancer cases detected at repeat screening, and one of these was in a never smoker. The significance of the nearly double the rate of lung cancers detected at baseline in never smokers compared to smokers is of uncertain significance. If screening were to be done in never smokers, it would appear that one could not rely heavily on lack of smoking as a means to direct nodule evaluation in a less suspicious fashion.

NODULE CHARACTERISTICS

There are a number of nodule characteristics that can indicate that a nodule is more likely malignant or more likely benign. These include calcification, nodule size, edge characteristics, solid versus ground glass attenuation, single versus multiple nodules, and nodule growth.

Calcification

Calcified nodules detected at CT screening are considered by convention to be benign and generally not tabulated. The patterns of calcification that have well stood the test of time as indication of benign nodules certainly apply in the screening context. Many current screening protocols on multi-detector scanners call for thin sections and allow for retrospective reconstruction so that sensitivity for calcification is significantly enhanced and the need for additional scanning to detect calcification may be obviated. Nodules with eccentric calcification remain indeterminate and require follow-up.

Nodule size

Nodule size has long been recognized as an important feature in estimating likelihood of malignancy. Non-screening CT studies in which nodules were greater than 3 cm and indeterminate indicated a 93–99% likelihood of malignancy.[21,22] A recent article on evaluating solitary pulmonary nodules indicated that a nodule was of low risk of cancer if it were less than 1.5 cm.[23] Clearly, CT screening requires a paradigm shift in thinking in regard to our evaluation of detected nodules. The median diameter of non-small-cell lung cancers detected by CT in the Mayo study was 15 mm for prevalence cancers and 12 mm for incidence cancers.[20] In the Sobue study, baseline or prevalence cancers had a mean diameter of 19.8 mm and incidence cancers had a mean diameter of 14.6 mm.[6] In

the ELCAP study, incidence cancers had a mean of 10.7 mm.[10] The appropriate evaluation of screen-detected nodules needs to reflect nodule size; however, we cannot afford to wait until a nodule is 15 mm before raising concern that it is malignant.

In the ELCAP study, 1% of the nodules detected at 2–5 mm were malignant; 24% of the nodules 6–10 mm were malignant; 33% of nodules 11–20 mm were malignant; and 80% of nodules 21–45 mm were malignant.[3] A similar relationship of size to likelihood of malignancy was seen in the Mayo study.[24] Among baseline nodules ≤3 mm, 0.2% were malignant; for nodules 4–7 mm, 0.9% were malignant; nodules 8–20 mm, 21% were malignant; and of nodules greater than 20 mm, 33% were malignant. A screen-detected nodule that is greater than 10 mm likely needs to be considered as large and suspicious for malignancy.

Edge characteristics

A spiculated nodule edge has long been recognized as an indication that a nodule is more likely malignant. The small size of most screen-detected nodules does not allow detailed edge characteristic evaluation. Edge distinction may be seen in nodules that are nearly a centimeter or more in size and can assist in evaluation decision-making.

Single versus multiple

Chest X-ray series and non-screening CT series have focused on the solitary pulmonary nodule as the nodule of concern. Again, a change in our thinking is required. The finding of a malignant nodule on screening will not uncommonly be in the situation of other nodules detected. In the ELCAP baseline evaluation, 30% of the cancers identified had multiple nodules at time of detection.[3] The majority of prevalence cancers in the Mayo study had other (likely benign) nodules detected as well. It appears to be appropriate to consider each nodule individually rather than being complacent by assuming that a benign diagnosis explains the genesis of each of the nodules in a multiple nodule situation. Some algorithms assume that if more than six nodules are present, then the CT is 'negative.'[16] There may be a limit to the number of nodules that can be easily and accurately followed in an individual participant, but multiple nodules require attention. Our own practice is to identify the six largest nodules but still consider it a 'positive' scan if more nodules are present.

Nodule growth

Nodule growth remains an excellent indicator of malignancy in the screen-detected setting (Figure 14.3). Baseline scanning is the usual initial detection point for a nodule, but old radiographs could still be extremely helpful in identifying nodules that are new, nodules that have

diminished in size, or nodules that are growing. One needs to be sure that the patient has not had a prior chest CT for another reason or may have had a CT of the abdomen or even of the heart that might include the lung windows showing the nodule.

The vast majority of nodules detected by CT screening are too small for further evaluation with contrast enhancement, PET scanning or needle biopsy. In the Mayo study, 89% of the nodules were ≤7 mm.[4] In the Diederich study, 73% of the non-calcified nodules detected were ≤5 mm.[7] In the ELCAP study, 58% of participants with nodules had nodules measuring 2–5 mm,[3] and in the McWilliams study, 73% of the non-calcified nodules detected were ≤4 mm.[9] Consequently observation is an increasingly useful tool for nodule evaluation; one is primarily looking for growth as the indicator of malignancy and lack of growth or shrinkage as the indicator that a nodule is benign. Occasionally benign nodules do grow –

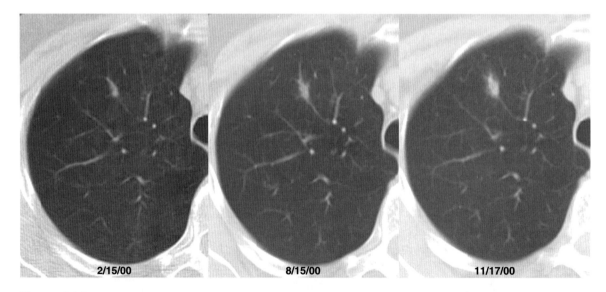

2/15/00   8/15/00   11/17/00

Figure 14.3
Nodule growth is an excellent indicator of malignancy. (A) Screening CT scan shows a 3 × 3-mm RUL nodule. (B) At 6-month follow-up the nodule was thought to be 'perhaps slightly larger'. (C) Further increase in size was noted after an additional 3-month follow-up. Resection showed a 1.3 × 0.7-mm adenocarcinoma.

just to make matters more difficult. Prior chest X-ray studies of nodule growth patterns estimated doubling times for lung cancer in the range of 3 weeks to 400 days.[25] Nodules growing faster or slower than this were suspected to be benign. CT screening has changed these parameters. Hasagawa et al reported more prolonged doubling times among nodules that were ground-glass opacities or semi-solid compared to solid nodules.[26] Retrospective doubling times for solid nodules had a mean of 149 days and significantly shorter than for semi-solid nodules at 457 days and a mean of 813 days for ground-glass nodule cancers. Some cancers grow exceedingly slowly. The corollary to this would be lesser reassurance that a nodule that is unchanged at 2 years is in fact benign if it is a semi-solid or solid nodule (Figure 14.2). Nodules indicating growth within these broadened parameters should prompt needle biopsy or resection.

GROUND-GLASS OPACITIES

The majority of nodular opacities detected with screening CT will be solid nodules. Nodules that are semi-solid or pure ground-glass attenuation deserve special consideration. Both the semi-solid and ground-glass opacities (GGO) appear to be more likely malignant than solid nodules and have a better prognosis than solid nodular carcinomas (Figure 14.4). The ELCAP study reported that among 233 baseline non-calcified nodules detected, there were 189 solid nodules, 16 semi-solid nodules, and 28 pure GGO.[27] Only 7% of the solid nodules were malignant in contrast to 63% of the semi-solid nodules and 18% of the pure GGO. The index of suspicion for malignancy may need to be raised when evaluating semi-solid and GGO. The majority of the partial or pure GGO will be bronchoalveolar cell carcinomas or adenocarcinomas with bronchoalveolar cell features. Focal fibrosis, atypical adenomatous hyperplasia, lymphoid hyperplasia and lymphoproliferative disorders may also present as focal, non-solid nodular opacities.[28] The prognosis from BAC and adenocarcinoma with BAC features presenting in this fashion is reported to be excellent. Suzuki reported that there were 47 bronchoalveolar cell carcinomas among 69 lung cancers with a large GGO component; all were stage I, only two showed vascular invasion, and

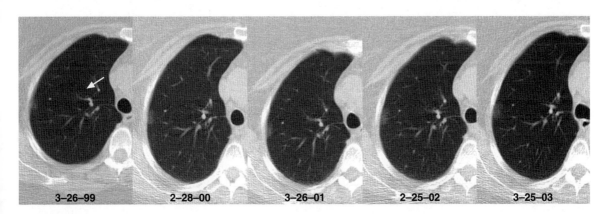

| 3–26–99 | 2–28–00 | 3–26–01 | 2–25–02 | 3–25–03 |

Figure 14.4
Ground-glass opacity (GGO). Baseline and annual screening CT scans show a slowly enlarging GGO in the RUL. The nodule was first called on the 3-25-03 film. Resection revealed a 1.7 × 1.0 mm, stage IA, bronchoalveolar cell carcinoma.

there was no evidence of local or distant recurrence after a median of 35 months of follow-up.[29] Similarly, Watanabe reported no evidence of recurrence after median follow-up of 32 months in 17 patients with malignancies presenting as GGO with all having resection by wedge or segmentectomy.[30] Whether or not cancers presenting GGO would also represent over-diagnosis is unclear. Given the apparent excellent overall prognosis of pure GGO cancers, it would appear appropriate to alter the approach to pure GGO from that of solid-type nodules of the same size. Perhaps longer observation intervals would be appropriate.

WHAT TO DO?

The detection of a non-calcified nodule by CT screening raises the question of what the appropriate evaluation is. Each of the single-arm prospective studies had algorithms for nodule evaluation. These algorithms are more similar than different, but the nuances may be of some practical significance (Table 14.3). To our knowledge, there have not been any studies comparing different algorithms for the evaluation of screen-detected nodules. Based on the current literature and our experience with CT screening we would propose the algorithm in Figure 14.5 for management of screen-detected nodules.

OBSERVATION

Clearly, the most appropriate intervention for most screen-detected non-calcified nodules of small size is no intervention at all. As difficult as it often is for physicians to do nothing but observe, follow-up CT is the mainstay of evaluation for the majority of nodules. Studies differ on what nodule size is considered positive. Some studies have considered nodules <5mm to be negative. This may be appropriate as long as it is recognized that the next annual scan is really done in follow-up and that it is important to note any change in a nodule of any size.

The ELCAP study recommended broad-spectrum antibiotics for all participants with positive scans.[31] Thin-section CT (TSCT) was then performed at 1 month. Nodules that were ≤5mm were recommended to have TSCT at 3, 6, 12 and 24 months. Nodules of 6–10mm were pursued on a case-by-case basis with the recommendation of either biopsy or follow-up. Nodules of 11mm were recommended to have a biopsy.

In the Mayo study, nodules ≤3mm were recommended to have TSCT at 6 months with follow-up at 12–24 months for stable nodules.[4] Nodules 4–7mm had TSCT at 3 and 6 months with additional annual follow-up at 12 and 24 months. Nodules 8–20mm were recommended to have contrast-enhanced CT and/or PET scanning with suspected malignant lesions having biopsy or removal. Biopsy was recommended for nodules >20mm.

The Anti-Lung Cancer Alliance recommendations were reported by Sobue and these included no additional evaluation for nodules <5mm.[6] For those ≥5mm, TSCT was recommended with biopsy for suspicious lesions. In the Nawa study, those with nodules ≤7mm were recommended to have annual follow-up.[5] Nodules 8–10mm were recommended to have TSCT at 1 month with follow-up at 3 and 6 months and annual follow-up thereafter. Nodules ≥11mm were recommended to have biopsy.

In the Pastorini study, 12-month follow-up was recommended for nodules ≤5mm.[8] Those >5mm had TSCT at 1 month with CT enhancement if their density was greater than 0

Table 14.3 Nodule evaluation	
Study	**Evaluation algorithm**
ELCAP[3,31]	All participants with positive results received broad-spectrum antibiotics and TSCT at 1 month Nodules ≤5 mm had TSCT at 3 and 6 months 6–10 mm case-by-case evaluation with biopsy or follow-up ≥11 mm biopsy recommended
Mayo[4]	Nodules ≤3 mm follow-up TSCT at 6 months 4–7 mm TSCT 3 and 6 months 8–20 mm CT enhancement study and/or PET >20 mm biopsy recommended
ALCA[6]	Nodules <5 mm no interval follow-up ≥5 mm TSCT and biopsy if suspicious
Nawa[5]	Nodules <8 mm no interval follow-up 8–10 mm TSCT at 1 month, 3 and 6 months ≥11 mm biopsy recommended
Diederich[7]	≤5 mm TSCT 3 and 6 months 6–10 mm TSCT 3 and 6 months >10 mm TSCT and biopsy for suspicious-appearing lesions
Pastorini[8]	≤5 mm non-suspicious no interval follow-up >5 mm TSCT at 1 month and CT enhancement if density >0 Hounsfield units, follow-up at 6 months if negative CTE If positive CTE or PET, biopsy recommended >20 mm biopsy recommended
McWilliams[9]	≤4 mm TSCT 6 months 5–9 mm TSCT 3 and 6 months 10 mm evaluation on an individual basis

Hounsfield units. Follow-up at 6 months was recommended for non-suspicious lesions. Lesions that were positive by CT enhancement or PET were recommended to have biopsy. Those >20 mm also were recommended to have biopsy.

In the McWilliams study, nodules of ≤4 mm had follow-up at 6, 12 and 24 months; those 5–9 mm had follow-up in 3, 6, 12 and 24 months; and those 10 mm and greater had additional evaluation on an individual basis.[9]

These studies differ in the specific millimeter size of the nodule that defines the interval of follow-up. However, in all, the smallest and by far and away the majority of nodules are simply observed.

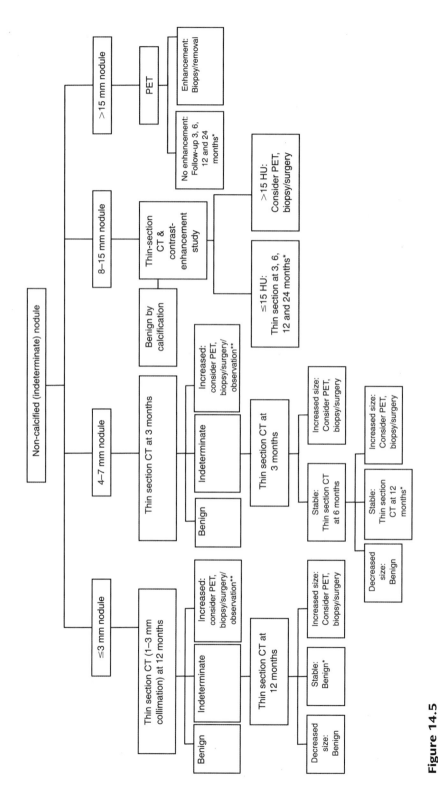

Figure 14.5

Algorithm for screen-detected nodule evaluation. (Recommendation is based on the size of the largest nodule.)

* Solid nodules that are stable for 24 months are considered benign.

** Suggestion of a millimeter or two of growth may be due to CT slide differences.

FURTHER IMAGING

Advances in radiologic techniques help to provide direction in management of nodules detected at CT screening. These techniques may be applied immediately following detection or at follow-up.

TSCT (1–3 mm collimation) is more sensitive than standard CT (collimation 7–10 mm) in recognizing calcification and, if in a benign pattern, may obviate further nodule evaluation. As the algorithm descriptions in the previous section demonstrate, TSCT may be applied immediately following detection with low-dose spiral CT or at follow-up. Our preference for nodules 4–7 mm would be to perform TSCT at 3 months rather than immediately (if screening protocol did not involve a multi-detector scanner with reconstruction capability). Although an immediate thin-section evaluation may identify calcification and identify the nodule as benign, most will not be calcified; one interval CT may be avoided by performing TSCT at interval follow-up. The interval scan then provides the value of TSCT but also the important added feature of time and the possibility of identifying nodule growth. Immediate TSCT may then be obviated if the management plan would be to follow a non-calcified nodule anyway.

Volumetric assessment of nodule size with TSCT is under development. Preliminary data support that repeat CT within as short a period as 1 month may detect growth in most malignant nodules as small as 5 mm.[32] The availability of volumetric nodule measurement may well help detect growth much sooner than with two-dimensional CT.

CT enhancement is a technique in which a patient weight-dependent amount of iodinated contrast material is injected at a fixed rate. Thin-section scans through the nodule are obtained at 1, 2, 3 and 4 minutes after the onset of injection. Enhancement is defined as the maximum nodule density in Hounsfield units (HU) following contrast injection minus the pre-contrast injection value of density. A nodule that enhances more than 15 Hounsfield units is indeterminate and has a higher likelihood of being malignant than benign. Nodules that enhance less than 15 Hounsfield units are highly likely benign and direct a course of observation. CT enhancement is readily available and easily applied and can be performed at the same setting as thin-section CT when a benign calcification pattern is not identified. The technique requires that a nodule be 7 mm in diameter on a mediastinal window to allow for accurate measurement of enhancement in a region of interest. Consequently it is not applicable for nodules that are <7 mm on lung windows. In a multicenter study, Swensen et al showed that CTE had a sensitivity of 98%, specificity of 58%, and overall accuracy of 77%.[33] The mean nodule size in this study was only 15 mm and supports that the technique may be helpful in determining likelihood of benignancy in nodules of a size that is often detected at CT screening.

POSITRON EMISSION TOMOGRAPHY

PET scanning uses the injection of the glucose analog 18F-2-fluorodeoxyglucose (FDG) and identifies nodules with high metabolic activity. Nodule enhancement is an indication that a nodule is more likely malignant than benign, and absence of enhancement is a strong predictor that a nodule is benign (Figure 14.6). A growing nodule that shows no enhancement on PET should still be considered suspicious for malignancy and prompt needle biopsy or resection (Figure 14.7). In a meta-analysis, Gould

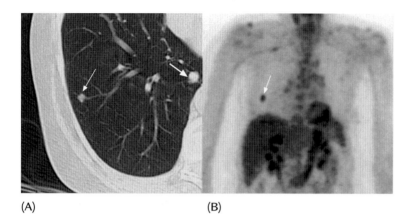

(A) (B)

Figure 14.6
PET-positive lung cancer. (A) CT shows a small peripheral nodule in the RLL that was enlarging (small arrow) and a larger, stable nodule medially (large arrow). (B) PET shows the smaller peripheral nodule to be metabolically active. At resection, the peripheral nodule was a 9 × 7-mm adenocarcinoma and the larger, medial nodule was a granuloma.

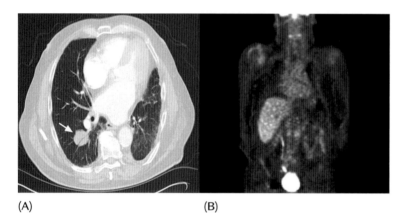

(A) (B)

Figure 14.7
PET-negative lung cancer. (A) CT shows a 3-cm nodule in the RLL. (B) PET scan shows the nodule is not metabolically active. In retrospect the nodule was enlarging. Resection showed a stage 1B adenocarcinoma with bronchoalveolar features.

et al showed that in the evaluation of a solitary pulmonary nodule PET had a sensitivity of 94% and a specificity of 86%.[34] Within this meta-analysis, there were only eight cases in which the nodule was <1 cm in size. The lower limit of nodule size for PET applicability using current techniques is about 7 or 8 mm. This had prompted recent reviewers to recommend that PET not be applied in nodules <1 cm.[35] In a multicenter prospective study of 89 patients with SPNs, Lowe et al reported that FDG-PET had an overall sensitivity of 92% and a specificity of 90% for detecting malignant nodules.[36] The sensitivity fell to only 80% when nodules of 15 mm or smaller were analyzed. Weber et al reported a sensitivity of 97% using FDG-PET to

identify a malignancy; however, the mean nodule size in this study was 34 mm, and the results do not apply to the nodules of screen-detected size.[37]

Further limitation of PET for evaluation of nodules of the size detected by CT has been reported.[38] Of 47 proven malignant lesions that were ≤1 cm in size, 37 had positive PET scans and ten had false-negative PET scans (overall sensitivity 79%). For cancers 1.0–1.5 cm in diameter, 26 of 31 were positive at PET (sensitivity 84%) and for cancers <1.0 cm, 11 of 16 were PET-positive (sensitivity 69%). There was no difference in the median size of the PET-positive and PET-negative cancers (10–11 mm). Of the ten PET-negative cancers, six were non-small-cell (four bronchoalveolar cell), three were metastatic and one was a small cell lung cancer.

Pastorino reported that of 42 PET scans done on screen-detected nodules there were four false-positive and two false-negative scans for a sensitivity of 90% and a specificity of 82%.[8] In the Mayo study, 15 of the participants with 16 proven non-small-cell lung cancers were evaluated by PET.[39] Five of the cancers were false negative on PET scanning. The size of the PET-negative cancers was 7–11 mm versus 7–13 mm for the PET-positive non-small-cell cancers. Three of the five PET-negative cancers were bronchoalveolar cell cancers and two were adenocarcinomas. PET scanning has been shown to be cost-effective in the evaluation of pulmonary nodules; however, the fact that the majority of the screen-detected nodules are <8 mm indicates that current PET techniques should not be applied to most nodules and that PET is often negative in bronchoalveolar cell carcinomas. In a study of cost effectiveness for 2-cm nodules, Gould et al showed that PET was most cost effective when selectively used. Cost effectiveness for PET was greatest when clinical suspicion for malignancy was high and CT nodule appearance was benign and, conversely, when clinical suspicion of malignancy was low and CT suggested the nodule was malignant.[40] In a study assessing the impact of CT enhancement on the cost effectiveness of PET, Comber et al reports that adding CTE before PET improved the cost-effectiveness strategies for the management of pulmonary nodules.[41] We consider PET to play a central role in nodule evaluation and staging for most patients with known or suspected non-small-cell lung cancer.

MAGNETIC RESONANCE (MR)

There is relatively little information regarding the use of MR to evaluate small pulmonary nodules compared to the amount of information available for CT enhancement and PET. Ohno et al reported on 58 patients with pathologically proved pulmonary nodules with a diameter of <30 mm.[42] Patients underwent dynamic MR imaging using a standard dose (0.1 mmol/kg body weight) of gadopentetate dimeglumine contrast material. The authors found that the slope of enhancement enabled more accurate differentiation between malignant and benign nodules than did the maximum relative enhancement ratio. The sensitivity, specificity and positive predictive value of the slope enhancement for distinguishing malignant nodules were 100%, 85% and 93% respectively. Fifteen of the nodules in this study were <10 mm. None of the screening studies to date have applied MR evaluation to pulmonary nodules as a routine. MR will not in the foreseeable future play a major role in nodule evaluation or staging.

BIOPSY

The role of biopsy in evaluating screen-detected lesions is another area of controversy. To some degree, pursuit of biopsy is dependent on philosophy (such as whether or not a lesion needs to be diagnosed prior to surgical removal), and dependent on feasibility (as to a lesion's size, location, and the local expertise in pursuing such a lesion). The role of biopsy has varied considerably in different screening trials. In the ELCAP study, essentially every nodule was needle biopsied prior to surgical removal.[3] Similarly, in the Pastorini study, lesions that were positive by CT enhancement or by PET were candidates for biopsy.[8] In the Mayo study, only a few nodules were needle biopsied; most malignancies were removed without tissue confirmation prior to resection. We would consider a surgical nodule removal as a resection rather than a biopsy, and the varying use of these terms can lead to confusion.[43]

When considering biopsy for a screen-detected lesion, one has either transthoracic needle aspiration (TTNA) or bronchoscopy from which to choose. Although bronchoscopy is an excellent tool for sampling central airway lesions, mediastinal nodes, and parenchymal masses, for the vast majority of screen-detected small peripheral nodules, the bronchoscope has no role. Diagnostic yields with bronchoscopy for peripheral pulmonary nodules less than 2 cm in diameter have consistently been in the range of 10–20%.[44–46] The likelihood of obtaining a specific benign diagnosis is even lower. Studies from Japan have shown higher yield, but these results have not been widely reproduced. Aoshima reported that the likelihood of diagnosis by bronchoscopy was nearly 50% in lesions less than 2.5 cm in size.[47] Bandoh et al reported that using flexible bronchoscopy with multiplanar reconstruction images and Ultrafast Pap smear was 82% for lesions ≤2 cm in size.[48] Although these are excellent results, they are still not comparable to recent series evaluating small peripheral nodules with TTNA. There are very little data within bronchoscopy use for nodules ≤10 mm. The presence of an air bronchogram in a pulmonary nodule, especially if this gives a specific road map as to the bronchial location, will increase yield to an acceptable level for bronchoscopy.[49,50]

Given the ability of low-dose screening to detect cancers when they are at a mean of 15 mm, acceptable yield with biopsy is almost only achieved in nodules of this size with CT-guided needle biopsy. Ohno et al reported TTNA had an accuracy of 52% for nodules ≤10 mm, 74% for nodules 11–15 mm and 91% for nodules 16–20 mm.[51] This paper reported an overall pneumothorax rate of 28%, but only 2.5% required chest tubes. Wallace et al reported on 61 patients with lung nodules 1.0 cm or smaller who underwent CT-guided TTNA.[52] Adequate samples for diagnosis were obtained in 77%, and the overall sensitivity was 82% and specificity 100% with a diagnostic accuracy of 88% based on 57 patients being evaluable. Results for nodules 8–10 mm (sensitivity 88%, accuracy 92%) were better than those for nodules 5–7 mm in size (sensitivity 50%, accuracy 70%). Similarly impressive results were reported by Yamagami et al using an automated cutting needle with CT fluoroscopic guidance.[53] TTNA for nodules ≤10 mm gave an adequate sample in 96% and an accurate diagnosis in 88%. These impressive results are unequaled in bronchoscopic series for similar-size lesions. Until significant further progress is made in bronchoscopy, nodules ≤2 cm requiring biopsy and not having a CT-bronchus sign should be pursued with TTNA.

Whether or not a lesion should be biopsied remains controversial. Needle biopsy would appear appropriate for newly detected lesions at screening that are 8 mm and greater. Although it may be appropriate to biopsy smaller lesions, the yields at present do not justify the expense and risk. Although it may be desirable to needle a nodule that has grown from 3 mm to 5 mm on sequential scanning, this is not practical in most radiologists' hands. Perhaps a more difficult issue is whether or not, in the high-risk screen-detected situation, the lesion that grows from 10 mm to 15 mm requires needle biopsy. Our own bias would be to pursue PET scanning in this situation. If the PET were positive with no evidence of nodal disease, then we would directly pursue resection. A positive needle biopsy would result in surgery – due to the high likelihood of malignancy, a non-specific benign diagnosis would result in the same, and so we would usually obviate biopsy in this situation.

SURGICAL RESECTION

Resection for cure is the desired outcome for every non-small-cell lung cancer detected by screening CT. The reality is that some advanced-stage cancers will be detected for which surgical resection is no longer appropriate. The more frequent problem is deciding which of the myriad of nodules detected by screening CT should be surgically removed. The increasing ability to diagnose small nodules as malignant by needle aspiration or high probability of malignancy by enhanced radiologic techniques helps to identify the few cancers among the many benign nodules. In the absence of a non-surgical test that distinguishes malignant from benign nodules with perfect accuracy, benign nodules will be removed. However, an aggressive surgical approach for the indeterminate nodule with the mentality of 'when in doubt, take it out' simply cannot apply to the screened situation.[54] Screening trials to date have benign nodule resection rates of between 13% and 33%.[3–5,7–9] Keeping benign nodule resections to a minimum is preferred, though caution in removal is in obvious conflict with the desire to expediently resect malignant lesions. We are frequently unable to know they are benign prior to resection.

We need to balance the benefit of potentially curable resection for the malignant lesion to the risk and unnecessary resection of removing benign lesions. A new lesion that is greater than 15 mm and positive on PET may be biopsied to confirm malignancy or resection directly. Similarly, a lesion that has shown significant growth in follow-up, that is also enhancing, may be

appropriate to resect if no evidence of metastasis is present. Improvements in nodule localization techniques have facilitated video-assisted thoracoscopic resections, but this improved ability to remove a nodule should not replace appropriate radiographic evaluation. Recent series of VATS resection have reported that benign nodules comprised 50% or more of the nodules removed.[55–57] The small size and often the ground-glass character of these nodules may require preoperative localization. Localization is not only necessary for the surgeon to remove the nodule but also for the pathologist to find the lesion in the resected specimen. Suzuki et al suggested that pre-VATS localization techniques should be used when the lesion is more than 5 mm from the nearest pleural surface or is 10 mm or less in size.[56]

FUTURE DIRECTIONS

Although much has been learned in pursuit of the pulmonary nodule detected by CT screening, much remains to be known. Applying CT in the screening situation leads to detection of many small nodules, and the optimal management of these nodules is gaining in clarity at certain points and remains muddled in others. Given that the majority of nodules detected by CT screening are but a few millimeters in size, observation of these minor abnormalities is appropriate, though the interval necessary for follow-up remains unclear. Studies specifically looking at different follow-up strategies are needed. In other words, if a single 3 mm nodule is detected, would follow-up at 24 months be appropriate or does this need to be imaged at 12 months? Similarly, the optimal follow-up for nodules of 4–7 mm or so in size is not clear.

For nodules of 8–10 mm, some would pursue PET scanning first; others would pursue needle biopsy first. The subsequent evaluation is dependent on many factors and the most effective and perhaps most cost-effective approach needs to be defined. Routine use of PET scanning does not currently appear appropriate for most nodules of ≤1 cm. This may change with advancements in PET technology.

The preliminary data with CT volumetric assessment suggests that malignant nodules may be identified by growth within as short as 1 month.[32] Further availability and experience with volumetric assessment of nodules may significantly change the algorithms of follow-up. A nodule that is stable at 1 month by volumetric assessment might not need additional sampling for another 6 months or longer. Investigators are now reporting excellent results in pursuit of nodules <1 cm with transthoracic needle aspirate. Whether or not there is a size below which TTNA is not feasible or practical is not clear. Improvements in CT-directed bronchoscopy may also facilitate biopsy of small nodules with less risk of pneumothorax than by TTNA.

The ground-glass opacity presents its own series of challenges. Determining which of these lesions is atypical adenomatous hyperplasia versus bronchoalveolar cell carcinoma is evolving. These GGO lesions appear to have a much better prognosis and may not only allow for limited resection but also a more protracted evaluation course due to an apparent low risk of metastasis.

Imaging improvements continually occur. Multigated scanners allow for better resolution and better detection of pulmonary nodules. Whether or not this leads to more rapid detection of malignant lesions is uncertain. The evolution of screening has gone from 10 mm collimation to as low as 1.25 mm collimation. Which is the best balance of sensitivity and specificity is not clear. Computer-assisted detection and surface evaluation of nodules will likely assist the radiologist in determining presence of a nodule and likelihood of malignancy in the near future.[58,59] Further advances in radiologic techniques will hopefully allow earlier identification of malignant nodules with greater specificity; this would greatly ease some of the difficult decision making currently facing participants and physicians who choose to screen with CT. Use of serum or sputum biomarkers may also be an important future tool in enriching the screening population by identifying those at highest risk for cancer or, alternatively, to help identify which of those with nodules detected on CT are the ones with cancer.

REFERENCES

1. Sone S, Takashima S, Li F, et al, Mass screening for lung cancer with mobile spiral computed tomography scanner. Lancet 1998; 351:1242–5.
2. Kaneko M, Eguchi K, Ohmatsu H, et al, Peripheral lung cancer: screening and detection with low-dose spiral CT versus radiography. Radiology 1999; 201:798–802.
3. Henschke CI, McCauley DI, Yankelevitz DF, et al, Early lung cancer action project: overall design and findings from baseline screening. Lancet 1999; 354:99–105.
4. Swensen SJ, Jett JR, Sloan JA, et al, Screening for lung cancer with low-dose spiral computed tomography. Am J Respir Crit Care Med 2002; 165:508–13.
5. Nawa T, Nakagawa T, Kusano S, et al, Lung cancer screening using low-dose spiral CT: results of baseline and 1-year follow-up studies. Chest 2002; 122:15–20.
6. Sobue T, Moriyama N, Kaneko M, et al, Screening for lung cancer with low-dose helical computed tomography: Anti-Lung Cancer Association project. J Clin Oncol 2002; 20:911–20.
7. Diederich S, Wormanns D, Semik M, et al, Screening for early lung cancer with low-dose

spiral CT: prevalence in 817 asymptomatic smokers. Radiology 2002; 222:773–81.

8. Pastorino U, Bellomi M, Landoni C, et al, Early lung cancer detection with spiral CT and positron emission tomography in heavy smokers: Two-year results. Lancet 2003; 362: 593–7.

9. McWilliams A, Mayo J, MacDonald S, et al, Lung cancer screening: A different paradigm. Am J Respir Crit Care Med 2003; 168:1167–73.

10. Henschke CI, Naidich DP, Yankelevitz DF, et al, Early lung cancer action project: initial findings on repeat scanning. Cancer 2001; 92:153–9.

11. Swensen SJ, Jett JR, Hartman TE, et al, Screening for lung cancer with CT: Mayo Clinic experience. Radiology 2003; 226:756–61.

12. Frost JK, Ball WC, Levin ML, et al, Early lung cancer detection: results of the initial (prevalence) radiologic and cytologic screening in the Johns Hopkins Study. Am Rev Respir Dis 1984; 130:549–54.

13. Rusinek H, Naidich DP, McGuinness G, et al, Pulmonary nodule detection: Low-dose versus conventional CT. Radiology 1998; 209:243–9.

14. Tillich M, Kammerhuber F, Reittner P, et al, Detection of pulmonary nodules with helical CT: comparison of cine and film-based viewing. AJR 1997; 169:1611–14.

15. Selzer SE, Judy PF, Adams DF, et al, Spiral CT of the chest: comparison of cine and film based viewing. Radiology 1995; 197:73–8.

16. Henschke CI, Yankelevitz DF, McCauley DI, et al, Guidelines for the use of spiral computed tomography in screening for lung cancer. Eur Respir J 2003; 21:45S–51S.

17. Swensen SJ, CT screening for lung cancer. AJR 2003; 180; 1736–7.

18. Hillman BJ, ACRIN, Economic, legal and ethical rationales for the ACRIN National Lung Screening Trial of CT Screening for Lung Cancer. Academic Radiology 2003; 10:349–50.

19. Website: Seer.cancer.gov.

20. Swenson S, Jett J, Mandrekar S, et al, CT screening for lung cancer: five-year prospective experience. Radiology 2005; 235:259–65.

21. Zerhouni EA, Stitik FP, Siegelman SS, et al, CT of the pulmonary nodule: A cooperative study. Radiology 1986; 160:319–27.

22. Siegelman SS, Khouri NF, Leo FP, et al, Solitary pulmonary nodules: CT assessment. Radiology 1986; 160:307–12.

23. Ost D, Fein AM, Feinsilver SH, The solitary pulmonary nodule. N Engl J Med 2003; 348: 2535–42.

24. Midthun DE, Swensen SJ, Jett JR, Hartman TE, Evaluation of nodules detected by screening for lung cancer with low-dose spiral computed tomography. Lung Cancer 2003; 41:S40.

25. Nathan MH, Collins VP, Adams RA, Differentiation of benign and malignant pulmonary nodules by growth rate. Radiology 1962; 79: 221–31.

26. Hasegawa M, Sone S, Takashima S, et al, Growth rate of small lung cancers detected on mass screening. Radiology 2000; 73:1252–9.

27. Henschke CI, Yankelevitz DF, Mirtcheva R, et al, Screening for lung cancer: frequency and significance of part solid and non-solid nodules. AJR 2002; 178:1053–7.

28. Kodama K, Higashiyama M, Yokouchi H, et al, Natural history of pure ground-glass opacity after long-term follow-up of more than two years. Ann Thorac Surg 2002; 73:386–93.

29. Suzuki K, Asamura H, Kusumoto M, Kondo H, Tsuchiya R, 'Early' peripheral lung cancer: prognostic significance of ground-glass opacity on thin-section computed tomographic scan. Ann Thorac Surg 2002; 74:1635–9.

30. Watanabe S, Watanabe T, Arai K, et al, Results of wedge resection for focal bronchioloalveolar carcinoma showing pure ground-glass attenuation on computed tomography. Ann Thorac Surg 2002; 73:1071–5.

31. Henschke CI, Yankelevitz DF, Libby D, et al, Computed tomography screening for lung cancer. Clinics Chest Med 2002; 23:49–57.

32. Yankelevitz DF, Gupta R, Zhao B, Henschke CI, Small pulmonary nodules: evaluation with repeat CT – preliminary experience. Radiology 1999; 212:561–6.

33. Swensen SJ, Viggiano RW, Midthun DE, et al, Lung nodule enhancement at CT: multicenter study. Radiology 2000; 214:73–80.

34. Gould MK, Maclean CC, Kuschner WG, Rydzak CE, Owens DK, Accuracy of positron emission tomography for diagnosis of pulmonary nodules and mass lesions: a meta-analysis. JAMA 2001; 285:914–24.

35. Tan BB, Flaherty KR, Kazerooni EA, Iannettoni MD, The solitary pulmonary nodule. Chest 2003; 123:89S–96S.

36. Lowe VJ, Fletcher JW, Gobar L, et al, Prospective investigation of positron emission tomography in lung nodules. J Clin Oncol 1998; 16:1075–84.

37. Weber W, Young C, Abdel-Dayem HM, et al, Assessment of pulmonary lesions with 18 F-fluorodeoxyglucose positron emission imaging using coincidence mode gamma cameras. J Nucl Med 1999; 40:574–8.

38. Daniels CE, Doerger KM, Jett JR, et al, Utility of FDG-PET in diagnostic evaluation of small pulmonary nodules. Lung Cancer 2003; 41:S14.

39. Lindell RM, Hartman TE, Swensen SJ, et al, PET imaging of non-small cell lung cancer detected by screening chest CT (in press – AJR).

40. Gould MK, Sanders GD, Barnett PG, et al, Cost-effectiveness of alternative strategies for patients with solitary pulmonary nodules. Ann Intern Med 2003; 348:1123–33.

41. Comber LA, Keith CJ, Griffiths M, Miles KA, Solitary pulmonary nodules: impact of quantitative contrast-enhanced CT on the cost-effectiveness of FDG-PET. Clin Radiol 2003; 58:706–11.

42. Ohno Y, Hatabu H, Takenaka D, et al, Solitary pulmonary nodules: potential role of dynamic MR imaging and management – initial experience. Radiology 2002; 224:503–11.

43. Yankelevitz DF, Wisnivesky JP, Henschke CI, Comparison of biopsy techniques in assessment of solitary pulmonary nodules. Seminars in Ultrasound, CT, and MRI 2000; 21:139–48.

44. Cortese DA, McDougall JC, Biopsy and brushing of peripheral lung cancer with fluoroscopic guidance. Chest 1979; 75:141–5.

45. Reichenberger F, Weber J, Tamm M, et al, The value of transbronchial needle aspiration in the diagnosis of peripheral pulmonary lesions, Chest 1999; 116:704–8.

46. Baaklinii WA, Reinoso MA, Gorin AB, Sharafkaneh A, Manian P, Diagnostic yield of fiberoptic bronchoscopy in evaluating solitary pulmonary nodules. Chest 2000; 117:1049–54.

47. Aoshima M, Chonabayashi N, Can HRCT contribute in decision-making on indications for flexible bronchoscopy for solitary pulmonary nodules and masses? J Bronchology 2001; 8: 161–5.

48. Bandoh S, Fujita J, Tojo Y, et al, Diagnostic accuracy and safety of flexible bronchoscopy with multi-planar reconstruction images and Ultrafast Papanicolaou stain: evaluating solitary pulmonary nodules. Chest 2003; 124: 1985–92.

49. Naidich DP, Sussman R, Kutcher WL, et al, Solitary pulmonary nodules. CT-bronchoscopic correlation. Chest 1988; 93:595–8.

50. Bilaceroglu S, Kumcuoglu Z, Alper H, et al, CT bronchus sign-guided bronchoscopic multiple diagnostic procedures in carcinomatous solitary pulmonary nodules and masses. Respiration 1998; 65:49–55.

51. Ohno Y, Hatabu H, Takenaka D, et al, CT-guided transthoracic needle aspiration biopsy of small (≤20 mm) solitary pulmonary nodules. AJR 2003; 180:1665–9.

52. Wallace MJ, Krishnamurthy S, Broemeling LD, et al, CT-guided percutaneous fine needle aspiration biopsy of small (≤1 cm) pulmonary lesions. Radiology 2002; 225:823–8.

53. Yamagami T, Iida S, Kato T, et al, Usefulness of new automated cutting needle for tissue core biopsy of lung nodules under CT fluoroscopic guidance. Chest 2003; 124:147–54.

54. DeCamp MM, The solitary pulmonary nodule: aggressive excisional strategy. Semin Thorac Cardiovasc Surg 2002; 14:292–6.

55. Mullan BF, Stanford W, Barnhart RTR, Galvin JR, Lung nodules: Improved wire for CT guided localization. Radiology 1999; 211:561–5.

56. Suzuki K, Nagai K, Yoshida J, et al, Video-assisted thoracoscopic surgery for small indeterminate pulmonary nodules. Chest 1999; 115:563–8.

57. Jimenez MF, Prospective study on video-assisted thoracoscopic surgery in the resection of pulmonary nodules: 209 cases from the Spanish Video-Assisted Thoracic Surgery Study Group. Eur J Cardio-Thorac Surg 2001; 19:562–5.

58. Awai K, Murao K, Ozawa A, et al, Pulmonary nodules at chest CT: effect of computer-aided diagnosis on radiologists' detection performance. Radiology 2004; 230:347–52.

59. Aoyama M, Li Q, Katsuragawa S, et al, Computerized scheme for determination of the likelihood measure of malignancy for pulmonary nodules on low-dose CT images. Am Assoc Phys Med 2003; 30:387–94.

15 The pathology of screen-detected lesions

Keith M Kerr, Masayuki Noguchi

Contents Introduction • Central bronchogenic disease • Peripheral disease • Future work • Conclusion

INTRODUCTION

Lung cancer is the most important cause of death from malignant disease worldwide, and is likely to remain so for many years, given projected estimates for global tobacco consumption. The disease is aggressive, yet presents with symptoms relatively late in its natural history, by which time most tumors have metastasized. This common disease, a major cause of cancer mortality, generally fatal once symptomatic, yet curable if detected early enough, is a prime target for screening.[1]

The rationale behind any cancer screening is that disease must be detected before there is a significant risk of metastases having developed. In general, a lung tumor must be over 1 cm in diameter and favorably sited to be visible on a plain PA chest radiograph (CXR). The great majority of tumors, however, present when symptomatic, over 3 cm in diameter and with metastases already present and clinically detectable. Yet even a 1 cm diameter cancer has undergone about 30 volume doublings, contains approximately 10^{10} cells and has probably been in existence for several years. For much of this time the disease will have been preinvasive, posing no risk of metastasis, but a considerable period of time elapses between the onset of invasion, with risk of metastases and conventional disease detection. Up to 15% of tumors

less than 1 cm diameter are accompanied by metastatic disease.[2] Although surgical resection of Stage IA disease can lead to up to 85% cure rate,[3] overall survival rates (5–15%) reflect the fact that most patients present only when symptomatic, with advanced disease. Thus it is essential to detect and treat this disease either at the preinvasive stage or as soon as possible after invasion has occurred.

There are two main pathways for the development of lung cancer. This may be an oversimplification, but reflects our current understanding of lung carcinogenesis. Central bronchogenic disease, mostly squamous cell and small-cell carcinoma, arises from the bronchial epithelium, while peripheral tumors, mostly adenocarcinomas, derive from the (bronchiolo)alveolar epithelium. The WHO classification of lung cancer recognized three preinvasive lesions, namely bronchial squamous dysplasia/carcinoma in-situ (SD/CIS), the (bronchiolo)alveolar lesion atypical adenomatous hyperplasia (AAH) and an extremely rare lesion called diffuse idiopathic pulmonary neuroendocrine cell hyperplasia (DIPNECH).[4] (DIPNECH is included due to its association with typical carcinoid tumors but is of no practical relevance to cancer screening and will not be considered further.) SD/CIS is the precursor lesion for invasive squamous cell carcinoma, while AAH is a putative precursor for localized non-mucinous bronchioloalveolar carcinoma (LNMBAC) and invasive adenocarcinoma. There is no morphologically recognizable precursor lesion specific for small-cell lung cancer (SCLC). While some genetic changes, key to the development of SCLC[5] may in the future allow early disease detection through a biomarker/molecular biology-based approach, SCLC is currently only recognizable at a cellular level when it is invasive, a particular problem given its notable aggressiveness. Saccomanno[6] previously suggested that SCLC might derive from SD/CIS due to a 'sudden chromosomal aberration', remarkably prescient, given that loss of *RB* or *P16* may in part respectively determine small- or non-small-cell carcinogenesis.[7]

This simplified partition of tumor development is useful in understanding the pathological findings and, perhaps, some of the problems with lung cancer screening to date. Reliance on CXR to detect lung cancer essentially means a tumor will be at least 1 cm in diameter, well-established and invasive when found. Such tumors will be peripheral lesions or, particularly in the prevalence setting, advanced central bronchogenic tumors, which have spread beyond the airway to replace aerated lung and/or distort the hilar shadow. Sputum cytology or fluorescence bronchoscopy can, de facto, identify bronchial SD/CIS and early invasive bronchogenic carcinomas, but also advanced peripheral tumors which invade bronchi. CT-based screening studies essentially identify nodules in the parenchymal compartment of the lung. CT scans, in common with CXR, generally cannot detect intrabronchial abnormalities.

The remainder of this chapter will consider these two pathways of lung carcinogenesis in the context of screen-detected disease and discuss the pathological findings of various screening studies; those using CXR plus sputum cytology, later augmented by fluorescence bronchoscopy, which mostly detect bronchogenic disease, and more recent work using high-resolution CT scanning to detect peripheral parenchymal disease.

CENTRAL BRONCHOGENIC DISEASE

The following discussion first considers the development of squamous cell carcinoma. As mentioned above, the origin of small cell carcinoma is unclear.

Bronchial epithelial reserve cell hyperplasia is probably the earliest change to occur during central bronchial carcinogenesis. On this background both squamous metaplasia and dysplasia may develop. The most frequent trigger is chronic exposure to tobacco smoke. The morphological changes reflect the sequential genetic changes which occur in the transforming cell population and drive the development of invasive malignancy. The WHO classification grades dysplasia which occurs in squamous epithelium as mild, moderate or severe.[4] This grading is based on the division of the squamous epithelium into lower, middle and upper thirds and takes account of the distribution of mitoses and the expansion into the more superficial layers of the epithelium of the population of mal-orientated basal cells, which acquire increasingly aberrant nuclear features. Details of this classification are reviewed in Chapter 5. Some studies group moderate and severe dysplasia together as high-grade dysplasia.

Carcinoma in-situ is the most advanced stage of this preinvasive disease progression and is distinguished from severe dysplasia by the lack of epithelial maturation and a completely chaotic, disorganized epithelium composed of very pleomorphic squamous cells whose cytological features signal malignancy, although, by definition, invasion is absent. Invasive disease is recognized when there is unequivocal infiltration of the tissue deep to the basement membrane. The tumor then becomes vascularized, progresses and both infiltrates the airway and the surrounding lung. With invasion comes the risk of metastases. From the very earliest stage of squamous metaplasia, superficial cells may be shed into the airway: thus on cytological grounds alone, the distinction between grades of SD/CIS, and between CIS and invasive squamous carcinoma is difficult,[6,8] and tissue biopsy is generally required if invasion is to be confirmed.[9]

Screening by chest radiograph and sputum cytology

Several studies have been reported on CXR and sputum cytology to detect lung cancer. The histological findings of the prevalent cancers found in the four earliest studies are shown in Table 15.1.[10–13] These studies differ from each other in significant ways, but the cancers detected showed certain characteristics. As would be expected from screening by sputum cytology

and CXR, tumors of all types were found and largely reflect the cell type distribution in the population in general, although in the three American studies, especially in that from Memorial Sloan-Kettering,[11] the proportion of small-cell tumors is low. Case numbers in the Czech study[13] are smaller, but the frequency of small-cell and lack of adenocarcinoma may reflect the different population studied; however, in another European study,[14] the cell-type distribution in screen-detected cases was almost identical to that of the Mayo Clinic study[12] and similar to their control non-screened group, except that again there were fewer small-cell tumors in the screened group. In two Japanese studies almost 50% of the cases were adenocarcinoma, 34% were squamous cell, while small-cell accounted for 16%, again appropriate for the source population.[15,16]

While CXR was, overall, more effective than sputum cytology in detecting cancers, even more were found when these modalities are employed together. Sputum cytology was

Table 15.1 Histological findings of prevalent cancers in selected chest radiograph/sputum cytology-based screening studies

	No of tumors (% screened population)	Squamous (% total)	Adenocarcinoma (% total)	Small cell (% total)	Others (% total)
Frost et al 1984[10] (Johns Hopkins)	79 (0.76%)	31 (39%)	22 (28%)	10 (12.6%)	16 (20.4%)
Flehinger et al 1984[11] (Memorial Sloan-Kettering)	53 (0.52%)	24 (45%)	24 (45%)	1 (2%)	4 (8%)
Fontana et al 1984[12] (Mayo Clinic)	91 (0.83%)	39 (43%)	25 (27%)	12 (13%)	15 (17%)
Kubik et al 1986[13] (Prague, Czech Republic)	19 (0.3%)	9 (47%)	–	7 (37%)	3 (16%)

effective in detecting squamous cell carcinomas, particularly in early disease, and some small-cell cancers, but insensitive for adenocarcinomas, most of which, like most large-cell carcinomas, were found by CXR only. Interestingly, interval symptomatic tumors which presented during the study, and those discovered in the cohorts post-screening, showed a much higher proportion of small-cell carcinomas,[17,18] reflecting the absence of a detectable preinvasive stage and rapid progression to symptomatic disease prior to or between screening tests.[6]

Screen-detected tumors tended to be of earlier stage than those in either the non-screened control groups[12-14] or in the general experience of symptomatic lung cancer, where 16–18% are stage I. In the Memorial Sloan Kettering study,[11] 40% of the cancers were stage I and just over 50% were resectable. In the Mayo Clinic[12] and Czech[13] studies about one half of the cases were of stage I or II compared with 32% and 21%, respectively, of controls.

These trials did not impact on mortality rates from lung cancer and were declared failures. In addition, the prolonged survival of patients with screen-detected cancer prompted claims that screening had overdiagnosed life-threatening cancer,[19] despite the rather obvious fact that, by detecting cancers earlier, even those patients who have metastases at the time of detection will live longer. A review of the Mayo study pathological material[20] showed no evidence that misdiagnosis of cancer could account for the excess of malignancy in the screened group, as previously suggested. However, a small proportion (no more than 14.5%) of cases were CIS, rather than invasive disease. Given that CIS has an excellent prognosis without inevitable progression to invasion, this could account for a degree of 'overdiagnosis' of life-threatening cancer. However, more compelling evidence against the 'overdiagnosis' hypothesis, or the suggestion that screen-detected cancer is less malignant than that seen in everyday clinical practice, comes from observations that patients with stage I screen-detected cancer do badly if not treated by radical surgery.[21] Furthermore, a review of tumor doubling times for screen-detected cases in the Mayo Lung Project and Memorial Sloan Kettering studies showed no tendency towards more slowly growing tumors.[22] Also, autopsy studies fail to show evidence of the clinically insignificant lung cancer, which the 'overdiagnosis' hypothesis would predict,[3] although this point has been challenged.[23]

Disease detection by sputum cytology

Sputum cytology has an average sensitivity of 65% for detecting all lung cancers, though the range is wide (22–98%). The chance of successful detection increases with central tumor, squamous cell type, large (advanced) tumors and increased number of specimens examined.[24] In screening studies the detection rate by cytology is lower since lesions are, in general, smaller. In the NCI trials about 30% of the screen-detected prevalent cancers gave positive cytology[25] and not surprisingly a significant number of patients with dysplasia were also detected. In a more recent Japanese study, 22% of detected cancers gave positive cytology, half of which were cytology positive/CT negative and, as expected, all were squamous cell cancers.[26]

That sputum cytology can detect lesions 18–36 months before the CXR is abnormal[24] is commensurate with the concept of radiographically occult squamous cell carcinoma (ROSCC) shedding cells into sputum before the tumor has invaded significantly beyond the bronchial wall. Dysplastic lesions may also be detected in this way. As well as reporting CIS or invasive carcinoma in 2% of their sputum cytology-screened population, the Denver SPORE study also found that 26% of their study cohort had moderate/severe dysplasia while 48% had mild dysplasia.[27] The study group was a targeted population of particularly heavy smokers who also had evidence of COPD and airflow limitation. In a community-based high-risk study group who had normal chest radiology, sputum cytology detected a carcinoma prevalence of 1.8%, with more cases found on follow-up of patients with high-grade dysplasia.[28] Of these cases, 14% were CIS, 74% were stage I tumors, 86% were squamous cell but only 6% were adenocarcinomas. These studies found relatively high rates of cancer, reflecting the influence of study group selection on the findings.

There are a number of descriptions of the pathology of ROSCC. In a small study of 20 cases found out with a screening program, five cases were classified as CIS, three were described as microinvasive, while four of the 12 resected invasive cancers had N1 disease.[8] Sixty-eight ROSCCs were detected and completely resected in the Mayo Lung Project.[29] Of these, 33% were CIS, 18% were microinvasive intramucosal cancers, 31% invaded further into, but not beyond the airway, while 18% invaded extrabronchially. Screening studies using CXR and sputum cytology in Miyagi prefecture, Japan have reported a total of 184 resected ROSCCs.[30] Two patterns of disease were described in this study, one called *creeping carcinoma*, the other *penetrating carcinoma*. The former was more common (85% of invasive tumors) and showed lateral extension of the tumor internal to the bronchial cartilage. Tumors less than 20 mm in maximum extent never showed nodal metastases. Only 8% of all creeping-type tumors measured over 20 mm and these showed nodal metastases in 24% of cases (2% overall). Penetrating-type tumors were less common, but 13% had nodal metastases.[31,32] Carcinoma in-situ accounted for 13% of resected ROSCCs. CIS lesions measured up to 12 mm, with just over one quarter invisible at normal bronchoscopy and none had nodal disease.[33] These authors speculated that the penetrating type of tumor was less common in this radiographically occult screen-detected group since most such tumors progress rapidly to invade beyond the bronchus and become visible on CXR earlier in their natural history. This implies that the creeping-type tumors may be biologically different and could be the non-life-threatening cancer, suggested by the 'over-diagnosis' hypothesis. The data from the Miyagi study and elsewhere suggest that 22–29% of patients with early central ROSCC will have further synchronous or metachronous cancers, reflecting the field cancerization present in these patients' airways. The 5 year survival for the Miyagi patients who had surgical resection was 80%.

Fluorescence bronchoscopy

Chest radiography is an insensitive tool, particularly for detecting bronchogenic (central) cancer and when 'positive', the disease is relatively advanced. Sputum cytology may detect ROSCC or preinvasive disease but is also relatively insensitive. When disease is detected, the risk of metastases is already high and sputum cytology cannot localize the lesion(s). Identification of preinvasive bronchial disease is difficult since most lesions are invisible at standard white light bronchoscopy (WLB). In one study only 29% of CIS detected by sputum cytology was visible at WLB.[34]

Autofluorescence bronchoscopy (AFB) has radically changed this situation. Using blue light, abnormal mucosa gives a much weaker green autofluorescence than normal mucosa (Figure 15.1). AFB was 6.3 times more sensitive than WLB in identifying high-grade SD or CIS and was even superior (2.7-fold) in detecting invasive disease.[34] In this study, however, 46% of biopsy specimens from areas deemed 'abnormal' at AFB were histologically normal and a further 34% showed hyperplasia, metaplasia or mild SD. In a later study, the same investigators found that males had more high-grade dysplasia than females.[35] In a review of fluorescence bronchoscopy studies, Lam and colleagues reported this technique identified CIS in 1.6% of over 1000 patients screened, but found moderate or severe dysplasia in a further 19% of individuals selected for screening on the basis of a heavy smoking history and atypical sputum cytology.[36] Overall, about 40% of the lesions found were seen at WLB, while the detection rate rose to 80% using AFB. The remaining lesions were found in random biopsy specimens.

The pathological findings of three AFB screening studies[36–38] are presented in Table 15.2. The inclusion of biopsy samples taken at random or from areas deemed 'borderline abnormal' at AFB added to the number of cases of dysplasia, but also considerably increased the number with insignificant pathology, thus

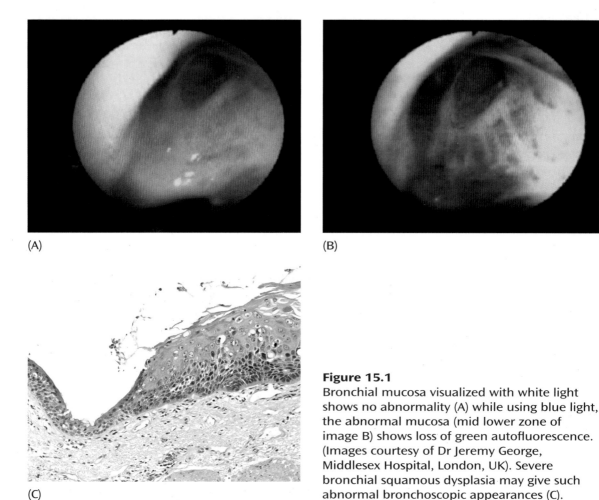

(A)

(B)

(C)

Figure 15.1
Bronchial mucosa visualized with white light shows no abnormality (A) while using blue light, the abnormal mucosa (mid lower zone of image B) shows loss of green autofluorescence. (Images courtesy of Dr Jeremy George, Middlesex Hospital, London, UK). Severe bronchial squamous dysplasia may give such abnormal bronchoscopic appearances (C).

Table 15.2 Histological findings after biopsy of abnormal mucosa detected at autofluorescence bronchoscopy

Worst case histology (per patient)	Lam et al 2000[36] (autofluorescence bronchoscopy)	Hirsch et al 2001[37] (autofluorescence or WL bronchoscopy)	Moro-Sibilot et al, 2002[38] (autofluorescence and WL bronchoscopy)
Normal	5%	9.1%	29%
Hyperplasia/metaplasia	30%	18.2%	38%
Mild dysplasia	44%	14.5%	
Moderate dysplasia	13%	50.9% (combined score for 'high-grade' dysplasia)	17%
Severe dysplasia	6%		
Carcinoma in-situ	1.6%	1.8%	
Invasive carcinoma	0.4%	5.5%	16%

increasing the false positive rate. The Denver[37] and French[38] studies examined very high-risk individuals, including some patients with previous lung cancer, perhaps explaining their high rates of high-grade disease. Hirsch et al[37] also found that AFB was more sensitive than WLB for detecting high-grade dysplasia (68.8% vs 21.9%) and for detecting angiogenic squamous dysplasia (75% vs 15%). (Angiogenic squamous dysplasia is a micropapillary lesion in the bronchial mucosa in which tufts of capillary vessels and fibroblasts are covered by a frequently thin dysplastic squamous epithelium.[39] This dysplasia is difficult to grade since the epithelium is thin and the relationship between this lesion and invasive disease has yet to be determined.) Despite the apparent improved sensitivity of AFB in detecting pre-neoplasia, the Denver group also reported that ten of the 32 foci of severe dysplasia in their study were not localized at AFB.[37]

Lam et al[36] measured the size of a small number of AFB-detected lesions and found that 55% measured 1.5 mm or less, 45% were between 1.6 and 3 mm. The largest lesion was the single CIS measured in the study. Woolner reported the median diameter of CIS at 8 mm,[40] while other studies showed that CIS lesions are only a few cells thick (mean five) in keeping with intraepithelial neoplasia.[41] Preneoplastic lesions are small, as well as multifocal.

Autofluorescence bronchoscopy allows localization of preinvasive disease, for which it has high sensitivity but lesser specificity. While it is superior to WLB in detecting these tiny lesions, it is not fool-proof.

Progression of preinvasive squamous lesions

Much has been learned about the molecular and genetic events which are associated with the progression of preinvasive bronchial disease.

This has been reviewed elsewhere.[42] What is far from clear, however, is what determines the rate or likelihood of progression within individual patients.

Longitudinal studies of dysplasia were virtually impossible before AFB was developed. Studies using sputum cytology to detect atypical squamous cells suggested that about 10% of patients with moderate cellular atypia and 40–80% with severe cellular atypia will develop invasive disease.[43,44] Each of the stages of dysplasia and CIS probably lasts several years before invasion supervenes.[6] Sputum atypia does not, however, directly equate with dysplasia and may not reflect the range and degree of disease present.

Follow-up, using AFB over a minimum 6 month period, of six patients with biopsy-proven CIS and three with severe dysplasia, found that two of those with CIS and three with dysplasia developed invasive disease. However, the remaining four CIS patients did not, including three apparently reverting to normal histology.[45] However, subsequent follow-up, in some cases over 6 years, revealed that all patients eventually developed invasive carcinoma,[46] as did all four patients with severe dysplasia in another study.[47] A much larger study with a 2-year follow-up period using AFB[48] found much less disease progression (Table 15.3). Two other studies showed progression from CIS to invasive disease in 25%[49] and 29%[50] respectively. All studies are difficult to interpret since higher grade lesions are often treated. Clearly there are ethical issues in not doing so. Furthermore, there may well be instances in all those studies where biopsy resects the preneoplastic lesion, especially those lower-grade foci which tend to be smaller, thus giving a false impression of regression. Partial removal could also induce inflammatory regression. There are also potential problems with the consistency and accuracy of pathological diagnosis and grading of preinvasive lesions.[51]

There are interesting issues concerning morphologically normal bronchial mucosa. It is known that, in the type of high-risk patient targeted by screening trials, normal looking mucosa shows malignancy-associated genetic changes[52] and that these 'lesions' are very small. Some areas which are abnormal at AFB are histologically normal and this has prompted some to speculate that AFB may be able to detect abnormalities 'beyond the threshold of the microscopic abilities of the pathologist'.[45] While this is an intriguing thought, given the genetic studies, it is difficult to see what the biological basis of this idea might be, considering AFB 'sees' not only the epithelium but also subepithelial tissue and where biopsy sampling error is also an issue.

There are interesting data on molecular factors, which may influence and predict the likelihood of progression in preinvasive bronchial disease. Dysplasia associated with invasive carcinoma shows p53 positivity and/or loss of p16 expression whilst dysplasias in patients without invasive cancer do not.[53,54] Markers such as p53, p16INKA, bax, bcl2, Fhit and cyclins D1 and E may also have value in predicting disease progression.[54–57]

There are still insufficient data to allow clear statements about the risk of progression of preinvasive disease. Progression may take months to years but is not inevitable. Sputum cytology may underestimate the degree of disease present. Biopsy may remove the lesion, so giving a false impression of regression, or may miss the lesion, leading to overestimates of rapid progression. It is likely, however, that, as the disease becomes more severe, so does the likelihood of progression.

Table 15.3 Outcome of preinvasive lesions detected at autofluorescence bronchoscopy (modified from ref 48)

| Initial histology n = no of lesions | Findings on follow-up after 2 years | | | |
	Stable lesion	Regression to lesser grade	Disease progression	Invasive disease
Normal or inflammatory n = 36	83%		17% developed SD	
Hyperplasia or metaplasia (Hyp/Met) n = 152	32%	37% became normal	30% became MMD 2% became CIS	One lesion became invasive carcinoma
Mild/moderate dysplasia (MMD) n = 169	37%	37% became Hyp/Met 23% became normal	3.5% became severe dysplasia	
Severe dysplasia (SD) n = 27	37%	22% became MMD 41% became normal	*	
Carcinoma in-situ (CIS)** n = 32	87.5%	9% became normal		

This study involved 104 patients, up to four AFB examinations and over 1000 biopsy samples.
*Three cases of severe dysplasia were graded CIS at 3 months and were treated. No CIS was present at 2 years.
**78% remained SD or CIS at 3 months and were treated. None progressed to invasive disease.

PERIPHERAL DISEASE

While most squamous cell carcinomas arise from the bronchial epithelium in central airways, some will develop in smaller subsegmental bronchi or bronchioles, presumably by the same mechanism, and present as 'peripheral' tumors. Most peripheral carcinomas of lung are, however, adenocarcinomas which arise from bronchioloalveolar epithelium. While CXR will again detect relatively advanced cases, bronchoscopy and sputum cytology are essentially useless, especially in the screening setting, for detecting adenocarcinoma.

This section discusses the development of lung adenocarcinoma, highlights the preinvasive lesions involved and examines the findings of those CT-based screening studies, for which this pathway of lung carcinogenesis is so relevant.

Peripheral adenocarcinogenesis

Previous concepts of peripheral adenocarcinoma arising in scars have, for most cases, been refuted.[58] More recently, attention has focused on atypical adenomatous hyperplasia (AAH) and localized non-mucinous bronchioloalveolar carcinoma (LNMBAC) as preinvasive precursors of peripheral invasive adenocarcinoma.[58–60] Thus peripheral adenocarcinoma probably develops from AAH (the equivalent stage of hyperplasia and dysplasia in the central airway), through an intermediate stage of in-situ adenocarcinoma (LNMBAC), wherein invasion develops and invasive adenocarcinoma results: an adenoma–carcinoma sequence in the lung periphery. Many morphologic, molecular and genetic studies support the place of AAH in this pathway[61–64] and the work of Noguchi and colleagues on early adenocarcinoma[65] led to the fundamental change in the definition of BAC as a non-invasive lesion in the WHO classification of 1999.[4]

In comparison to central bronchogenic disease, less is known about the biology and progression of the preinvasive stages of adenocarcinoma, and AAH especially is very difficult to detect. This poses particular problems for screening.

Atypical adenomatous hyperplasia is a well-defined focal, usually centriacinar lesion in which alveoli are lined by a discontinuous heterogeneous population of round, cuboidal or columnar cells, including peg-shaped Clara cells (Figure 15.2). Ciliated or mucous cells are absent and nuclear pleomorphism is generally mild though binucleate cells are common. Mitoses are almost never seen. The alveolar walls show variable fibrous thickening and occasional lymphocytes. A more prominent inflammatory infiltrate is unusual and this and any fibrosis do not extend beyond the limits of the lesion delineated by the epithelial cells lining the alveoli. A small proportion of AAH lesions show a more continuous, but still heterogeneous layer of rather more atypical cells, relatively few of which are columnar. The subject of grading AAH is controversial and currently not recommended by the WHO panel though it is clear that within the spectrum of AAH there is a range of cellularity and atypia. Most AAH are very small lesions: 64% measure <3 mm, 17% measure 3–5 mm, but 10% measure over 10 mm. Of the more cellular, atypical AAH lesions, 67% measure over 5 mm.[66] AAH is commoner in the upper lobes, in the subpleural zone and is generally always present as multiple foci.

Prior to CT screening, AAH was found incidentally in lung resected for another reason, most often lung cancer, especially adenocarcinoma.[67,68] AAH is reported in up to 35% of adenocarcinoma-bearing lungs, is commoner in females than in males (including those with adenocarcinoma),[68] but has also been reported,

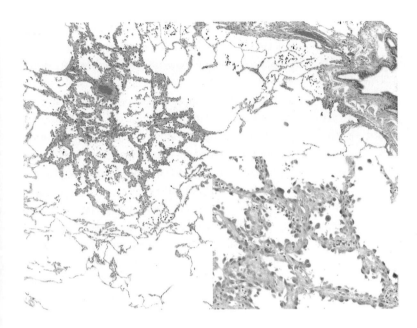

Figure 15.2
Localized lesion of atypical adenomatous hyperplasia in a centriacinar location. This lesion is approximately 1.5 mm in diameter. The high-power inset shows the typical cytological features (see text).

in autopsy studies, in 2–4% of patients without lung cancer.[69,70] Any relationship between AAH and smoking is unclear as is a link between any previous or family history of malignancy.[70]

There is a morphological continuum between AAH and BAC yet until recently the lack of clear criteria for making the distinction led to confusion. Each lesion still retains an intact alveolar architecture with a replacement-pattern of growth of cells displacing the normal alveolar cells lining mild to moderately thickened alveolar walls. This is of crucial importance in determining the CT features of these lesions detected during screening (see below). Although Miller proposed that all lesions over 5 mm should be considered carcinoma (LNMBAC),[71] it is clear that this is not appropriate and Noguchi and colleagues have made a useful proposal for classifying BAC, which now appears in the most recent 2004 revision of the WHO classification of lung cancer.[72] If the lesion fulfills three or more of the following five histological criteria, it may be deemed a LNMBAC of pure type (ie adenocarcinoma in situ or type A adenocarcinoma, see below): (1) marked cell stratification; (2) high cell density and marked overlapping of nuclei; (3) coarse nuclear chromatin and presence of nucleoli; (4) tumor cells growing in a wooden-peg-like arrangement or in a true papillary pattern; and (5) a tumor cell height greater than the height of the epithelial cells in the surrounding terminal bronchioles. AAH rarely shows more than one of these features. Most pure LNMBAC lesions are over 10 mm in diameter and the cell population tends to be more homogeneous than that in AAH. Both AAH and pure LNMBAC have an excellent prognosis, commensurate with their status as preinvasive disease.

Amongst early adenocarcinomas of the peripheral lung up to 2 cm in maximum dimension, tumors with a BAC component are commonest and can be classified into three subtypes as follows: type A, localized or pure bronchioloalveolar carcinoma (LNMBAC) type; type B, LNMBAC with alveolar collapse; and type C, LNMBAC with active fibroblastic prolif-eration. Type C adenocarcinomas constitute the largest group among the three subtypes. Type A and B show excellent prognosis (100%, 5-year survival), but the 5-year survival rate for type C is less than 80%. Therefore, types A and B are thought to be adenocarcinoma in-situ of the peripheral lung.

Type C carcinoma shows a peripheral BAC component and a central scarred area with active fibroblastic proliferation within which invasive tumor cells are invariably found. Inter-estingly, if this central fibrotic focus is 5 mm or less in size, 5-year survival is still 100%,[73] as with type A and B lesions. As the central, solid, fibrotic focus, with invasive disease, increases in size, prognosis become poorer. Such lesions are designated mixed-type adenocarcinoma includ-ing a BAC component in the WHO classifica-tion.

Those few sub-2 cm adenocarcinomas without a BAC component show an expansive growth pattern which compresses the surround-ing lung and may be subdivided into three subtypes: type D, poorly differentiated adeno-carcinoma; type E, tubular adenocarcinoma; and type F, the so-called true papillary adeno-carcinoma. These are considered small but advanced carcinomas with a less favorable prog-nosis, and would be classified under the WHO classification according to the pattern(s) of acinar (tubular), papillary or solid mucin-secret-ing carcinoma present. Such patterns of invasive tumor are likely to appear solid on CT scanning (see below).

Nodules detected by CT scan

While the CXR can detect relatively advanced cancer (masses of at least 1 cm diameter) in both central and peripheral lung, it has no role in detecting preinvasive lesions. For all practical purposes AAH and most localized BAC are invisible on CXR. Thus detecting early periph-eral disease has been a major challenge, partly addressed by the use of high-resolution thin-section CT scans to detect small pulmonary nodules. The relative fall in the incidence of squamous cell carcinoma and the rise of adeno-carcinoma, which is now the commonest lung cancer type in many countries, emphasizes the importance of effective screening for adenocarci-noma and its precursors.

High-resolution CT scans can detect nodules of a few mm in size in the lung, but there are many possible causes of such tiny nodules; normal anatomy and both neoplastic and non-neoplastic processes. Calcified nodules are assumed to be inflammatory and ignored. The shape of lesion and the nature of the margin are assessed and, for smaller lesions, evidence of growth on repeat scan is suspicious of malig-nancy. The internal structure of nodules may also be determined. A non-solid, so-called 'ground glass opacity' (GGO) pattern within small nodules, either in all or part of the lesion is a direct result of the lesion retaining an alve-olar architecture and correlates with the struc-ture of AAH and BAC, either in pure form or as part of mixed-type invasive adenocarcinoma.

CT screening studies detect much larger numbers of non-calcified nodules and cancers, in a larger proportion of the screened popula-tions (up to two thirds), when compared with chest radiography.[74] Most nodules (88–99%) are deemed benign on the basis of small size (5 mm or less), lack of growth or benign CT appearances. Criteria for radiological 'suspicion' vary but anything between 3–23% of such nodules have been investigated further and consequently, biopsy rates also vary widely and depend on study protocol.

Pathological findings of CT-screening studies

Pathological data on the prevalent lung cancers detected by CT screening in eight comparable studies[26,74–80] are shown in Table 15.4. After screening around 20 790 people, 150 prevalent lung cancers were reported (0.7%). Of these, 99 (66%) were adenocarcinoma and a further 22 (15%) were BAC. Of the remaining 30 cases, 19 were squamous cell carcinomas (12.5% of total). Sone et al[76] included two AAH lesions under 'other carcinoma' while Nawa et al[79] also report finding five AAH lesions incidentally, although it is unclear as to whether or not these were CT-detected lesions. The majority of the cancers were relatively small and 75% were stage I. Twenty-six percent of detected tumors measured less than 10 mm[26,74,76,78,79] and half of these 30 cases were from one study.[74] In one of the studies, nodules less than 10 mm were assumed to be benign and ignored.[77] The dominance of adenocarcinoma reflects screening of the parenchymal zone of the lung and the predominance of Japanese in the population screened. As with CXR/sputum screening, small early-stage cancers are detected. In a recently reported study comparing CT and CXR for screening a high-risk population, more cancers were detected in the CT-screened arm.[81] However, in this study only 48% of CT-detected cases were stage I. Furthermore, although a bias towards adenocarcinoma was seen in the CT-detected group, the difference was not significant. This study differs from the previously reported studies listed in Table 15.4, probably due to substantial differences in study design.

The data on incidence cancers found on repeat screening are limited and variable but, in general, incident cancers seemed to be smaller, more often stage I and are fewer in number when compared to their respective prevalent cases.[26,78–80,82,83] Adenocarcinoma is still the dominant cell type; however, small-cell lung cancers were found in three of the five incident groups,[26,78,82] in contrast to only one prevalent cohort.[78] Sobue postulated that prevalent cancers should be a mixture of large tumors and slowly growing cases with a long pre-clinical detectable phase whilst incident lesions should be small early tumors or rapidly growing cancers.[26] To a large extent the available published data support this suggestion.

Some studies give data on a few so-called false positive cases, coming to biopsy (nodules suspicious/likely to be malignant on CT but benign after histology). In some the lesions are simply reported as 'benign',[74,80] or inflammatory[75] but in those others, granulomas, scars, intrapulmonary lymph nodes, hamartoma and pulmonary embolus are the more specific pathologies responsible for the nodules.[78,79] As the size of the screened population rises, so may the number and variety of non-malignant lesions removed. CT diagnosis may be refined to limit the false-positive rate but in order to remove as many cancers as possible, some benign lesions will inevitably be resected. To date the vast majority of lesions designated benign on the basis of radiological features in the screening studies have not been biopsied.

'Ground-glass' opacities

Pathologists have long appreciated the importance of a retained alveolar structure in peripheral lung neoplasia, this being a defining characteristic of BAC and AAH. As CT scan resolution improved, so the fine structure of small peripheral lung nodules, detected within and outside screening studies, has been characterized. So called 'ground-glass' opacities (GGO) refer to hazy foci in which the lung architecture is not completely obscured, since some alveolar structure and air are retained in the nodule.

Table 15.4 Pathological findings in CT screen-detected prevalent cancers

Reference	% of screened population with cancer	No of tumors	Adenocarcinoma	BAC	Squamous carcinoma	Other	Stage I	Mean size mm (range)	No, false +ve biopsies
Kaneko et al, 1996[75]	0.3%	15	11	–	4	–	93%	16 (8–35)	1
Sone et al 1998[76]	0.48%	19	12	2	2	3 a	84%	17 (6–47)	3
Henschke et al 1999[74]	2.7%	27	18	3	1	4	85%	b (5–45)	4 c
Diererich et al 2002[77]	1.5%	12	5	–	5	1	58%	25 d (11–60)	3
Swenson et al 2002[78]	1.38%	21	11	4	3	3	62%	18 (7–55)	8
Sobue et al 2002[26]	0.81%	13	10	–	3	–	77%	19.8 (10–<30)	No data
Nawa et al 2002[79]	0.45%	37	22	13	–	2	86%	17 e	10
Pastorino et al 2003[80]	1.1%	11	10	–	1	–	55%	21 f	6

BAC – Bronchioloalveolar carcinoma.
Stage I – % of tumors of AJCC stage I.
a – Two of these lesions were AAH.
b – Data not given to allow calculation. 52% of cases measured 6–10 mm.
c – Three of these were carried out against ELCAP protocol recommendations.
d – All nodules <10 mm considered benign.
e – Range not given though largest tumor was 26 mm.
f – Range not given.

In a detailed study of 104 peripheral adeno-carcinomas less than 2 cm in diameter, HRCT evidence of GGO within the lesion showed a strong correlation with BAC histology and cancers with a greater GGO component had a better prognosis.[84] Other studies have shown similar findings and noted close correlation between solid areas within a GGO and alveolar collapse, fibrosis and invasive tumor on histology (Figure 15.3).[85,86] A recent study of 96 incident GGOs showed all pure GGOs 1 cm or less were either LNMBAC (70%), AAH (27%) or rarely invasive adenocarcinoma (3%), while larger GGOs and those with a mixed, part-solid

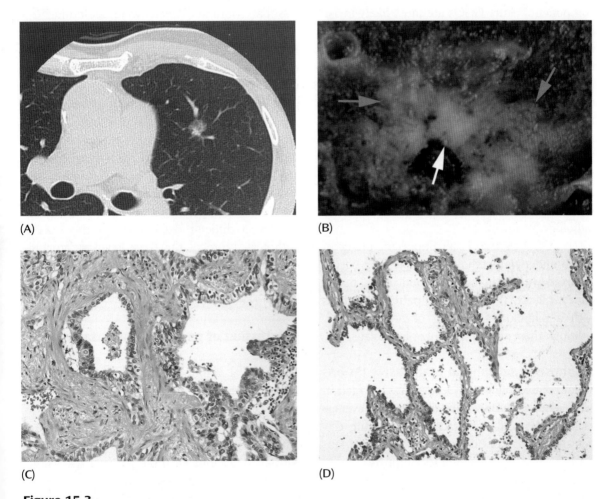

(A)   (B)

(C)   (D)

Figure 15.3
This tumor was detected during screening using spiral CT imaging. The lesion is a part-solid, part-ground-glass nodule in the left upper lobe (A). The gross cut surface of this lesion in the resection specimen showed a solid white central nodule (B, white arrow) surrounded by softer gray/white tissue (B, red arrows). Histology showed invasive acinar pattern of adenocarcinoma in the central solid area (C), while the peripheral zones showed bronchioalveolar carcinoma (D). Case courtesy of Dr R Kakinuma, National Cancer Centre Hospital, Tokyo, Japan.

CT-structure were adenocarcinoma in 38.5% of cases.[87] In a study of mostly screen-detected subcentimeter cancers, all those cases with a pure or mixed GGO CT pattern were LNMBAC, whilst solid nodules showed various histologies.[88]

CT screen-detected nodules with a GGO pattern and which show growth are highly likely to be either AAH, LNMBAC (type A/B) or mixed type (type C) adenocarcinoma with a BAC component.[89] Pure GGOs are most likely invisible on CXR.[90] Review of the ELCAP scans for a GGO pattern in the nodules found that 18% of non-solid (pure GGO) nodules and 7% of solid nodules but 63% of part-solid (mixed GGO) nodules were malignant (including LNMBAC).[91] In a review of those cancers which were initially missed on CT screening, the pathological/radiological findings were predictable: lesions were mostly subcentimeter well-differentiated adenocarcinomas, pure GGOs and obscured by normal structures or underlying disease on radiology.[92]

The GGO pattern is an important predictor of the underlying pathology and when it occurs admixed with radiologically solid areas, malignancy is likely. The pure GGO pattern correlates with a pathological finding of AAH or BAC, although there are also non-neoplastic causes.[93]

Diagnosis of peripheral preinvasive lesions

So far relatively few AAH lesions are reported in CT screening studies, though given the average size of AAH and the practice of ignoring CT-detected lesions of under 5 mm, this is not surprising. As HRCT technology improves, more smaller nodules, especially GGOs will be identified. The pathological evidence suggests that most GGOs less than 5 mm will be AAH, non-specific fibroinflammatory lesions or bronchiolar metaplasia while most solid sub-5 mm lesions are unlikely to be malignant. In a prospective pathological study, looking for AAH in 554 lung cancer resection specimens, careful examination of well-prepared 5–10 mm thick slices of inflated lung identified many AAH but also numerous scars and inflammatory foci. About 2% of these cases showed clinically undetected synchronous primary parenchymal tumors, almost all of which were over 10 mm in diameter and mixed (type C) adenocarcinoma with a predominant BAC pattern. Solid cancers less than 5 mm in diameter were not found.[68]

The histological distinction between AAH and BAC is difficult. Interestingly, in a small number of resected AAH and LNMBACs, while size was not a discriminator, CT density was less in the AAHs.[94] Sensitivity and specificity rates for CT-guided transthoracic aspiration or needle biopsy of solitary pulmonary nodules are generally over 90% but for lesions under 15 mm the results are much poorer and thoracoscopic excision biopsy has been recommended.[88,94,95] AAH cannot be diagnosed on aspiration cytology and BAC may also be a difficult diagnosis.[96] In the ELCAP pathology protocol the term 'atypical bronchioloalveolar cell proliferation' is recommended when features on aspiration cytology fall short of those needed to diagnose BAC.[97]

Progression of peripheral preinvasive disease

The clinical implication of detecting AAH is unclear given our lack of knowledge of the rates and risk of progression of this lesion. Follow-up of patients with AAH has failed to show any difference in prognosis when compared to those without AAH, but all these patients had surgically resected lung cancer, which is likely to have determined outcome more quickly than AAH progression.[98,99] Anecdotally, however, the authors know of several patients who have re-presented with metachronous adenocarcinomas years after their first cancer and AAH was diagnosed. A 20-year-old study of unresected stage I so-called BAC showed progression of all 48 tumors in 2 years and a frequently fatal outcome in 3 years, about 10% of cases progressing more slowly but with the same eventual outcome.[100] Again, interpretation of these findings is difficult in the absence of a histological diagnosis; the term BAC was used to include invasive cancers prior to the WHO 1999 definition, and in this study, mucinous BAC may also be included. Given the relationship between the GGO pattern, particularly in its pure form, and AAH/BAC, HRCT has potential as a tool for conducting longitudinal studies,[101] though combining this with histologic and molecular studies will be well-nigh impossible.

Larger, more atypical AAH lesions are more likely to express p53 and c-erbB2 or have K-RAS mutations[62] and loss of Fhit expression is associated with invasion.[102] Sequential progression from type A and B to type C carcinoma is characterized by a significant rise in MMP-2 activation and allelic losses at 3p (FHIT), 17p (p53), 18q (Smad 4) and 22q.[103,104] The value of these or other markers, as predictors of progression, is unknown.

FUTURE WORK

Further refinements are needed to improve both sensitivity and specificity of the tools available to detect early bronchial and peripheral disease. More also needs to be learned about the biology and risk of progression of preinvasive lesions since, if more such individuals are discovered, informed decisions need to be made regarding their management. Pathologists must become more familiar with criteria for classifying these lesions so that consistent data are gathered. For the foreseeable future expert pathological review of screen-detected and resected lesions will be essential.

To date the majority of sputum-based screening studies have used traditional cytopathologic morphology to detect abnormal cells, but new approaches using automated image analysis and monoclonal antibodies may improve test sensitivity.[105,106]

Proteins such as heterogeneous nuclear riboprotein A2/B1 and p53 may be detected in sputum and sputum DNA can be examined for malignancy-associated alterations, all potential surrogate markers for use in screening.[24] A sputum-based approach will, intuitively, be better at detecting bronchial disease, yet it is peripheral adenocarcinoma which is increasing in frequency. The chances of finding an effective marker for this pathway of carcinogenesis will hinge on better understanding of the biology of the early disease.

CONCLUSION

This chapter has discussed the two known pathways of lung carcinogenesis (specifically in relation to squamous cell and adenocarcinoma), the preinvasive lesions involved and how this is reflected in the findings of various screening studies. Knowledge of the pathology of early lung cancer and preinvasive lesions is crucial to the understanding of lung cancer screening and the results obtained. Different screening modalities target different areas of the lung, find different patterns of disease and pose different problems both for those detecting the abnormality and for the pathologist who must diagnose the preinvasive or malignant disease. As radiological advances and biomarker-based methods to detect disease are introduced, pathologists must ensure that developments are underpinned by the gold standard of a tissue diagnosis. As more people elect to participate in screening, more early and preinvasive lesions will be sampled and resected. This will provide an important and rare opportunity for research in an area crucial to our attempts to improve treatment of this most common and deadly malignant disease.

REFERENCES

1. Mulshine JL, Smith RA, Screening and early diagnosis of lung cancer. Thorax 2002; 57: 1071–8.
2. Yoshida J, Nagai K, Yokose T, et al, Primary peripheral lung carcinoma smaller than 1 cm in diameter. Chest 1998; 114:710–12.
3. Strauss GM, Randomized population trials and screening for lung cancer. Cancer 2000; 89: 2399–421.
4. Travis WD, Colby TV, Corrin B, et al (eds), Histological typing of lung and pleural tumours. WHO International Histological Classification of Tumours, third edn. Berlin, Springer, 1999.
5. Wistuba II, Berry J, Behrens C, et al, Molecular changes in the bronchial epithelium of patients with small cell lung cancer. Clin Cancer Res 2000; 6:2604–10.
6. Saccomanno G, Archer VE, Auerbach O, et al, Development of carcinoma of the lung as reflected in exfoliated cells. Cancer 1974; 33: 256–70.
7. Fong KM, Sekido Y, Gazdar AF, Minna JD, Molecular biology of lung cancer: clinical implications. Thorax 2003; 58:892–900.
8. Tao LC, Chamberlain DW, Delarue NC, et al, Cytologic diagnosis of radiographically occult squamous cell carcinoma of the lung. Cancer 1982; 50:1580–6.
9. Franklin WA, Diagnosis of lung cancer. Pathology of invasive and preinvasive neoplasia. Chest 2000; 117:80s–9s.
10. Frost JK, Ball WC, Levin ML, et al, Early lung cancer detection: Results of the initial (prevalence) radiologic and cytologic screening in the Johns Hopkins study. Am Rev Respir Dis 1984; 130:549–54.
11. Flehinger BJ, Melamed MR, Zaman MB, et al, Early lung cancer detection: Results of the initial (prevalence) radiologic and cytologic screening in the Memorial Sloan-Kettering study. Am Rev Respir Dis 1984; 130:555–60.
12. Fontana RS, Sanderson DR, Taylor WF, et al, Early lung cancer detection: Results of the initial (prevalence) radiologic and cytologic screening in the Mayo Clinic study. Am Rev Respir Dis 1984; 130:561–5.
13. Kubik A, Parkin DM, Khlat M, et al, Lack of benefit from semi-annual screening for cancer of the lung: follow-up report of a randomised controlled trial on a population of high-risk males in Czechoslovakia. Int J Cancer 1990; 45:26–33.
14. Salomaa E-RM, Does the early detection on lung carcinoma improve prognosis? The Turku study. Cancer 2000; 89:2387–91.
15. Okamoto N, Suzuki T, Hasegawa H, et al, Evaluation of a clinic-based screening program for lung cancer with a case-control design in Kanagawa, Japan. Lung Cancer 1999; 25: 77–85.
16. Nishii K, Ueoka H, Kiura K, et al, A case-control study of lung cancer screening in Okayama prefecture, Japan. Lung Cancer 2001; 34:325–32.
17. Fontana RS, Sanderson DR, Woolner LB, et al, Screening for lung cancer. Critique of the Mayo Lung project. Cancer 1991; 67:1155–64.
18. Melamed MR, Lung cancer screening results in the National Cancer Institute New York study. Cancer 2000; 89:2356–62.
19. Parkin DM, Moss SM, Lung cancer screening. Improved survival but no reduction in deaths – the role of 'overdiagnosis'. Cancer 2000; 89: 2369–76.
20. Colby TV, Tazelaar HD, Travis WD, et al, Pathologic review of Mayo lung project. Is there a case for misdiagnosis or overdiagnosis of lung carcinoma in the screened group? Cancer 2002; 95:2361–5.

21. Dominioni L, Imperatori A, Rovera F, et al, Stage I non-small cell lung carcinoma. Analysis of survival and implications for screening. Cancer 2000; 89:2334–44.

22. Yankelevitz DF, Kostis WJ, Henschke CI, et al, Overdiagnosis in chest radiographic screening for lung carcinoma; frequency. Cancer 2003; 97:1271–5.

23. Dammas S, Patz EF, Goodman PC, Identification of small lung nodules at autopsy: implications for lung cancer screening and overdiagnosis bias. Lung Cancer 2001; 33: 11–16.

24. Thunnissen FBJM, Sputum examination for early detection of lung cancer. J Clin Pathol 2003; 56:805–10.

25. Anonymous, Early lung cancer detection: summary and conclusions. Am Rev Respir Dis 1984; 130:565–70.

26. Sobue T, Moriyama N, Kaneko M, et al, Screening for lung cancer with low-dose helical computed tomography: Anti-lung Cancer Association project. J Clin Oncol 2002; 20: 911–20.

27. Kennedy TC, Proudfoot SP, Franklin WA, et al, Cytopathological analysis of sputum in patients with airflow obstruction and significant smoking histories. Cancer Res 1996; 56: 4673–8.

28. Petty TL, The early identification of lung carcinoma by sputum cytology. Cancer 2000; 89:2461–4.

29. Woolner LB, Fontana RS, Cortese DA, et al, Roentgenographically occult lung cancer: pathologic findings and frequency of multicentricity during a 10-year period. Mayo Clin Proc 1984; 59:453–66.

30. Fujimura S, Sakurada A, Sagawa M, et al, A therapeutic approach to roentgenographically occult squamous cell carcinoma of the lung. Cancer 2000; 89:2445–8.

31. Nagamoto N, Saito Y, Suda H, et al, Relationship between length of longitudinal extension and maximal depth of transmural invasion in roentgenographically occult squamous cell carcinoma of the bronchus (nonpolypoid type). Am J Surg Pathol 1989; 13:11–20.

32. Nagamoto N, Saito Y, Ohta S, et al, Relationship between lymph node metastasis to primary tumour size and microscopic appearance of roentgenographically occult lung cancer. Am J Surg Pathol 1989; 13:1009–13.

33. Nagamoto N, Saito Y, Sata M, et al, Clinicopathological analysis of 19 cases of isolated carcinoma in situ of the bronchus. Am J Surg Pathol 1993; 17:1234–43.

34. Lam S, Kennedy T, Unger M, et al, Localization of bronchial intraepithelial lesions by fluorescence bronchoscopy. Chest 1998; 113: 696–702.

35. Lam S, LeRichie JC, Zheng Y, et al, Sex-related differences in bronchial epithelial changes associated with tobacco smoking. J Natl Cancer Inst 1999; 91:691–6.

36. Lam S, MacAulay C, LeRichie JC, et al, Detection and localization of early lung cancer by fluorescence bronchoscopy. Cancer 2000; 89: 2468–73.

37. Hirsch FR, Prindiville SA, Miller YE, et al, Fluorescence versus white-light bronchoscopy for detection of preneoplastic lesions: a randomised study. J Natl Cancer Inst 2001; 93: 1385–91.

38. Moro-Sibilot D, Jeanmart M, Lantuejoul S, et al, Cigarette smoking, preinvasive bronchial lesions and autofluorescence bronchoscopy. Chest 2002; 122:1902–8.

39. Keith RL, Miller YE, Gemmill RM, et al, Angiogenic squamous dysplasia in bronchi of individuals at high risk for lung cancer. Clin Cancer Res 2000; 6:1616–25.

40. Woolner LB, Pathology of cancer detected cytologically. In: Atlas of Early Lung Cancer. National Cancer Institute co-operative early lung cancer group. Tokyo, Igaku-Shoin, 1983, pp. 107–213.

41. Auerbach O, Stout AP, Hammond EC, et al, Changes in bronchial epithelium in relation to cigarette smoking and in relation to lung cancer. N Engl J Med 1961; 265:255–67.

42. Hirsch FR, Franklin WA, Gazdar AF, et al, Early detection of lung cancer: Clinical perspectives of recent advances in biology and radiology. Clin Cancer Res 2001; 7:5–22.

43. Frost JK, Ball WC, Levin ML, et al, Sputum cytopathology: use and potential in monitoring the workplace environment by screening for biological effects of exposure. J Occup Med 1986; 28:692–703.

44. Risse EKJ, Voojis GP, van't Hof MA, Diagnostic significance of 'severe dysplasia' in sputum cytology. Acta Cytol 1988; 32:629–34.

45. Venmans BJ, van Boxem TJ, Smit EF, et al, Outcome of bronchial carcinoma in situ. Chest 2000; 117:1572–6.

46. Sutedja TG, Postmus PE (personal communication, 2004).

47. Satoh Y, Ishikawa Y, Nakagawa K, et al, A follow-up study of progression from dysplasia to squamous cell carcinoma with immunohistochemical examination of p53 protein overexpression in the bronchi of ex-chromate workers. Br J Cancer 1997; 75:678–83.

48. Bota S, Auliac J-B, Paris C, et al, Follow-up of bronchial precancerous lesions and carcinoma in situ using fluorescence endoscopy. Am J Crit Care Med 2001; 164:1688–93.

49. Thiberville L, Payne P, Vielkinds J, et al, Evidence of cumulative gene losses with progression of premalignant epithelial lesions to carcinoma of the bronchus. Cancer Res 1995; 55:5133–9.

50. Banerjee AK, Rabbitts PH, George J, Lung cancer 3: Fluorescence bronchoscopy: clinical dilemmas and research opportunities. Thorax 2003; 58:266–71.

51. Sutedja TG, Venmans BJ, Smit EF, et al, Fluorescence bronchoscopy for early detection of lung cancer. A clinical perspective. Lung Cancer 2001; 34:157–68.

52. Park IW, Wistuba II, Maitra A, et al, Multiple clonal abnormalities in the bronchial epithelium of patients with lung cancer. J Natl Cancer Inst 1999; 91:1863–8.

53. Brambilla E, Gazzeri S, Lantuejoul S, et al, p53 mutant immunophenotype and deregulation of p53 transcription pathway (bc12, bax and waf1) in precursor bronchial lesions of lung cancer. Clin Cancer Res 1998; 4:1609–18.

54. Brambilla E, Gazzeri S, Moro D, et al, Alterations of Rb pathway (Rb-p16INK4-cyclin D1) in preinvasive bronchial lesions. Clin Cancer Res 1999; 5:243–50.

55. Jeanmart M, Lantuejoul S, Fievet F, et al, Value of immunohistochemical markers in preinvasive bronchial lesions in risk assessment of lung cancer. Clin Cancer Res 2003; 9: 2195–203.

56. Ponticiello A, Barra E, Giani U, et al, P53 immunohistochemistry can identify bronchial dysplastic lesions proceeding to lung cancer: a prospective study. Eur Respir J 2000; 15: 547–52.

57. Sozzi G, Oggionni M, Alasio L, et al, Molecular changes track recurrence and progression of bronchial precancerous lesions. Lung Cancer 2002; 37:267–70.

58. Shimosato Y, Kodama T, Kameya T, Morphogenesis of peripheral type adenocarcinoma of the lung. In: Shimosato Y, Melamed MR, Nettesheim P (eds) Morphogenesis of Lung Cancer, Volume 1. Boca Raton, FL, CRC Press, 1982, pp. 65–90.

59. Miller RR, Nelems B, Evans KG, et al, Glandular neoplasia of the lung. A proposed analogy to colonic tumours. Cancer 1998; 61: 1009–14.

60. Shimosato Y, Noguchi M, Matsuno Y, Adenocarcinoma of the lung: its development and malignant progression. Lung Cancer 1993; 9: 99–108.

61. Kerr KM, Adenomatous hyperplasia and the origin of peripheral adenocarcinoma of the lung. In: Corrin B (ed.) Pathology of Lung Tumours. Edinburgh, Churchill Livingstone, 1997, pp. 119–34.

62. Kerr KM, Pulmonary preinvasive neoplasia. J Clin Pathol 2001; 54:257–71.

63. Kitamura H, Kameda Y, Ito T, et al, Atypical adenomatous hyperplasia of the lung. Implica-

tions for the pathogenesis of peripheral lung adenocarcinoma. Am J Clin Pathol 1999; 111: 610–22.

64. Mori M, Rao SK, Popper HH, et al, Atypical adenomatous hyperplasia of the lung: A probable forerunner in the development of adenocarcinoma of the lung. Mod Pathol 2001; 14: 72–84.

65. Noguchi M, Morokawa A, Kawasaki M, et al, Small adenocarcinoma of the lung. Histologic characteristics and prognosis. Cancer 1995; 75:2844–52.

66. Kerr KM, Morphology and genetics of preinvasive pulmonary disease. Curr Diag Pathol 2004; 10:259–68.

67. Noguchi M, Shimosato Y, The development and progression of adenocarcinoma of the lung. In: Hansen HH (ed.) Lung Cancer. Boston, Kluwer Academic, 1995, pp. 131–42.

68. Chapman AD, Kerr KM, The association between atypical adenomatous hyperplasia and primary lung cancer. Br J Cancer 2000; 83: 632–6.

69. Sterner DJ, Mori M, Roggli VL, et al, Prevalence of pulmonary atypical alveolar cell hyperplasia in an autopsy population: a study of 100 cases. Mod Pathol 1997; 10:469–73.

70. Yokose T, Doi M, Tanno K, et al, Atypical adenomatous hyperplasia in the lung in autopsy cases. Lung Cancer 2001; 33:155–62.

71. Miller RR, Bronchioloalveolar cell adenomas. Am J Surg Pathol 1990; 14:904–12.

72. Colby TV, Noguchi M, Henschke C, et al, Adenocarcinoma. In: Travis WD, Brambilla E, Muller-Hermelink HK, et al (eds), World Health Organisation Classification of Tumours. Pathology and Genetics of Tumours of the Lung, Pleura, Thymus and Heart. Lyon, IARC Press, 2004, pp. 35–44.

73. Suzuki K, Yokose T, Yoshida J, et al, Prognostic significance of the size of central fibrosis in peripheral adenocarcinoma of the lung. Ann Thorac Surg 2000; 69:893–7.

74. Henschke CI, McCauley DI, Yankelevitz DF, et al, Early lung cancer action project: overall design and findings from baseline screening. Lancet 1999; 354:99–105.

75. Kaneko M, Eguchi K, Ohmarsu H, et al, Peripheral lung cancer: screening and detection with low-dose spiral CT versus radiography. Radiology 1996; 201:798–802.

76. Sone S, Takashima S, Li F, et al, Mass screening for lung cancer with mobile spiral computed tomography scanner. Lancet 1998; 351:1242–5.

77. Diederich S, Wormanns D, Semik M, et al, Screening for early lung cancer with low-dose spiral CT: prevalence in 817 asymptomatic smokers. Radiology 2002; 222:773–81.

78. Swensen SJ, Jett JR, Sloan JA, et al, Screening for lung cancer with low-dose spiral computed tomography. Am J Respir Crit Care Med 2002; 165:508–13.

79. Nawa T, Nakagawa T, Kusano S, et al, Lung cancer screening using low-dose spiral CT. Results of baseline and 1-year follow-up studies. Chest 2002; 122:15–20.

80. Pastorini U, Bellomi M, Landoni C, et al, Early lung cancer detection with spiral CT and positron emission tomography in heavy smokers: 2-year results. Lancet 2003; 362: 593–7.

81. Gohagan JK, Marcus PM, Fagerstrom RM, et al, Final results of the Lung Screening Study, a randomised feasibility study of spiral CT versus chest X-ray screening for lung cancer. Lung Cancer 2005; 47:9–15.

82. Henschke CI, Naidich DP, Yankelevitz DF, et al, Early Lung Cancer Action Project. Initial findings on repeat screening. Cancer 2001; 92: 153–9.

83. Sone S, Li F, Yang Z-G, et al, Results of three-year mass screening programme for lung cancer using mobile low-dose spiral computed tomography scanner. Br J Cancer 2001; 84:25–32.

84. Kodama K, Higashiyama M, Yokouchi H, et al, Prognostic value of ground-glass opacity found in small lung adenocarcinoma on high-resolution CT scanning. Lung Cancer 2001; 33: 17–25.

85. Aoki T, Nakata H, Watanabe H, et al, Evolution of peripheral lung adenocarcinomas: CT findings correlated with histology and tumour doubling time. Am J Roengenol 2000; 174: 763–8.

86. Takashima S, Maruyama Y, Hasegawa M, et al, Prognostic significance of high-resolution CT findings in small peripheral adenocarcinoma of the lung: a retrospective study on 64 patients. Lung Cancer 2002; 36:289–95.

87. Nakata M, Sawada S, Saeki H, et al, Prospective study of thoracoscopic limited resection for ground-glass opacity selected by computed tomography. Ann Thorac Surg 2003; 75: 1601–5.

88. Asamura H, Suzuki K, Watanbe S, et al, A clinicopathological study of resected subcentimeter lung cancers: a favourable prognosis for ground glass opacity lesions. Ann Thorac Surg 2003; 76:1016–22.

89. Takashima S, Sone S, Li F, et al, Indeterminate solitary pulmonary nodules revealed at population-based CT screening of the lung: using first follow-up diagnostic CT to differentiate benign and malignant lesions. Am J Roengenol 2003; 180:1255–63.

90. Yang Z-G, Sone S, Takashima S, et al, High-resolution CT analysis of small peripheral lung adenocarcinoma revealed on screening helical CT. Am J Roengenol 2001; 176:1399–407.

91. Henschke CI, Yankelevitz DF, Mirtcheva R, et al, CT screening for lung cancer: frequency and significance of part-solid and nonsolid nodules. Am J Roentgenol 2002; 178:1053–7.

92. Li F, Sone S, Abe H, et al, Lung cancers missed at low-dose helical CT screening in a general population: comparison of clinical, histopathologic and imaging findings. Radiology 2002; 225:673–83.

93. Vazquez MF, Flieder DB, Small peripheral glandular lesions detected by screening CT for lung cancer. A diagnostic dilemma for the pathologist. Radiol Clin North Am 2002; 38:579–89.

94. Nomori H, Ohtsuka T, Naruke T, et al, Differentiating between atypical adenomatous hyper-

plasia and bronchioloalveolar carcinoma using the computed tomography number histogram. Ann Thorac Surg 2003; 76:867–71.

95. Li H, Boiselle PM, Shepard JO, et al, Diagnostic accuracy and safety of CT-guided percutaneous needle aspiration biopsy of the lung: comparison of small and large pulmonary nodules. Am J Roentgenol 1996; 167:105–9.

96. Mitruka S, Landreneau RJ, Mack MJ, et al, Diagnosing the indeterminate pulmonary nodule: percutaneous biopsy versus thoracoscopy. Surgery 1995; 118:676–84.

97. Flieder DB, Screen-detected adenocarcinomas of the lung. Practical points for surgical pathologists. Am J Clin Pathol 2003; 119(suppl 1): s1–s19.

98. Vazquez M, Flieder DB, Travis WD, et al, Early lung cancer action project pathology protocol. Lung Cancer 2003; 39:231–2 (http://ISCreen. med.cornell.edu).

99. Takigawa N, Segawa Y, Nakata M, et al, Clinical investigation of atypical adenomatous hyperplasia of the lung. Lung Cancer 1999; 25: 115–21.

100. Hill CA, Bronchioloalveolar carcinoma: a review. Radiology 1984; 150:15–20.

101. Takashima S, Sone S, Li F, et al, Small solitary pulmonary nodules (1 cm or less) detected at population-based CT screening for lung cancer: reliable high-resolution CT features of benign lesions. Am J Roentgenol 2003; 180:955–64.

102. Kerr KM, MacKenzie SJ, Ramasami S, et al, Expression of Fhit, cell adhesion molecules and matrix metalloproteinases in atypical adenomatous hyperplasia and pulmonary adenocarcinoma. J Pathol 2004; 203:638–44.

103. Iijima T, Minami Y, Nakamura N, et al, MMP-2 activation and stepwise progression of pulmonary adenocarcinoma. Analysis of MMP-2 and MMP-9 with gelatin zymography. Pathol Int 2004; 54:295–301.

104. Aoyagi Y, Yokose T, Minami Y, et al, Accumulation of losses of heterozygosity and multistep carcinogenesis in pulmonary adenocarcinoma. Cancer Res 2001; 61:7950–4.

105. McWilliams A, Mayo J, MacDonald S, et al, Lung cancer screening. A different paradigm. Am J Resp Crit Care Med 2003; 168:1167–73.
106. Kennedy TC, Miller Y, Prindiville S, Screening for lung cancer revisited and the role of sputum cytology and fluorescence bronchoscopy in a high-risk group. Chest 2000; 117:72S–9S.

16 Surgical approaches to screen-detected lesions and tissue acquisition for translational research

Harvey I Pass

Contents Introduction • Historical perspectives • Recent evidence for limited resection • Recommendations and future directions • Tissue acquisition for translational research

INTRODUCTION

With the advent of lung cancer screening, many nodules are being detected which have different radiographic appearances. Some of these nodules will be lung cancer depending on the study reviewed, and it is being recognized that the appearance of the nodules may be a harbinger for different biologic characteristics regarding their invasiveness and propensity for metastases. Surgeons are now considering whether these solid and part-solid nodules should have lung sparing if they prove to be early lung cancer, and these decisions are being guided not only by the size of the nodules but also by their radiographic appearance.

When there is no medical contraindication to operative intervention, patients with stage IA and B should have complete surgical excision of the tumor with negative margins by a surgeon who is trained, board certified and does a sufficient number of cases per year. Until recently, it was felt that the 5-year survival of pathologic stage IA and IB disease are 70% and 55% respectively independent of the histology of the tumor. Tumor differentiation and vascular invasion, however, seem to be significant prognostic factors. On average, about a third of the patients with stage I lung cancer will recur, with two thirds of these recurrences being systemic and one third local. Approximately 5% of patients with Stage I lung cancer will develop a second primary at the rate of 2% per year.

One of the controversies for the treatment of stage IA and IB lung cancer has been the resurfacing of the debate of whether an anatomic resection should be preferred to a wedge resection or less than a lobar anatomic resection, i.e. segmentectomy, and whether these operations can be performed by thoracoscopic techniques. Since lung cancer screening studies are detecting smaller lesions which are either solid or part solid, data which guide the thoracic surgeon to the management of these new radiographic entities have not really existed for this subclassification of early lung cancers. Moreover, a number of studies have now revealed that the stage I category criterion which segregates IA and IB, i.e. 3 cm, may be outdated and in fact misleading. Any modern day discussion of sublobar resections and their role in the management of non-small cell lung cancer must not only refer to older studies which explored the use of wedge and segmentectomy, but must also segregate the patient population by their functional status, whether they already have had a lobar resection for lung cancer, as well as integrate the data arising from the newest studies of screen-detected lesions. These newest studies may not have the power or evidence based proof to change the present algorithm but at least they may stimulate the construction of new clinical trials which investigate lung-sparing techniques.

HISTORICAL PERSPECTIVES

Feasibility of sublobar resection for T1N0 NSCLC

Only a few studies in the 1980s and early 1990s investigating the use of segmentectomy or wedge resection for compromised and non-compromised individuals actually stratified the results based on lesion size.[1-5] The studies demonstrated the feasibility of limited resection with 5-year survivals ranging from 31–69%, and, in general, lobectomy had higher survival rates than lesser resections, and two- to four-fold fewer recurrences than lesser resections. The Lung Cancer Study Group (LCSG) designed and published in 1995 a randomized trial of 247 patients with T1 tumors who intraoperatively had dissection of N1 and N2 nodes to rule out nodal metastases. Limited resection (segmentectomy, 80; wedge resection, 42) was carried out in 122 patients.[6] The trial revealed a survival trend at 5 years for the lobectomy group (73%) compared to the limited resection group (56%, $P = 0.06$); and a significant improvement in the recurrence rate for the lobectomy patients (1.9% per patient year for lobectomy compared to 5.4% for limited resection, $P = 0.009$). From these data, it was generally concluded that lobectomy was the only appropriate operation for stage I lung cancer patients who could tolerate anatomic resection.

Do these studies, however, apply to what is actually being investigated in the 2000s specifi-cally with nodules that are found in lung cancer screening studies? Perhaps not, since there are issues of size stratification and qualitative morphologic differences among lesions seen on present-day computed tomography which has given insights into the biology of small lung cancers that we did not have in the 1990s.

The influence of size

There are studies which have questioned whether the 3 cm cutoff between T1 and T2 may be artificial. Warren published a retrospective study of 173 patients with stage I (T1 N0, T2 N0) non-small-cell lung cancer who underwent either a segmental pulmonary resection ($n = 68$) or lobectomy ($n = 105$) from 1980 to 1988. The rate of local/regional recurrence was 22.7% (15/66) after segmental resection versus 4.9% (5/103) after lobectomy. Nevertheless, when the data were analyzed according to lesion size less than or equal to 2 cm in diameter, it was found that the 34 lobectomies had a 5-year survival of 75%, which was not significantly different from the 65% 5-year survival of the 38 patients with tumors less than or equal to 2 cm who had had segmentectomies ($P = 0.2$).[5] Kodama performed limited resection with curative intent in 63 patients with T1 N0 M0 non-small-cell lung cancer, of which 46 normal functional status patients had segmentectomy as an intentional limited resection. The average size of these tumors was 1.6 cm. The other 17 patients underwent wedge resection or segmentectomy as a compromised limited resection because they would not tolerate anything but a lung-sparing option. The 5-year survival of 93% in the intentional resection group was not different from that for 77 patients who underwent lobectomy plus complete mediastinal lymph node dissection for T1 N0 M0 non-small-cell lung cancer during the same period. Local/regional recurrence occurred in 8.7% (4/46) of the segmentectomies. Of note, mediastinal lymph node sampling or dissection was not uniformly performed and the majority of these recurrences were in the mediastinum.[7]

Based on these and other retrospective evaluations there has been a call for the subdivision of stage IA into further categories based on size. In a recent publication by Gajra,[8] reviewing 246 consecutive, surgically treated patients with pathologic stage IA NSCLC, 86 patients had tumors ≤1.5 cm with an improved outcome compared to 160 patients with tumors 1.6–3.0 cm. The 5-year disease-free survival (DFS) was 81.5% and 70.9%, respectively ($P = 0.03$), and the 5-year overall survival was 85.5% and 78.6%, respectively ($P = 0.05$). In the multivariate analysis, tumor size was an independent prognostic factor for survival. Similarly, Port[9] reviewed the experience from New York Hospital for 244 stage I resections. For 161 patients with tumor sizes ≤2.0 cm, the 5-year survival probability was 77.2% (95% CI, 68.6–85.8%) compared to 60.3% (95% CI, 46.7–73.8%) in 83 patients with tumor size >2.0 cm ($P = 0.03$ by log-rank test). The overall 5-year disease-specific survival was 74.9% (95% CI, 67.6–82.2%). Disease-specific survival was 81.4% (95% CI, 73.3–89.4%) for patients with tumors ≥2.0 cm and 63.4% (95% CI, 49.6–77.1%) for patients with tumors >2.0 cm. These papers certainly would give further credibility to stratification of surgical procedure on the basis of size; however, they are retrospective, deal with mainly solid nodules, and are a different population than patients who are detected in screening programs. Moreover, as detailed below, simply because a tumor is less than 2 cm does not insure that lobar, hilar or mediastinal lymph nodes are not involved.

The influence of size and nodal involvement

Obviously, any thoughts of performing a limited resection should be entertained for the groups with the least chance of angioinvasion or lymph node metastases, and from the improved survivals of pathologic, small stage IA tumors, it seems to follow that the smaller the lesion, the better the chance for a good result with lung sparing. Our degree of comfort for limited resections as thoracic surgeons, however, would be greater if the size of the lesion correlated with the chance of nodal disease. A number of studies have been published in the last 10 years which specifically have examined the issue of tumor size and lymph node involvement, and the majority of these studies were large retrospective reviews based on pathologic stage of resected lung cancers of given sizes.[10–15] Table 16.1 demonstrates that the proportion of patients with positive nodes with tumors less than or equal to 2 cm was approximately 20%, while Table 16.2 reveals that close to 10% of individuals with tumors less than 1 cm will have lymph node involvement. There seemed to be a difference in metastatic potential of small tumors depending on the histology. In

Table 16.1 Nodal disease stage IA, tumors <2 cm

	n	% Positive nodes	% N2
Naruke (1993)	287	40	50
Assamura (1998)	174	20	60
Konaka (1998)	171	17.5	66
Takizawa (1998)	157	17	NS
Sugi (1998)	115	19	66
Wu (2001)	136	22	NS

NS, not significant.

Table 16.2 Nodal disease stage IA, tumors <1 cm

	n	Patients with positive nodes
Naruke (1993)	20	8 (40%)
Oda (1998)	22	0 (0%)
Suzuki (1998)	10	2 (20%)
Miller (2002)	100	7 (7%)
Cornell (2003)	56	6 (11%)

Asamura's study,[11] squamous cell carcinomas 2.0 cm or less in diameter rarely involved lymph nodes and thus were thought to be appropriate for future trials of limited resection. Konaka[12] found that lymph node metastasis was significantly more common in tumors 1.5–2.0 cm in diameter (22%) than in those 1.5 cm or less in diameter (14.0%, $P = 0.0490$), and there were no lymph node metastases in tumors 1.0 cm or less in diameter. Both Asamura and Konake felt that systematic mediastinal and hilar lymph node dissection is necessary even for cases with

tumor diameter less than 2 cm, but questions regarding the role of mediastinal lymph node dissection for tumors less than 1 cm were being raised. Takizawa[13] noted that there seemed to be less lymph node metastases with tumors less than 2 cm that were well-differentiated adenocarcinoma. Nevertheless, Wu[15] pointed out that even in peripheral adenocarcinomas less than 2 cm, there was a 20% chance for micrometastases, but that bronchoalveolar carcinomas seemed to have extraordinarily low rates of lymph node metastases when this size. When even smaller tumors (i.e. less than 1 cm) were examined, caution was warned when considering wedge or segmentectomy, as the Mayo experience revealed a trend towards decreased survival with limited resection.[21]

The likelihood of finding mediastinal lymph node metastases with tumors less than 3 cm has been also reported by those few studies which comment on preoperative mediastinoscopy for stage I disease.[17–19] Three studies, seen in Table 16.3, reveal that approximately 10% of patients with stage IA disease will have disease detected by mediastinoscopy and a proportion of the

Table 16.3 Studies of limited resection in compromised individuals

Author	Year	N	OR	LN staging	pT1 (%)	pN0 (%)	5-year survival (%)
Landreneau	1997	102	W	Yes	100	100	61
Errett	1985	100	W	Yes	12	45	69
Strauss	1998	58	W/S	NA	90	100	48
Miller	1987	32	W	NA	87	97	31
Kutschera	1984	30	S	No	NA	NA	20
Pastorino	1991	28	W/S	Yes	56	100	53
Average							47

LN, lymph node; pT1, pathologic T1; pN0, pathologic N0; N, number of cases; OR, operative resection; W, wedge; S, segmentectomy.

patients not found to have disease at the time of mediastinoscopy will be found to have unforeseen N2 disease at pathologic examination of the mediastinal dissection.

One must conclude that although there seemed to be a trend for less lymph node metastases as the tumor size decreased possibly making these small early lung cancers candidates to challenge whether a lobectomy must be performed for all stage I lung cancers, there were no guarantees that a smaller tumor was not associated with lymph node metastases. Moreover, only after pathologic examination of the lymph node basins could the surgeon be absolutely sure that the limited resection or lobectomy accomplished for the 'early lung cancer' was N0. Hence, further stratification of preoperative characteristics besides nodule size seemed to be necessary for the development of new limited-resection strategies.

Morphologic variations in early lung cancer

With the advent of low-dose helical CT for lung cancer screening, small peripheral nodules are detected that cannot be detected with conventional radiography, and a number of recent studies have demonstrated an increased incidence of small peripheral lung cancer using CT screening. This is of great concern because there has been a great increase in the number of lung cancers which are adenocarcinomas, and of the adenocarcinomas, bronchoalveolar carcinomas represent the fastest-increasing subset. The CT screening studies have now defined a whole spectrum of radiographic abnormalities which are either solid or non-solid. The non-solid entities are referred to as ground glass opacities (GGO), and a focal GGO is a finding on high-resolution CT that is defined as hazy increased attenuation of the lung with preservation of bronchial and vascular margins. It is caused by the combined effects of diminished intra-alveolar air and increased cellular density, with alveolar cuboidal cell hyperplasia, thickening of alveolar septa and partial filling of the terminal airspaces. A GGO can be the radiographic picture of inflammatory diseases, focal fibrosis, adenomatous alveolar hyperplasia, and adenocarcinoma, and as such, is non-specific.

Parallel with the discovery of these lesions on CT screening studies, data were accumulating that there were pathologic subtypes of adenocarcinoma which, based on their growth pattern, may influence survival. Noguchi is credited with classifying these tumors by reviewing 236 surgically resected 2 cm or less small peripheral adenocarcinomas.[20] Six types of tumor growth patterns were described; type A (localized bronchioloalveolar carcinoma (LBAC) with replacement growth of alveolar-lining epithelial cells with a relatively thin stroma; type B (LBAC with foci of structural collapse of alveoli resulting in fibrotic foci); type C (LBAC with foci of active fibroblastic proliferation); type D (poorly differentiated adenocarcinoma); type E (tubular adenocarcinoma); and type F (papillary adenocarcinoma with a compressive growth pattern). Noguchi reported that types A and B had no lymph node metastasis and the most favorable prognosis (100% 5-year survival).

It has now been recognized that 'pure GGO' might represent an early stage of bronchoalveolar carcinoma (BAC) (i.e. Noguchi A) and that BAC potentially progresses to 'GGO mixed with consolidation'. BAC itself represents a non-invasive lesion as a pure GGO, but progression of the nodular opacity from a 'pure GGO' to a more solid center surrounded by a 'GGO halo' may be due to the increasing cellular proliferation, causing increased CT density. This interaction of appearance and size being interlinked is being confirmed by both retrospective and prospective studies. Nakata[21,22] found that 93% of pure GGOs less than 1 cm were BAC or atypical alveolar hyperplasia (AAH) while 40% of pure GGOs greater than 1 cm were adenocarcinoma. Part-solid lesions were usually BAC if they were less than 1 cm but if larger than 1 cm, these lesions were adenocarcinomas 66% of the time. Kondo[23] found that, in Japan, early lung cancers that were less than 1 cm were Noguchi A or B in 85% of the cases with 14% being types C, D, E or F. Nodules greater than 1 cm were Noguchi types C–F in two thirds of the cases.

Hence, in any decision regarding limited resection or lobectomy when dealing with the small peripheral lung cancer, one must not only take into consideration the size of the lesion, but its CT appearance and then attempt to correlate this with the Noguchi classification, or more simply, whether it is non-solid, or part-solid. Moreover, one must be convinced that the pure GGO represents a neoplastic phenomenon either by documenting its lack of regression by antibiotics, or spontaneous disappearance on subsequent CT scans. If interventional radiology techniques can document abnormal cells compatible with BAC by needle biopsy, further intervention would be justified.

Impact of nodule heterogeneity on lesser resection planning

Armed with the new glossary of terms which define early lung cancer including GGO, solid, part-solid nodules and the Noguchi classification, as well as the impact of unsuspected lymph node involvement, the thoracic surgeon is confronted with a new algorithm for the use of lesser resection that is just now beginning to be constructed. The utility of lesser resection in individuals with compromised pulmonary functions, as depicted in Table 16.3 has been well established when lobectomy is not an option.[24–27] In these situations there is not a choice of an anatomic resection which encompasses regional lymphatic drainage, and margins must be dictated to a certain extent by the size of the lesion, and the underlying pulmonary deficit. With the recognition of an early lung cancer in a fit individual, the extent of the resection now must consider whether a given subtype of nodule has a higher propensity for local recurrence or more aggressive behavior, and which lesser resection will be appropriate based on the known natural history of the subtypes.

Localization of the lesion and 'adequate' margins

Issues regarding the localization of the lesion, especially in the smaller size GGOs or partial GGOs, become important since the surgeon must be able to feel the lesion in order to resect it, and a pure GGO may have few external characteristics or give tactile clues to not only find it but to decide what its extent is (Figures 16.1 and 16.2). The small lesions not only become difficult to locate but present problems in regard to the margin criteria especially if they have a large non-solid component. In order to aid in the localization of these lesions, the radiologist has assisted the surgeon by placing a hookwire under CT guidance into or near the lesion on the day of the operation. The hookwire technique is especially useful when approaching the lesion thoracoscopically without the benefit of feeling the lesion. Other techniques include having the radiologist mark the visceral pleura overlying the lesion for the surgeon using indocyanine green, or the injection of a semisolid material such as agar under CT guidance in order to assist the surgeon for intraoperative palpation.

In order to confirm that the margins of the lesions are free of disease, the Japanese have

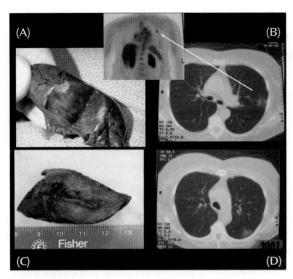

Figure 16.1
(A) Pure ground-glass opacity in the superior segment of a specimen of left upper lobe which matches the CT scan seen in (B). Note that there is subpleural puckering and a grayish zone of consolidation around the lesion. This proved to be invasive squamous cell carcinoma surrounded by atypical adenomatous hyperplasia treated by segmentectomy.
(C) Resection specimen of superior segmental lesion which matches pure GGO on CT (D). This proved to be a Noguchi B bronchoalveolar carcinoma which was treated by large wedge resection. Inset reveals that the PET scan was only suspicious for the upper lobe part solid nodule.

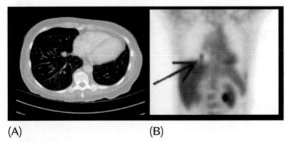

Figure 16.2
Same patient as Figure 16.1 who presented 2 years later with a solid nodule. (A) CT scan reveals right lower lobe nodule which reflects the high SUV area seen on the PET scan in (B). This proved to be a well-differentiated 1.5 cm adenocarcinoma without lymph node metastases and was treated by lobectomy.

described novel intraoperative techniques which will deliver an answer within 15–30 minutes. A 'run across' technique described by Sawabata[28] or a 'lesion soaking' technique[29] with evaluation of the cells by cytospin in the surrounding soaking solution have been shown to correlate with recurrence of the disease if found to be positive for cells. These techniques may assume greater importance in determining the extent of the limited resection or whether limited resection is feasible at all, as they are further validated prospectively by other centers. In the absence of these techniques, it is difficult to set criteria for the size of the resection if it is a simple wedge; nevertheless there are some data which state that the distance from lesion to margin should be at least as large as the maximum tumor diameter.[28]

RECENT EVIDENCE FOR LIMITED RESECTION

There are no phase III trials which have been designed to incorporate and validate the aforementioned lessons from screen-detected or small-size lung cancers in order to justify that 'lesser may be better' in early lung cancer. In order to rationally distill all this information to at least establish a strategic plan for future studies, a review of the most recent investigations which not only detail the surgical management of small peripheral lung cancers, but specifically comment on the demographics of the nodules excised may be helpful. Such a review should include studies of resections of small lesions which are T1 of 2 cm or smaller which have been resected by lobectomy in order to establish a gold standard for lymph node involvement, margin positivist, survival and recurrence. In the majority of these papers, however, especially if they are not from Japan, it is difficult to correlate the size with the radiologic characteristics of the lesions, and subsequent results of resection. Hence, much of the insightful data arises from a growing literature dealing with GGO of various solid consistencies which have been resected, and those studies which are especially useful are those which will have consistent data on lymph node dissection, standardization of surgical approach, and comment on recurrence and survival. The majority of these papers have been published since 2001, and originate from Japanese Institutions.

In a series of 94 patients resected by lobectomy for tumors less than 3 cm, Yamanaka[30] found that adenocarcinomas less than 2 cm had a 10% chance of metastases to segmental lymph nodes while tumors greater than 2 cm had a 15% chance of such spread (Table 16.4). Hence, in the adenocarcinoma situation, intraoperative sampling of the segmental lymph nodes with verification of their disease-free status may be a prerequisite before considering limited resection. In contrast, as also documented by Asamura,[11] squamous cell carcinomas less than 2 cm were not found to involve segmental lymph node. This predilection for a segmental involvement as well as micrometastases for adenocarcinomas was validated by Ohta[31] who found that squamous cancers less than 2 cm had no micrometastases to lymph nodes while adenocarcinomas between 1–2 cm had a 24% chance of micrometastases, and those less than 1 cm had a 36% chance of occult nodal metastases. Moreover, the patients with micrometastases had a 55% 5-year survival compared to 82% for those without micrometastases. In a smaller series of patients with tumors less than 2 cm, Nonaka[32] found a much higher propensity for lymph node disease with adenocarcinomas compared to squamous cell carcinomas.

From these studies which did not segregate on the basis of radiologic appearance, it appears that small, peripheral (<2 cm) SCCs are rarely, if at all, associated with lymph node metastases and may be amenable for trials of limited resection, but adenocarcinomas less than 2 cm could be associated with significant local recurrence if limited resection is not stratified by intraoperative hilar and segmental pathologic examination. Koike[33] performing a retrospective review limited resection in 74 patients who were resected for lung cancers less than 2 cm at his institution from 1992–2000. The majority of the patients (68) had adenocarcinoma. All of these patients had hilar lymphadenectomy with intraoperative verification of N0 status. The criteria for the 14 wedge resections was that there had to be at least a 2-cm-free surgical margin, and 60 patients had one or more segmentectomies. These limited resections were compared to a group of 159 lobectomy patients who refused limited resection. The 3-year and 5-year survivals were slightly higher in the lobectomy group (97.0% at 3 years and 90.1% at 5 years) than in the limited resection group (94.0% and 89.1%, respectively), but the differences were not statistically significant. There were no significant differences in the 3-year and 5-year disease-free survivals (limited resection group, 92.7% at 3 years and 88.7% at 5 years; lobectomy group, 94.2% at 3 years and 89.8% at 5 years).

A series of other papers have already reported results of limited resections for early lung cancers either by stratifying their results by Noguchi types or by the degree of ground-glass opacity in the lesions (Table 16.5). In general it was felt that the pure ground-glass opacity lesions represented a good cohort for limited resection because the mean volume doubling time in pure GGO tumors had been estimated to be 813 days, which is significantly longer

Table 16.4 Demographics of early lung cancers, solid nodules

Reference	Year	2<T <3cm	1<T <2cm	<1cm	SCC	Ad	LR	Lymph node disease	Nodal micro	Survival
30	2000	54	39	1	5<2cm 17>2cm	32<2cm 35>2cm	Lobe	Ad=10% SCC=0 Ad=15% SCC=11%	NA	NA
31	2001	All 3cm or less			26	155	Lobe		SCC<2cm (0%) SCC>2cm (50%) Ad>2cm (20%) 1cm<Ad<2cm (24%) Ad<1cm (36%)	+micro=55% −micro=82%
32	2003		46<2cm				Lobe	28% for <2cm	SCC=1 Ad=8	62% <2cm 5yr
33	2003		74<2cm 159<2cm				74 LR 60 seg; 14 wedge: 159 Lobe	All 74 had hilar sampling		LR: 89% 5yr Lobe: 90% 5yr

T, tumor size; Ad, adenocarcinoma; SCC, squamous cell carcinoma; Micro, micrometastases; LR, limited resection.

Table 16.5 Demographics of recent early lung cancer studies, non-solid and part-solid GGOs

Ref	Year	Size and GGO categorization	Resection type	LN total	Micrometastases	Survival
34	2001	42 < 2 cm (all A or B)	Wedge 34 Seg 2 Lobe 6	0%		>30 months without recurrence
35	2002	96 < 3 cm having HRCT	Solid component: I = 0%; II, 1–25%; III, 26–50%; IV, 51–75%; V, 76–100%	Lobe 79 Segment 11 Other 5	GGO > 50% No LN, invasion, or recurrence All BAC	GGO 26–50%: 22% GGO 1–25%: 18% GGO 0%: 31%	NA
36	2002	19 pure GGOs, 4–18 mm (observed more than two years) 39 pGGOs without waiting; 34 BAC (13.3 mm); 4 mixed (27 mm)	9 observation 10 LR 4 BAC; 1 Ad, 3 PLD; 1 AAH; 1 Fibrosis			All alive median 30 months without recurrence
37	2002	69 GGOs, 6–41 mm	Lobectomy 43 Segment 10 Wedge 16			>35 months median f/u without death or recurrence
38	2002	17 < 1.5 cm	All had wedge resection; no LN dissection	NA		No deaths, recurrence at 32 months
39	2003	54 < 2 cm	All lobectomy	A, B: LN = 0 C = 31% DEF = 50%	26% in pN0; 32% of all CDEF	AB: 10 yr 100% DEF: 10 year 75% No difference in micrometastases

Table 16.5 continued

Ref	Year	Size and GGO categorization	Resection type	LN total	Micrometastases	Survival
40	2003	19 pGGO <1 cm 9 part solid <1 cm 20 solid <1 cm	LR if outer 1/3 and palpable	28 pure or part GGO <1 cm without LN; 2 with vasc/lym invasions; 18% multicentric	20 solid: 16 Ad, 2 SCC, 1 SCLC, 1 carcinoid; 15% LN, 10 vas/lym invasion	Pure, part GGO 100% 5 yr No recurrences; Solid: 94% 5 yr
21	2003	57 <1 cm; (93% were BAC or AAH) 39 >1 cm but <2 cm 39% were adenocarcinoma	33 with wedge resection if <1 cm			No recurrences or deaths at median 18 months
41	2003	57 <1 cm		0/57 LN, invasion, or intrapulmonary metastases		97% 5 yr
		49 A, B; 8 DEF				
		26 >1 <1.5	11 A, B; 21 DEF	1/32 LN, 7/32 invasion, 0/32 intrapulmonary metastases		75% 5 yr
		34 >1.6 <2	9 A, B; 23 DEF	8/35 LN, 13/35 invasion, 3/35 intrapulmonary metastases		78% 5 yr
42	2004	27 pure (mean size 9.3 mm) 49 non-GGO adeno (mean size 21 mm)	All limited resection by segment or wedge	NA		GGO 5 yr 94% No recurrence or metastases; for 60 adenos <2 cm 60 adenos <2 cm 4/60 recurrences

A–F, Noguchi classifications; BAC, bronchoalveolar carcinoma: GGO, ground-glass opacity; Ad, adenocarcinoma, AAH; atypical adenomatous hyperplasia; LR, limited resection.

than in partly GGO tumors with a solid central component (457 days) or in entirely solid nodules (149 days).[43] Hypothetically, this higher growth rate of part-solid nodules could reflect an increased risk of invasiveness and potential for metastases during the development of adenocarcinoma.

Yamato[34] was one of the first investigators to actually perform a prospective study of limited resection for Noguchi A and B lung cancers, based on the intraoperative frozen section confirmation of Noguchi type and absence of lymph node metastases. Of the 42 patients in the study from 1996–99, 34 had wedge resections and two had segmentectomies. The remaining six patients had lobectomies for various reasons. These were small tumors with an average diameter of 12.3 mm. Although the study needs greater maturation, there were no recurrences at a median follow-up of 30 months. Confirmation of the indolent nature of Noguchi types A and B was also reported by Ishiwa[39] in a study of 54 patients with 2 cm or less adenocarcinomas who had resection by lobectomy. The A and B subtypes had no lymph node metastases, while 31% of the C subtype and 50% of the D, E and F subtypes had lymph node involvement. Moreover, 32% of the C–F categories were found to have unsuspected micrometastases. Ten-year survival estimates for the A and B types was 100% which decreased to 75% with the other subtypes. Most recently, Kondo[23] retrospectively analyzed the results of resection for early lung cancers with a stratification not only by Noguchi type but by size (i.e. less than 1 cm, between 1 cm and 1.5 cm and between 1.6 cm and 2 cm). As seen in Table 16.5, none of the lesions less than 1 cm ($n = 57$) had lymph node invasion or intrapulmonary metastases, and 5-year survival was 97%. As lesion size increased, the degree of lymph node involvement increased, and 5-year survival

decreased to 75–78%. From these data, Kondo suggests that types A and B adenocarcinomas that demonstrate pure GGO on CT could be considered for thoracoscopic resection without lymph node dissection. However, type C and non-alveolar replacement-type adenocarcinoma (types D, E and F) should have lobectomy with systematic lymph node dissection even if the tumor is less than 10 mm in diameter. The majority of these A and B small lesions occurred in non-smoking females, curiously the same group which has the greatest response to Iressa.

Other investigators have attempted to stratify early lung cancer suitability for limited resection by examining the proportion of the nodule that is GGO vs. solid. Matsuguma[35] reviewed stage IA resected lung cancers at his institution from 1994–99 who had high resolution computed tomography (HRCT) preoperatively. He divided GGOs by solid-component quartiles, and correlated their appearance with pathologic findings from their resection. When the GGO was more than 50% non-solid, all were bronchoalveolar cancers and none had involved lymph nodes or vascular invasion; however, as the solid component increased above 50%, the percentage of cases with micrometastases increased. By stratifying clinical stage IA patients according to percentage of solid and non-solid components, Matsuguma argues that one could use HRCT to aid in identifying those patients who would be ideal for limited resection by indirectly predicting those individuals with a higher chance of lymph node involvement.

Both Kodama[36] and Suzuki[37] confirmed that small peripheral GGOs were virtually 100% BAC; however, the natural history of the GGOs is variable, with some lesions not changing in size for over 2 years. Both observed that as the GGO increases in size and develops any solid component, the chance for an invasive adenocarcinoma increases. They recommended that if a GGO persisted on follow-up CTs or was growing, and had no solid component, the patients with such lesions may be candidates for limited resection. This type of management was indirectly validated by Watanabe who, after performing wedge resections for 17 GGOs less than 1.5 cm, reported no deaths or recurrence at 32 months. With a similar protocol, Nakata performed thoracoscopic wedge resection on 33 pure GGOs less than 1 cm prospectively. There were one adenocarcinoma, nine AAHS and 23 BACs which reinforces that not all stable or screen-detected GGOs are malignant.

Asamura[40] reinforced the importance of small size and location in reporting his experience with pure and part solid GGOs. Lymph node metastasis was seen in three (15%) of 48 patients with subcentimeter lung cancers emphasizing that 'tumor size less than 1 cm' does not simply mean the absence of the tumor spread through lymphatic or hematogenous pathways. Asamura, however, pointed out the importance of distinguishing between GGO-BAC type and solid type of lesions as lung cancer because lymph node metastases and recurrences were seen exclusively for solid lesions. In his series, resection was performed for patients with 1 cm or less tumor in the periphery of the lung, and for the pure and part solid GGOs with the solid component less than 50%, the 5-year survival with this approach was 100% without recurrences. Considering the extremely low chance of invasive features in these GGO type of 'small' lung cancers, in which the solid part occupies less than 50% of the entire area of the nodule, these data argue that limited resection might well be justified. Moreover, the GGO type of lung cancer in the Asamura series was documented to be multicentric since in five of 28 GGO types of subcentimeter lung cancers (18%), the lesions were

multiple. Hence, one should expect that the surgical candidate with GGO type of lung cancer may develop another one after some years, and preservation of lung parenchyma could be a priority.

The most recent data which comment on limited resection in the era of screen-detected lung cancers was reported by Nakamura[42] who analyzed 100 consecutive patients with primary NSCLC (83 stage IA and 17 stage IB) treated by wedge resection or segmentectomy without systematic dissection of lymph nodes between 1981 and 2002. By HRCT scanning, 27 tumors (27%) showed pure GGO. These all were diagnosed histologically as localized bronchiolo-alveolar carcinoma in the resection specimens, and none of these showed microscopic blood vessel or lymph vessel invasion. The pure GGOs included 18 type A, six type B and three type C in Noguchi's classification. Moreover, none encountered a locoregional recurrence or a distant metastasis after wedge resection. Accordingly, as echoed by Asamura and Watanabe, among others, Nakamura believes that patients with GGOs without a solid component on the HRCT scan are good candidates for wedge resection without lymphadenectomy.

RECOMMENDATIONS AND FUTURE DIRECTIONS

With maturation of studies for screen-detected lung cancers, as well as the publication of selected series regarding the natural history and surgical management of small (i.e. less than 2 cm), it is reasonable to consider designing novel intervention protocols which will once again, but in a more stratified population, explore the efficacy of intentional limited resection in good-performance stage IA lung cancer victims.

Although the natural history of the pure GGO has not been fully elucidated, it is generally agreed that these lesions, when resected and proven to be bronchoalveolar lung cancer, have the potential for a 100% cure rate, no recurrence, and do not metastasize to lymph nodes. These data, confirmed in a number of Japanese studies, lend credibility to the design of a trial of 'lesser resection' for the pure GGO. Although not totally evidence based, the Japanese studies imply that the pure GGO 15 mm or greater could be resected with a 'wide wedge resection' without lymph node sampling. For those pure GGO lesions less than 15 mm, close surveillance may be indicated and if the lesion remains a pure GGO but increases in size to 15 mm or greater, the individual would be a candidate for the lesser resection protocol. The pure GGO lesser resection trial could be a phase II trial design, and considerations for such a trial include: (1) 100% confidence that the lesion is a pure GGO, (2) method of resection, i.e. VATS vs. open thoracotomy and (3) preoperative localization of the lesion at the discretion of the surgeon. The role and need for lymph node sampling or dissection in this trial remains an issue, but based on data from limited studies revealing no recurrence of disease after resection, lymph node investigation could potentially be optional or at the surgeon's discretion.

For the solid and part-solid nodules, a randomized trial of lesser resection vs. lobectomy could be considered. Lesion size as a cutoff for such a trial is an issue for discussion, and more information from large lung cancer screening databases which involve resected solid and partially solid nodules should be reviewed with regard to: (1) type of resection, (2) lymph node status, (3) tumor size, (4) histologic findings and (5) survival and recurrence in order to possibly influence parameters for this trial, and decide whether lesion size should be 1.0 cm or 1.5 cm. Preoperative stratification would involve tumor size and percentage of solid component. It is preferable that the lesion is located in the peripheral third of the lung parenchyma, and the choice of the lesser resection, i.e. segmentectomy, 'extended' segmentectomy, or wide wedge resection would be at the discretion of the surgeon. Ideally, randomization to either lobectomy or lesser resection would be preformed intraoperatively after segmental lymph node dissection and frozen section examination to insure N0 status. Mediastinal lymph node sampling must be performed, and a systematic mediastinal lymph node dissection is preferred. This trial would clearly require a multi-institutional effort.

A multi-institutional trial is now underway with the sponsorship of the Japan Clinical Oncology Group (JCOG 0201). In that study, nodal status in clinical stage IA adenocarcinoma including PGGO is being examined by standard lobectomy and systematic lymphadenectomy. If there are no lymph node metastases in PGGO tumors in this trial, wedge resection for these lesions could be justified as standard therapy.

TISSUE ACQUISITION FOR TRANSLATIONAL RESEARCH

The ability to study the biology of early as well as late lung cancer with regard to molecular genomic and proteomic pathways requires the investigator to procure tissue. This is especially true when the goal is to study mechanisms of the newer biological agents. In studying such agents, the clinician must establish that the observed preclinical activity can be attributed to modulation of the target and that the biochemical/biological modulatory dose should be based on relevant target inhibition.[44] These issues usually require tissue, and become more relevant when one realizes that the dose for target modulation may not necessarily be the maximum tolerated dose of the agent. It is recognized that obtaining relevant tumor during clinical trials of these novel agents for laboratory analyses of the putative markers of drug effects, and the necessity to validate the laboratory assay for the marker are obstacles to drug development. These obstacles are even more difficult in patients with lung cancer, and investigators must make decisions regarding the validation tests to be done and the tissue requirements for such tests, the sites for biopsy, the methods of biopsy and their safety/efficacy, and their cost.

A variety of tests to determine intermediate biomarker status exist including immunohistochemical staining, DNA amplification, RNA amplification, and proteomics using two-dimensional gels, SELDI, or MALDI-TOF, or ELISAs, and a variety of sites can be analyzed including fluids (pleural effusions, ascites, cerebrospinal fluid, serum or urine) or tissue (primary tumor or metastatic tumor in the mediastinal lymph nodes or visceral deposits).

Cavities are the easiest to biopsy and usually yield cells from fluid; tissues accessible in 'tubular structures' like the bronchus require more invasive biopsy techniques and will sometime yield very little tissue, while having to access the primary lung cancer or nodes remains the hardest job when dealing with safety and efficacy concerns. Fortunately, minimal tissue is required for proteomic and genomic testing usually on the order of 1000 cells for DNA and RNA studies, while tissue proteomic studies will allow the identification of approximately 700 proteins with an abundance of 50 000–1 000 000 copies per cell from 50 000 acquired cells. From cavitary disease, one can obtain solid tumor via computerized tomographic-guided biopsy or thoracoscopy, or one can preserve tumor cells from malignant pleural effusions or ascites. The advantage of using malignant fluids, obviously, is the ability to do serial sampling for pharmacogenomics if one has an indwelling catheter, i.e. Pleurex, which permits longitudinal sampling while the patient is on or off therapy.

Acquisition of tissue from 'tubes' in lung cancer will center on endobronchial biopsy techniques including sputum sampling, bronchoalveolar lavage, bronchial brush, or endobronchial biopsy. Sputum can be difficult to deal with because of the associated mucus which must be removed using dithiothreitol or other agents. Moreover, a minority of respiratory cells are actually harvested. Preservation techniques also vary with regard to their utility in that cell architecture and immunohistochemical studies are best accomplished using Saccomannos reagent of 2% polyethylene glycol in 50% ethanol, while the rescuing of usable DNA and RNA from the respiratory cells may require cryopreservation after mucus removal or other specialty reagents including Cytech® solutions, RNA-later®, Trizol®, etc. Bronchoalveolar lavage (BAL) will usually recover between 100–200 000 cells/ml but numerous mononuclear and other inflammatory cells will be present.[42] Enrichment of the epithelial cellular component of the lavage is desirable and, in general, the first aliquot of BAL solution is enriched for ciliated epithelial cells when compared with subsequent aliquots. Respiratory cells are efficiently harvested in large numbers using bronchial brush techniques, and approximately 90 000 respiratory cells/brushing can be accomplished. For bronchial biopsy techniques, the largest forceps available should be used such that one can recover as many as 10 000 000 cells from a 10 mm^3 biopsy, and whenever possible, the biopsy should be guided using newer endobronchial techniques including autofluorescence technologies (see Chapter 11). If autofluorescence technology is not available, repetitive biopsies at the same site over time must be performed with the most common biopsy sites being the carina, bifurcation of the right upper lobe with the main bronchus, the bifurcation of the right middle lobe with the lower lobe, the bifurcation of the lingual with the left upper lobe, the medial basilar bronchus on the right lower lobe and the anterior basilar bronchus of the left lower lobe.

The most difficult situations to obtain useful tissue for translational studies are those which do not allow for the direct visualization of lesions to biopsy and one is required to use ultrasonography, fluoroscopy or computerized tomographic guidance to access the tissue. These situations become more difficult as the size of the lesion decreases and the location becomes more inaccessible or the tissue abuts critical organs.

Ultrathin bronchoscopes are being tested with external diameters of 2.8 mm in external diameter which have a working channel for brushings or BALs. These scopes will allow very peripheral GGOs or small nodules to be samples under fluoroscopic control. In the meantime, however, investigators looking for small lesions only seen on radiographic studies must rely on 'probing needles' either as aspiration biopsies or cores of easy-to-reach areas like the liver, skin or supraclavicular lymph nodes or more difficult harvest sites including lung parenchyma, mediastinal lymph nodes, pleural masses or adrenal lesions. Endoscopic ultrasonography of the subcarinal, paraesophageal and occasionally paratracheal lymph nodes are now being routinely sampled with minimal toxicity using the endobronchial or endoesophageal route.[45] Percutaneous biopsies using fluoroscopy remain a useful method for harvest however, the sensitivity approaches 89%, specificity 95%, positive predictive value of 99% and

negative predictive value of 70%, and a 0.02% mortality rate from air embolus or hemorrhage is reported in the most recent series. For lung cancer biopsies, the rate of pneumothorax approaches 20%, with 1.6–17% requiring a chest tube. Hemoptysis occurs in 5–10% and tumor implants from needle sites occur in 0.012%.[46] It is difficult to justify repeated percutaneous transthoracic biopsies for translational harvesting of lung cancer tissue, even in the protocol situation, and the yield is certainly intervention operator dependent. There are few trials which have commented on or used longitudinal transthoracic aspirations for research purposes.

The economic price of intervention harvesting of translational tissues has not been formally analyzed; however, in the literature, FNA is the most cost-effective way of retrieving diagnostic material compared to sputum analyses or bronchoscopy. For the biopsy of nodal basins, endoscopic ultrasonography via the esophagus is the most cost efficient compared to mediastinoscopy, transbronchial fine needle aspiration, and CT-guided fine needle aspiration, and EUS has the greatest sensitivity for all the techniques if metastases are suspected by radiographic data.

One must conclude that standard biopsy techniques can be used for sequential monitoring of the effects of new agents in lung cancer, but novel technologies are required to supplement the biopsy techniques to insure safe, relatively non-invasive but accurate tissue yields. Moreover, improvement in these novel biopsy techniques could potentially limit overall cost.

REFERENCES

1. Errett LE, Wilson J, Chiu RC, Munro DD, Wedge resection as an alternative procedure for peripheral bronchogenic carcinoma in poor-risk patients. J Thorac Cardiovasc Surg 1985; 90: 656–61.

2. Jensik RJ, Miniresection of small peripheral carcinomas of the lung. Surg Clin North Am 1987; 67:951–8.

3. Miller JI, Hatcher CR Jr, Limited resection of bronchogenic carcinoma in the patient with marked impairment of pulmonary function. Ann Thorac Surg 1987; 44:340–3.

4. Pastorino U, Valente M, Bedini V, et al, Results of conservative surgery for stage I lung cancer. Tumori 1990; 76:38–43.

5. Warren WH, Faber LP, Segmentectomy versus lobectomy in patients with stage I pulmonary carcinoma. Five-year survival and patterns of intrathoracic recurrence. J Thorac Cardiovasc Surg 1994; 107:1087–93.

6. Ginsberg RJ, Rubinstein LV, Randomized trial of lobectomy versus limited resection for T1 N0 non-small cell lung cancer. Lung Cancer Study Group. Ann Thorac Surg 1995; 60:615–22.

7. Kodama K, Doi O, Higashiyama M, Yokouchi H, Intentional limited resection for selected patients with T1 N0 M0 non-small-cell lung cancer: a single-institution study. J Thorac Cardiovasc Surg 1997; 114:347–53.

8. Gajra A, Newman N, Gamble GP, et al, Impact of tumor size on survival in stage IA non-small cell lung cancer: a case for subdividing stage IA disease. Lung Cancer 2003; 42:51–7.

9. Port JL, Kent MS, Korst RJ, et al, Tumor size predicts survival within stage IA non-small cell lung cancer. Chest 2003; 124:1828–33.

10. Naruke T, Significance of lymph node metastases in lung cancer. Semin Thorac Cardiovasc Surg 1993; 5:210–18.

11. Asamura H, Nakayama H, Kondo H, et al, Lymph node involvement, recurrence, and prognosis in resected small, peripheral, non-small-cell lung carcinomas: are these carcinomas candidates for video-assisted lobectomy? J Thorac Cardiovasc Surg 1996; 111:1125–34.

12. Konaka C, Ikeda N, Hiyoshi T, et al, Peripheral non-small cell lung cancers 2.0 cm or less in diameter: proposed criteria for limited pulmonary resection based upon clinicopathological presentation. Lung Cancer 1998; 21:185–91.

13. Takizawa T, Terashima M, Koike T, et al, Lymph node metastasis in small peripheral adenocarcinoma of the lung. J Thorac Cardiovasc Surg 1998; 116:276–80.

14. Sugi K, Kaneda Y, Esato K, Video-assisted thoracoscopic lobectomy achieves a satisfactory long-term prognosis in patients with clinical stage IA lung cancer. World J Surg 2000; 24:27–30.

15. Wu J, Ohta Y, Minato H, et al, Nodal occult metastasis in patients with peripheral lung adenocarcinoma of 2.0 cm or less in diameter. Ann Thorac Surg 2001; 71:1772–7.

16. Miller DL, Rowland CM, Deschamps C, et al, Surgical treatment of non-small cell lung cancer 1 cm or less in diameter. Ann Thorac Surg 2002; 73:1545–50.

17. De LP, Vansteenkiste J, Cuypers P, et al, Role of cervical mediastinoscopy in staging of non-small cell lung cancer without enlarged mediastinal lymph nodes on CT scan. Eur J Cardiothorac Surg 1997; 12:706–12.

18. Tahara RW, Lackner RP, Graver LM, Is there a role for routine mediastinoscopy in patients with peripheral T1 lung cancers? Am J Surg 2000; 180:488–91.

19. Choi YS, Shim YM, Kim J, Kim K, Mediastinoscopy in patients with clinical stage I non-small cell lung cancer. Ann Thorac Surg 2003; 75:364–6.

20. Noguchi M, Morikawa A, Kawasaki M, et al, Small adenocarcinoma of the lung. Histologic characteristics and prognosis. Cancer 1995; 75: 2844–52.

21. Nakata M, Sawada S, Saeki H, et al, Prospective study of thoracoscopic limited resection for ground-glass opacity selected by computed tomography. Ann Thorac Surg 2003; 75: 1601–5.

22. Nakata M, Saeki H, Takata I, et al, Focal ground-glass opacity detected by low-dose helical CT. Chest 2002; 121:1464–7.

23. Kondo T, Yamada K, Noda K, Nakayama H, Kameda Y, Radiologic-prognostic correlation in patients with small pulmonary adenocarcinomas. Lung Cancer 2002; 36:49–57.

24. Landreneau RJ, Sugarbaker DJ, Mack MJ, et al, Wedge resection versus lobectomy for stage I (T1 N0 M0) non-small-cell lung cancer. J Thorac Cardiovasc Surg 1997; 113:691–8.

25. Strauss G, Kwiatkowski, DJ, De-Camp M, Extent of surgical resection influences survival in stage IA non-small-cell lung cancer. Proc ASCO 1998; 17:462A.

26. Kutschera W, Segment resection for lung cancer. Thorac Cardiovasc Surg 1984; 32:102–4.

27. Pastorino U, Valente M, Bedini V, et al, Limited resection for stage I lung cancer. Eur J Surg Oncol 1991; 17:42–6.

28. Sawabata N, Matsumura A, Ohota M, et al, Cytologically malignant margins of wedge resected stage I non-small cell lung cancer. Ann Thorac Surg 2002; 74:1953–7.

29. Higashiyama M, Kodama K, Takami K, et al, Intraoperative lavage cytologic analysis of surgical margins in patients undergoing limited surgery for lung cancer. J Thorac Cardiovasc Surg 2003; 125:101–7.

30. Yamanaka A, Hirai T, Fujimoto T, Ohtake Y, Konishi F, Analyses of segmental lymph node metastases and intrapulmonary metastases of small lung cancer. Ann Thorac Surg 2000; 70: 1624–8.

31. Ohta Y, Oda M, Wu J, et al, Can tumor size be a guide for limited surgical intervention in patients with peripheral non-small cell lung cancer? Assessment from the point of view of nodal micrometastasis. J Thorac Cardiovasc Surg 2001; 122:900–6.

32. Nonaka M, Kadokura M, Yamamoto S, et al, Tumor dimension and prognosis in surgically treated lung cancer: for intentional limited resection. Am J Clin Oncol 2003; 5:499–503.

33. Koike T, Yamato Y, Yoshiya K, Shimoyama T, Suzuki R, Intentional limited pulmonary resection for peripheral T1 N0 M0 small-sized lung cancer. J Thorac Cardiovasc Surg 2003; 125:924–8.

34. Yamato Y, Tsuchida M, Watanabe T, et al, Early results of a prospective study of limited resection for bronchioloalveolar adenocarcinoma of the lung. Ann Thorac Surg 2001; 71:971–4.

35. Matsuguma H, Yokoi K, Anraku M, et al, Proportion of ground-glass opacity on high-resolution computed tomography in clinical T1 N0 M0 adenocarcinoma of the lung: A predictor of lymph node metastasis. J Thorac Cardiovasc Surg 2002; 124:278–84.

36. Kodama K, Higashiyama M, Yokouchi H, et al, Natural history of pure ground-glass opacity after long-term follow-up of more than 2 years. Ann Thorac Surg 2002; 73:386–92.

37. Suzuki K, Asamura H, Kusumoto M, Kondo H, Tsuchiya R, 'Early' peripheral lung cancer: prognostic significance of ground glass opacity on thin-section computed tomographic scan. Ann Thorac Surg 2002; 74:1635–9.

38. Watanabe S, Watanabe T, Arai K, et al, Results of wedge resection for focal bronchioloalveolar carcinoma showing pure ground-glass atenuation on computed tomography. Ann Thorac Surg 2003, 4:1071–5.

39. Ishiwa N, Ogawa N, Shoji A, et al, Correlation between lymph node micrometastasis and histologic classification of small lung adenocarcinomas, in considering the indication of limited surgery. Lung Cancer 2003; 39:159–64.

40. Asamura H, Suzuki K, Watanabe S, et al, A clinicopathological study of resected subcentimeter lung cancers: a favorable prognosis for ground glass opacity lesions. Ann Thorac Surg 2003; 76:1016–22.

41. Kondo D, Yamada K, Kitayama Y, Hoshi S, Peripheral lung adenocarcinomas: 10 mm or less in diameter. Ann Thorac Surg 2003; 3:250–5.

42. Nakamura H, Saji H, Ogata A, et al, Lung cancer patients showing pure ground-glass opacity on computed tomography are good candidates for wedge resection. Lung Cancer 2004; 44: 61–8.

43. Hasegawa M, Sone S, Takashima S, et al, Growth rate of small lung cancers detected on mass CT screening. Br J Radiol 2000; 73: 1252–9.

44. Dowlati A, Haaga J, Remick SC, et al, Sequential tumor biopsies in early phase clinical trials of anticancer agents for pharmacodynamic evaluation. Clin Cancer Res 2001; 7:2971–6.

45. Gress FG, Hawes RH, Savides TJ, Ikenberry SO, Lehman GA, Endoscopic ultrasound-guided fine-needle aspiration biopsy using linear array and radial scanning endosonography. Gastrointest Endosc 1997; 45:243–50.

46. Laurent F, Montaudon M, Latrabe V, Begueret H, Percutaneous biopsy in lung cancer. Eur J Radiol 2003; 45:60–8.

17 Non-surgical approaches to early-stage non-small-cell lung cancer (NSCLC)

Laurie E Gaspar, Tracey Schefter

Contents   Introduction • External beam radiation treatment • Brachytherapy • Radiofrequency ablation • Cryotherapy • Electrocautery • Nd:Yag laser • Photodynamic therapy • Conclusion

INTRODUCTION

The standard treatment of early-stage non-small-cell lung cancer (NSCLC) is surgery, usually lobectomy or pneumonectomy. Whether surgery should also be the standard of care for very small lesions detected by current screening programs is more controversial. The majority of these screened patients have extensive smoking histories and resultant cardiovascular and pulmonary disease, making surgery a relative or absolute contraindication in many cases. Furthermore, many patients have poor pulmonary function, sometimes due to prior surgery or radiation therapy for a prior, more advanced lung cancer. Synchronous or metachronous primary NSCLC are common in these patients so that lung-sparing strategies for very early lesions might be desirable.

Non-surgical approaches to early NSCLC rely on bronchoscopy reports and imaging studies to determine the local extent of disease. Computerized tomography (CT) scans may underestimate the size and local extension of small NSCLC.[1] In a phase II study by the CALGB, 58 patients with clinical T1N0M0 NSCLC were to proceed to a video-assisted thoracoscopic resection (VATS) followed by external beam radiation therapy targeted to the tumor bed. The final pathology report indicated that 14 tumors

(24%) were upstaged, 13 to T2 and one tumor to T4 (multiple lesions).

Despite the current limitations in assessing local tumor extension, there are many studies of non-surgical approaches to early NSCLC. This chapter will discuss the following approaches.

- External beam radiation with conventional fractionation or stereotactic body radiation therapy
- Brachytherapy
- Radiofrequency ablation
- Cryotherapy
- Electrocautery
- Nd:YAG laser therapy
- Photodynamic therapy.

EXTERNAL BEAM RADIATION TREATMENT

Conventional fractionation

Retrospective single-institution reports of conventionally fractionated radiotherapy for medically inoperable lung cancer (MILC) have shown local control rates of 30–60% and overall 5-year survival rates of 5–30%.[2–14] Selected recent studies are summarized in Table 17.1.[5,11–14] Unfortunately it is difficult to select data for

Table 17.1 Definitive fractionated radiotherapy

Author	Number of patients	Total dose/dose per fraction	Stage (%)	Nodal failure	Local failure	Survival
Graham 1995[5]	103	56.8 Gy (mean dose)/ 2–2.5 Gy	T1N0(31), T1N1(3), T2N0(59), T2N1(7)	NS	NS	Overall 35% at 2 yrs, 14% at 5 yrs
Sibley 1998[12]	141	64 Gy (median dose)/ 1.2 Gy BID or 3 Gy QD	T1N0(54%), T2N0(46%),	4(7%)	29%	Overall 39% at 2 yrs 13% at 5 yrs. DSS 62% at 2 yrs, 39% at 5 yrs
Roswell 2001[11]	2003 (pooling of 26 non-randomized studies)	40–90 Gy (range)/ 1.5–2 Gy	T1–2, N0–1, or T3N0	NS	6–70%	Overall 22–72% at 2 yrs, 17–55% at 3 yrs, 13–39% at 5 yrs. DSS 54–94% at 5 yrs. DSS 54–94% at 2 yrs, 22–56% at 3 yrs
Cheung 2000[14]	105	52.5 Gy/2.625	T1(33), T2(57), T3(9), T4(4), N1(5)	6.60%	68.90%	Overall 35% at 3 yrs. DSS 43.5% at 3 yrs
Langerwaard 2002[13]	113	60–72 Gy (median 66 Gy/2–3 Gy	T1N0(58), T2N0(42)	NS	15% at 1 yr, 57% at 3 yrs	Overall 71% at 1 yr, 25% at 3 yrs, 12% at 5 yrs. DSS 70% at 1 yr, 30% at 3 yrs

DSS, Disease specific survival.

small tumors alone since patients with T1–T3 primary lesions were often reported together. Several authors observed improved local control rates for smaller lesions.[4,5,7,12,15]

Elective nodal irradiation for clinically uninvolved nodal regions was not employed in several studies, with a low reported rate of isolated nodal relapse of only 6–7%.[12,14,16] In 2001, a more formal systematic review of published studies of 26 non-randomized studies of radical radiotherapy for early-stage NSCLC was published by Rowell et al.[11] The pooled isolated local failure rate was approximately 50%. In contrast, surgical series of operable stage I lung cancer have reported local failure rates of only 10–20%.[17,18] This observed difference in outcome is likely to be partially attributable to selection bias and differences in staging. However local failure rates of 50% with conventional radiation therapy support the concept that more aggressive local therapy is needed.

Recognizing the importance of total dose in determining local control and of volume of normal lung in determining complications, investigators from University of Michigan performed a phase I dose-escalation study with conventionally fractionated external beam radiation.[15] Patients with stage I or II were eligible, in addition to patients with locally advanced stage IIIA and IIIB NSCLC. Eighteen of the 48 patients had stage I or II disease. The preliminary report indicates that at total doses of 92.4 Gy there have been no cases of severe pneumonitis observed in the patients with small lesions in which a small amount of normal lung was encompassed in the radiation field. No toxicity or local control data are available as of this time. Rosenzweig and colleagues from MSKCC reported the toxicity and preliminary local control results of a phase I 3D dose-escalation study in 52 patients.[19] The majority of patients were considered ineligible for surgery because of

locally advanced disease (71%). No new adjuvant or adjuvant chemotherapy was given. The primary endpoint was grade 3 pulmonary toxicity defined as toxicity requiring corticosteroids or oxygen. Following one case of fatal pneumonitis following 70.2 Gy, the protocol was amended to include only the gross disease in the target volume, i.e. no elective nodal coverage. Doses have been escalated from 70.2 Gy to 75.6 Gy using conventional fractionation. There were no cases of radiation pneumonitis in patients in which the amount of normal lung encompassed in the radiation field was very small. The rate of grade 3 or greater pulmonary toxicity was 27% for patients with larger target volumes in which more normal lung was included. Overall 2 year local control was 37%. Overall survival at 2 years was 19% and 38% for the 70.2 Gy and 75.6 Gy group, respectively ($P > 0.05$). The authors concluded that it is safe to treat to 70.2 Gy and 75.6 Gy in selected patients with relatively small target volumes. Further dose escalation to 81 Gy is ongoing.

The Radiation Therapy Oncology Group (RTOG) is currently conducting a phase II study in which the radiation regimen is 74 Gy in 37 once-daily fractions of 2 Gy. This is given concurrent with weekly carboplatin and paclitaxel. Patients are eligible if they have stage I–IIIB NSCLC that can be encompassed with a radiation field that keeps the total lung dose receiving 20 Gy to less than 30%. The objective of the study is to determine the maximally tolerated dose of radiation that can be given with concurrent paclitaxel and carboplatin, and to estimate the complete response rate as defined by diagnostic CT performed 3 months after completion of all therapy.

Stereotactic body radiation therapy

Swedish investigators pioneered the application of stereotactic techniques, originally developed for brain tumors, to extra-cranial sites such as lung and liver.[20,21] Stereotactic body radiation therapy (SBRT), sometimes called extracranial stereotactic radiosurgery or extracranial stereotactic radioablation involves the application of high-dose, tightly focused external beam irradiation to target volumes in the lung, liver or other extracranial sites. Radiation dose and overall treatment time have been shown to be important in NSCLC[22] and by giving only 1–5 fractions

with a large dose per fraction, SBRT takes advantage of both of these factors (Figures 17.1–17.3).[23,24]

Stereotactic localization means that internal tumor locations are identified with reference to an external, three-dimensional frame of reference. There are many different commercial and non-proprietary stereotactic systems. High-precision patient immobilization and repositioning are required to administer 1–5 fractions of

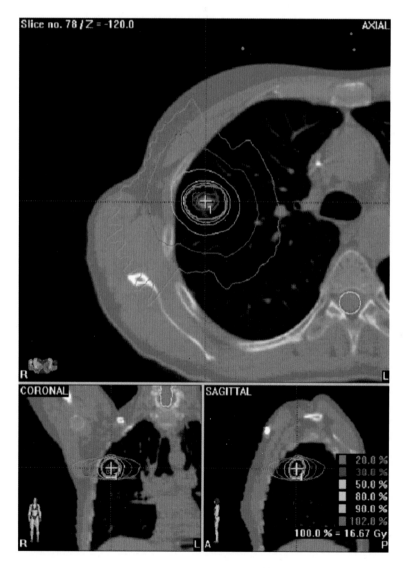

Figure 17.1
Stereotactic radiation therapy dose distribution. Dose distribution obtained using Brainlab™ stereotactic planning system (dynamic conformal arcs). The ABC™ gated breathing device was employed. The gross tumor volume (GTV) is outlined in purple and the planning target volume (pink) is an expansion volume obtained by adding 5 mm radially and 1 cm craniocaudally to the GTV. Notice the sharp fall-off in dose (distance between the prescription isodose of 90% and the 50% isodose line is very small).

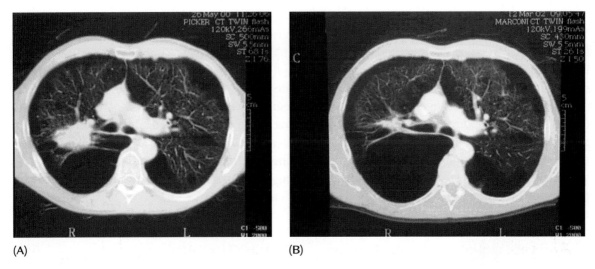

(A)   (B)

Figure 17.2
CT scans of a patient with severe bullous emphysema who was treated with stereotactic radiation therapy to 36 Gy in 3 fractions; before treatment (A) and 2 years after treatment (B).[31] with permission.

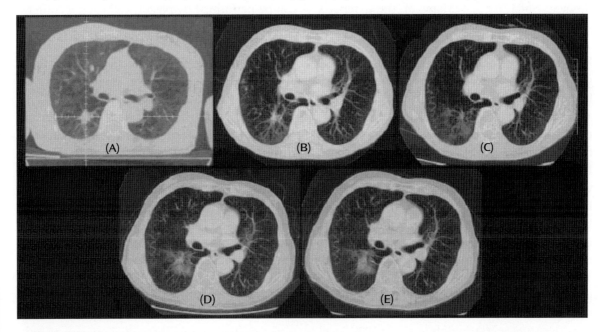

Figure 17.3
T1N0M0 adenocarcinoma of the lung. (A) A 2.5-cm tumor is seen in the center image of the positioning CT scan on the first treatment day. This CT image was scanned slowly (4 s/scan) with shallow respiration. SRT of 50 Gy in five fractions during 1 week was given at the 80% isodose line of 3.5 cm in diameter. (B) Two months after SRT, the tumor had shrunk. (C) Fifteen months after SRT, the tumor disappeared. (D) Thirty-three months after SRT, a limited volume of radiation fibrosis was seen. (E) Forty-three months after SRT, the volume of the fibrosis looked somewhat smaller.[28] with permission.

high dose radiation, typically in the range of 10–20 Gy per fraction. The margins to account for uncertainty in target position and intra- and inter-fractional target movement are kept small to minimize the risk of toxicity. Typical margins are 1 cm in the superior–inferior direction and 0.5 cm in all other directions. Given the very tight margins utilized during SBRT, respiration-related movement of lung tumors during daily treatment is an area of great concern. Numerous publications regarding breathing control during radiotherapy, utilizing respiration-gated radiotherapy or real-time tumor tracking radiotherapy with implanted fiducials, have been conducted but an in-depth review of these issues is beyond the scope of this chapter.[25–28]

Table 17.2 summarizes selected reports of thoracic SBRT.[23,24,29–32] Many of these reports grouped together primary and metastatic lung and liver tumors, but the results of treatment for NSCLC are separated wherever possible. In general, local control has been in the range of 90% with few reported complications.

Timmerman et al reported the preliminary results of a prospective phase I study of stereotactic radiotherapy in medically inoperable stage I NSCLC.[23] Pretreatment pulmonary function was generally poor with a mean FEV1 of 1.24 liters (range 0.4–2.53) or 46% of predicted FEV1 (range 19–94%). Within each stratified group (T1 and T2) doses of 60 Gy in three fractions (20 Gy per fraction) were safely achieved. There were early changes in FEV1, FVC, DLCO and PO_2 but these parameters returned to baseline at 3–6 months. The maximum tolerated dose was never reached but the 100% local control observed following 48–60 Gy prompted the investigators to go on to a phase II study utilizing a total dose of 60 Gy.

SBRT is an evolving field and further clinical studies are needed to determine the optimal dose and fractionation schedule to achieve high rates of local control with low complication rates. The Radiation Therapy Oncology Group (RTOG) is currently conducting a limited institution phase II study of SBRT for medically inoperable NSCLC using the schedule established by Timmerman et al of 60 Gy in three fractions.[23] It is hoped that the encouraging local tumor control and low associated toxicity observed in Timmerman et al's experience will be demonstrated in the RTOG multi-institutional study.

BRACHYTHERAPY

Brachytherapy is the direct application of radioactive sources near, or into, a tumor bed. It can be performed by placing radioactive sources into a lumen (intraluminal or endobronchial brachytherapy), or by implanting sources directly into the mass (interstitial brachytherapy). Brachytherapy may be done as early as 24–48 hours following laser therapy.[33,34]

As compared to conventional external beam radiation, brachytherapy offers the potential advantage of providing a very high dose of radiation to the tumor-bearing area relative to the dose to the surrounding normal structures. This is due to the 'inverse square law' that governs the dose falloff from point sources of radioactivity, i.e. the dose emitted declines as a function of the inverse square of the distance from the source. The unavoidable consequence of brachytherapy is the high dose delivered to normal structures immediately adjacent to the tumor such as normal bronchial mucosa or pulmonary vasculature (Figure 17.4).[35] Centering of the radioactive source within the bronchial lumen helps reduce the dose to any one portion of the bronchial wall. Various centering techniques including spacer catheters and specially designed catheters have been utilized.[35–37]

Table 17.2 Stereotactic radiotherapy							
Author	Number of patients	Total dose/ dose per fraction	Stage	Tumor size or volume	Toxicity	Local control	Overall survival
Blomgren 1998[29]	3 primary NSCLC (75 total tumors including primary and metastatic tumors in lung and liver)	30 Gy/15 Gy	T1–2N0	3–198 cc (mean 48 cc)	Fatigue, fever	100%	NA
Wulf 2001[30]	12 primary NSCLC (51 primary and metastatic tumors of lung and liver)	30 Gy/10 Gy (one patient 14 Gy/7 Gy)	Not reported	57–72 cc median/mean for all lung tumors (n = 27)	Grade I pneumonitis (1 patient) – fatal pulmonary bleed (1 patient)	Actuarial local control at 12 months 76% (primary and metastatic)	NA
Uematsu 2001[24]	50	50 Gy/10 Gy*	T1–T2, N0	0.8–5.0 cm (median 3.2 cm)	Rib fracture (1 patient), mild transient pleuritis (6 patients)	94%	66% at 3 yrs

continued

Table 17.2 continued

Author	Number of patients	Total dose/ dose per fraction	Stage	Tumor size or volume	Toxicity	Local control	Overall survival
Fukomoto 2002[31]	22–48–60 Gy/XGy	48–60 Gy/ 6–7.5 Gy given in 8 fractions	T1–T2, N0	1.42–5.95 cm (medium 2.67 cm)	Radiation pleuritis (2 patients), pericarditis (1 patient), pneumonitis (2 patients)	16 patients at 2–3 months, 71% at 1 yr, 67% at 2 yrs	NA
Hof, Herfarth 2003[32]	10	19–26/19–26 (single dose)	Not reported	5–19 cc (median 12 cc)	None serious	88.9% at 1 yr, 71.1% at 2 yrs (median follow-up 14.9 months)	80% at 1 yr, 64% at 2 yrs
Timmerman 2003[23]	37	24–60 Gy/ 8–20 Gy given in 3 fractions	19 T1N0, 18 T2N0 (≤7 cm)	1.5–157 cc (median 22.5 cc)	Asymptomatic pericardial effusion (1 patient), pneumonitis requiring steroids and/or oxygen (9 patients)	100% in patients treated to ≥54 Gy	50% DFS 64% overall (median survival follow-up 15.2 months)

Doses – prescribed to varying isodose curves; NA, not available; DFS, disease-free survival.
*2 patients with T1N0 and 16 patients with T2N0 had conventional RT 40–60 Gy in 2 Gy fractions before SRT.

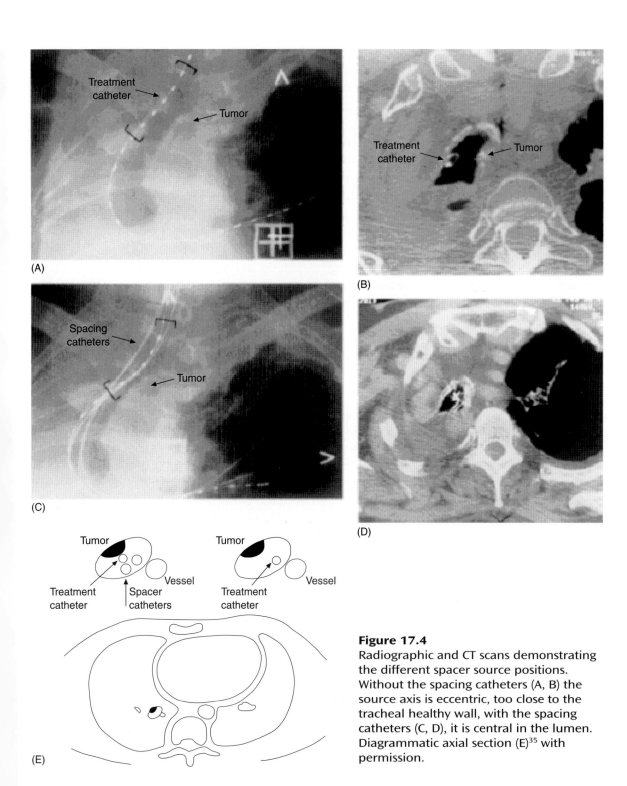

Figure 17.4
Radiographic and CT scans demonstrating the different spacer source positions. Without the spacing catheters (A, B) the source axis is eccentric, too close to the tracheal healthy wall, with the spacing catheters (C, D), it is central in the lumen. Diagrammatic axial section (E)[35] with permission.

Endobronchial or interstitial brachytherapy for lung cancer can be categorized as temporary or permanent. Temporary implants are placed with the intention of removing them at a predetermined time in the future which may be minutes, hours or days. Temporary implants can deliver low, intermediate or high dose rate radiation which is defined as follows: low dose rate (LDR) less than 2 Gy per hour, intermediate dose rate (IDR) 1–12 Gy per hour, and high dose rate (HDR) greater than 2 Gy per minute. LDR brachytherapy takes 1–4 days and is usually done on an inpatient basis in one or two sessions. A typical LDR system utilizes iridium wire or iridium-192 seeds embedded in a vicryl strand to deliver 0.4–1.0 Gy per hour or approximately 10 Gy per day. IDR brachytherapy, often utilizing cesium-137 sources, is completed within several hours and is frequently given in several fractions of 5–10 Gy separated by 1–2 weeks. HDR brachytherapy treatment is completed within minutes, and like IDR is frequently given in two to three fractions of 5–10 Gy. Brachytherapy is referred to as 'permanent' if the irradiation is delivered over an infinite period of time. This technique is most appropriate for very LDR interstitial treatment, i.e., the placement of a radioactive source into the tumor or target region where no lumen exists.

Endobronchial brachytherapy

Clinical results of endobronchial brachytherapy for early NSCLC are summarized in Table 17.3.[35-41] Brachytherapy can be used either as the sole treatment or in combination with external beam irradiation. In general, local control rates have been reported to be in the range of 55–95%, with higher local control rates following higher total doses. For example, Marsiglia et al reported excellent results following HDR brachytherapy as the sole treatment in 34 patients with early NSCLC.[35] Twenty-three of the patients had T1N0M0 disease. The 2-year actuarial survival was 74% with a local control rate of 85%. The relatively low complication rate observed in this series was attributed to the use of spacer catheters that centered the brachytherapy source within the airway, reducing the dose to the adjacent bronchial wall and large blood vessels (Figure 17.1). Saito et al[37] and Fuwa et al[36] also employed centering techniques and reported low complication rates.

Serious complications such as bronchial stenosis and hemorrhage have occurred following endobronchial brachytherapy. The median time to onset of complications was reported to be 7 months in one small series.[41] Tredaniel et al reported their experience with HDR endobronchial brachytherapy alone in 29 patients unable to undergo surgery for limited invasive endobronchial tumors.[38] All tumors were visible within the bronchial lumen, extended no more than 1 cm from the bronchial wall, and were without nodal involvement. The most common brachytherapy dose was 42 Gy prescribed at a 1 cm depth, given in six fractions of 7 Gy over 30 days. No other form of therapy was given. Bronchoscopy 2 months following completion of therapy demonstrated macroscopic complete response in 21 of 25 evaluable patients. Median overall survival had not been reached after 23 months of follow-up. Fatal massive hemoptysis occurred in five patients but recurrent disease was suspected in all. No autopsies were performed. Unfortunately, two patients died of massive bronchorrhea, prompting the authors to caution that the dose/fractionation utilized was likely at the upper limits of tolerance of the bronchial mucosa. This is further supported by the report from Perol et al in which there were six deaths possibly attributed to HDR brachytherapy; two due to hemoptysis, four due to unknown reasons. Perol et al[39] suggested that

Table 17.3 Endobronchial brachytherapy

Author	Number of patients	Brachytherapy dose	Stage	Complications	Local control	Survival
Tredaniel 1994[38]	29	HDR 28–42 Gy at 1 cm (7 Gy/fx over 4–6 wks)	Limited to bronchus, M0****	Massive bronchorrhea (2 patients)	78% at 14 months (62% histologic CR)	Median >23 months
Marsiglia 2000[35]	34	HDR 30 Gy at 0.5–1 cm (5 Gy/fx/wk)	T1 = 4, N0 = X, M0 (inoperable)	Pneumothorax (1 patient), massive hemorrhage post biopsy (1 patient)	85% 2 yrs 73% 3 yrs	Overall 78% 2 yrs
Perol 1997[39]	19	HDR 21–35 Gy at 1 cm (7 Gy/fx/wk)	<1 cm, N0, M0, R0	Massive hemorrhage (2 patients), severe bronchial wall necrosis (2 patients)	75% 1 yr	Overall 78%, 1 yr, 58% 2 yrs. Median 28 months
Lorchel 2003[40]	33 (35 lesions)	HDR 30 Gy (5 Gy/fx/3–4 days) at 1 cm	CIS or T1N0	Infections (6 patients), bronchial stenosis (12 patients)	55% at median follow-up of 9 months	Overall 71.4% 1 yr, 53.8% 2 yrs. DSS 69.5% 1 yr, 59% 2 yrs
Taulelle 1998[41]	22	HDR 30–35 Gy at 1 cm (7–10 Gy/ fx/week)	Small lesions strictly limited to bronchial lumen	17% serious non-fatal complications – hemoptysis, bronchial stenosis, soft tissue necrosis, fistula or pneumothorax. 7% fatal toxicity – massive hemoptysis or fistula**	NS	Overall 71% 1 yr, 46% 2 yrs

continued

Table 17.3 continued

Author	Number of patients	Brachytherapy dose	Stage	Complications	Local control	Survival
Fuwa 2001[36]	39	IDR 10–66 Gy at 1 cm (median 28 Gy) at 0.3–0.7 mm (4–6 Gy/fx/ 3–4 days)***	RO T1N0 38 T4N0 1	Bronchial ulcer (1 patient), bronchial stenosis (2 patients)	90% 3 yrs	87% 3 yrs, 87% 5 yrs
Saito 1996[37]	41	LDR 25 Gy at 0.3–0.9 cm (5 Gy/fx/1–2 fx per wk)*	T1N0M0	Pneumonitis, non-fatal (2 patients)	95% (median follow-up of 24.5 months)	39 patients alive at median follow-up of 24.5 months

*Also treated with 40 Gy conventionally fractionated external beam radiation therapy.
**Not stated separately for these 22 patients only. Stated complications are for entire group of 189 patients treated for cure or palliation.
***Also treated with 40–56 Gy conventionally fractionated external beam radiation therapy.
****Most frequent indication was new contralateral NSCLC following previous surgery and radiation for NSCLC.
RO, radiographically occult by CT scan; MS, median survival; Fx, fractions; CR, complete response; HDR, high dose rate; IDR, intermediate dose rate; LDR, low dose rate; DSS, disease-specific survival.

future studies utilize 5 Gy per fraction rather than 7 Gy and that the delivery system should center the brachytherapy source within the bronchus.

An alternative to brachytherapy alone is the combination of brachytherapy and external beam brachytherapy. The addition of external beam radiation allows a more regional approach as well as potentially less radiation-related bronchitis and hemoptysis since there is generally a lower dose of brachytherapy delivered. Saito et al[37] combined 40 Gy conventionally fractionated external beam radiation with 25 Gy endobronchial HDR brachytherapy and obtained excellent local control (95%) at a median follow-up of 24.5 months.

The American Brachytherapy Society (ABS) HDR consensus guidelines currently recommend that brachytherapy alone with curative intent be utilized in early-stage patients who are medically inoperable due to decreased pulmonary function, advanced age or refusal of surgery.[42] A total dose of 25 Gy in five fractions of 5 Gy, or a total dose of 22.5 Gy in three fractions of 7.5 Gy is recommended. The ABS recommends that the dose be prescribed to a depth of 1 cm from the central axis of the catheter.

Future studies of endobronchial brachytherapy utilizing CT planning may yield better results, particularly in terms of lower complications.[43] CT-assisted brachytherapy, particularly if combined with a centering catheter, has the potential to deliver a more uniform dose to the tumor and surrounding normal bronchial mucosa. However, the extra time required for CT-based planning may not make this a practical approach.[44]

Interstitial brachytherapy

Interstitial brachytherapy can be done intraoperatively, trans-bronchially or percutaneously. For temporary or permanent implants to adhere to radiation safety guidelines, sources such as iodine-125, palladium-103 and gold-193 are used. These isotopes have low-energy gamma rays, small physical size, and short half-lives measured in terms of days. The radioactive seeds can be inserted manually one-by-one into the target area using commercially available applicators. However, the risk of subsequent seed movement has led many experienced brachytherapists to recommend that the seeds be in the form of a strand with a vicryl carrier, which can be woven into a dexon mesh and secured to the tumor bed.[45–47]

Clinical results following interstitial brachytherapy for early NSCLC are summarized in Table 17.4.[46–48] Chen et al[46] looked at the feasibility and efficacy of permanent interstitial brachytherapy in 23 patients with stage I NSCLC who also underwent video-assisted thoracoscopic resection (VATR). At the time of VATR, I-125 impregnated mesh was placed in the cavity in order to deliver 100–120 Gy to the tumor bed and staple line with a 1 cm margin (Figures 17.5, 17.6).[46] Three patients died postoperatively secondary to problems not attributed to the brachytherapy. With a median follow-up of just 11 months (range 2–20 months) there were no local recurrences. Three patients developed distant metastases. The brachytherapy had no adverse effect on postoperative pulmonary function. This experience from Pittsburgh was reported in a larger group of patients with either T1A or T1B NSCLC.[47] The survival at 3–4 years was 60%. When the results were retrospectively compared to a large group of patients treated with sublobar resection only, the local recurrence was much less (2% versus 19%) but the incidence of distant metastases was similar, in the range of 22–29%.

HDR interstitial brachytherapy has been utilized to treat small peripherally situated

Table 17.4 Interstitial brachytherapy

Author	Number of patients	Brachytherapy dose	Stage	Complications	Local control	Survival
Chen 1999[46]	23	Permanent I-125 100–120 Gy at 0.5 cm	T1N0M0	None	100%**	NS
Santos 2003[47]	102	Permanent I-125 100–120 Gy at 0.5 cm	T1–2, N0M0	None	98%	60% 3–4 yrs
Lee 2003[48]	33 (19 T1N0M0)	Permanent I-125 125–140 Gy at 1 cm***	T1–2, N0–2 (only 1 patient N1, 1 patient N2), M0, not candidates for lobectomy or pneumonectomy	Postoperative death due to infection (1 patient), serious postoperative complications such as lobar or lung collapse, hemothorax, prolonged air leak, myocardial infarct (10 patients)		Median survival 45 months. Projected 5-yr survival 47%. Cancer-specific 5-yr survival 61%. Projected 5-yr cancer-specific survival 77% for T1N0M0.

*T1N0M0 NSCLC or pulmonary metastases.
**No recurrences locally but one intrathoracic recurrence.
***Brachytherapy to staple line at time of sublobar resection.
NS, not stated.

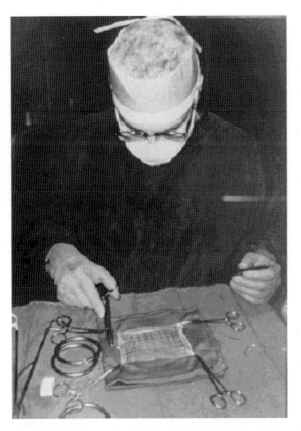

Figure 17.5
Attachment of I125 seeds in vicryl suture to a sheet of vicryl mesh utilizing sterile technique[45] with permission.

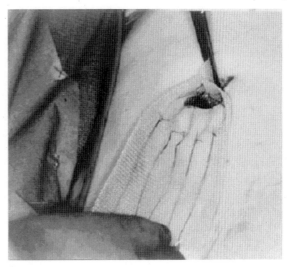

Figure 17.6
Insertion of the I125 seeds through the thoracoscopy port with video assistance[45] with permission.

short follow-ups of 18 and 10 months. CT-guided interstitial permanent placement of iodine-125 seeds has also been described.[50]

RADIOFREQUENCY ABLATION

Radiofrequency ablation (RFA) is a thermal energy delivery modality that results in cell death via coagulative necrosis. RFA delivers an alternating current supplied by a radiofrequency energy generator. The needle electrode is placed within the tissue and multiple tines or hooks are required to distribute the energy within the lesion (Figure 17.7).[51]

The ability of heat to cause cancer cell death has been known for some time.[52] This strategy has been applied extensively to primary and metastatic liver tumors.[53–55] CT-guided percutaneous (mostly by interventional radiologists) or open thoracotomy (by surgical oncologists) are the most common approaches for delivering

primary lung cancers, although the clinical experience is limited to small groups of patients. The reports are often technically oriented. For example, Kobayashi et al described the results of two patients following CT-guided bronchoscopic placement of a HDR applicator into small peripheral NSCLC.[49] One patient received a total dose of 24 Gy delivered in three fractions of 8 Gy 1 week apart. The other patient received a single dose of 15 Gy. All doses were prescribed at a 1 cm depth. The treatments were tolerated well and there was local control at

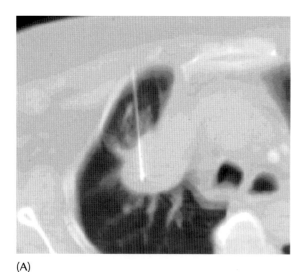

(A)

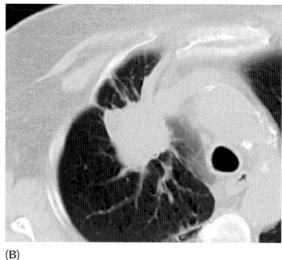

(B)

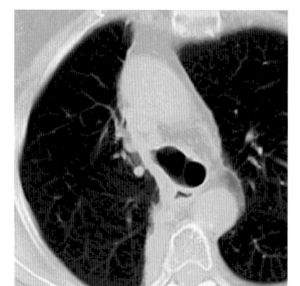

(C)

Figure 17.7
Results of RFA in a 78-year-old woman with emphysema and a right supra-hilar mass. Results of biopsy showed squamous cell carcinoma. The patient was a poor surgical candidate due to comorbid conditions (heart disease, emphysema). (A) CT scan obtained prior to external-beam radiation therapy shows an electrode inserted into the mass for percutaneous RFA. (B) CT scan obtained 3 months after RFA (6 weeks after radiation therapy) shows the mass with adjacent parenchymal stranding but no retraction. (C) CT scan obtained 27 months after RF ablation demonstrates shrinkage of the tumor with parenchymal fibrosis and contraction medially. Tissues treated with RF ablation become cicatricial, and the lesions may still be apparent at imaging.[54] with permission.

RFA. The procedure is done under either conscious sedation or general anesthesia.

Table 17.5 summarizes selected reports of thoracic RFA.[51,56] One of the largest experiences reported to date has come from Herrera et al at Rhode Island.[56] These investigators have been piloting the combination of RFA and radiation therapy, both external beam and brachytherapy,

for lung malignancies. The rationale behind this combination is predicated on the fact that tumors have a central area of relative hypoxia which is resistant to radiation, and that RFA for large lesions (>3 cm) is less likely to completely ablate tumor cells at the periphery. Incomplete ablation at the periphery is one of the limitations of a single treatment with RFA. Multiple

Table 17.5 Radiofrequency ablation

Author	Number of patients	Stage	RFA technique	Other therapy	Survival
Herrera 2003[56]	33 (5 primary NSCLC)	T1N0 (1 patient), T2N0 (2 patients), metastatic (1 patient)	CT guided percutaneous (28), mini-thoracotomy (5)	No	NS
Dupuy 2000[51]	3	Stage IV lung recurrence (1 patient), recurrence (1 patient), breast cancer lung metastases (1 patient)	Percutaneous CT guided (3)	1 patient with 5 cm lesion had RFA for cytoreduction followed by external beam radiotherapy	NS

NS, not stated.

overlapping treatments with RFA have been successfully applied to liver tumors and more recently to lung tumors.[57] However, the fact remains that the larger the lesion, the higher the risk of incomplete ablation, despite the use of overlapping or cluster electrodes. External beam radiation can successfully cover the periphery, while RFA can overcome the radiation-resistant central hypoxic region. The role of RFA for primary medically inoperable NSCLC will be determined as more studies are completed.

CRYOTHERAPY

Cryotherapy is another approach for the definitive treatment of small endobronchial NSCLC.[58] Cryotherapy causes cellular necrosis due to tissue freezing of the tumor cells as well as the feeding blood vessels. Nitrous oxide-driven cryoprobes are most often used. Cryotherapy is safe, with little risk of bronchial wall perforation, no radiation exposure, no risk of electrical accidents or fires, and does not require laser training and certification.[59] Disadvantages include delayed results and the requirement for multiple endoscopies to remove debris, or to retreat if there is less than a complete response.

There are very few reports of the clinical results of cryotherapy for early NSCLC. Deygas et al described good results utilizing this technique in 35 patients with carcinoma in situ (CIS) involving airways that could be visualized with bronchoscopy.[58] Nineteen percent of these patients had multifocal lesions. Most of these patients had previously undergone surgery or radiation for an earlier invasive lung cancer. Local control at 1 year was obtained in 72% of the patients. Forty-six percent of the patients were alive at 4 years. There were no serious complications attributed to the cryotherapy. Additional new primary NSCLC developed in

eight of the 35 patients, of which five were invasive and three were CIS, emphasizing the need to continue to follow these patients closely with bronchoscopy.

ELECTROCAUTERY

Electrocautery is the use of a high-frequency electrical current that generates heat due to tissue resistance, resulting in destruction of tissue.[60] It is generally done under direct bronchoscopic visualization. Clinical results of electrocautery for early NSCLC are summarized in Table 17.6.[61,62] Vonk-Noordegraaf et al described their experience with electrocautery in 24 patients treated over a 6-year period.[61] The results are presented combined with eight other patients treated with other bronchoscopic treatment (photodynamic therapy in five patients, NdYAG in one) that makes it somewhat difficult to interpret the results specifically for those treated with electrocautery. All patients had radiographically occult NSCLC 1 cm or less in diameter without evidence of extrabronchial extension. This series excluded patients with only carcinomas in situ. The most common reason for selecting electrocautery for treatment of these patients was poor pulmonary function due to prior lung cancer treated with surgery. The electrocautery was performed via bronchoscopy using under approximately 30 W of energy applied until coagulation became visible. The tumors were coagulated with a 0.5-cm margin of surrounding normal mucosa. Patients were followed closely with bronchoscopy and biopsies for at least 2 years or until death. The treatment was repeated if there was less than a complete response, i.e. negative histology by biopsy and brushing, without visible tumor. Patients went on to localized high-dose external beam radiation if there was

Table 17.6 Electrocautery

Author	Number of patients	Tumor extent	Complications	Local control	Survival
Vonk-Noordegraaf 2003[61]	24	RO, <1 cm maximum diameter, confined to bronchus, N0M0	Fatal hemoptysis (1 patient)	97%	NS
Van Boxem 1998[62]	13 (15 tumors)	RO CIS or T1, N0M0	None serious	54% local control with median follow-up of 22 months	NS

CIS, carcinoma in situ; NS, not stated; RO, radiographically occult.

less than a complete response after two electrocautery treatments. Three patients underwent repeat electrocautery at the time of recurrence and there was eventually a 97% local control. Eight patients developed distant metastases but it was suspected that these metastases could have arisen from the prior higher-stage lung cancers treated previously with surgery. No severe late toxicities related to electrocautery were reported but one patient had fatal hemoptysis following salvage external-beam radiation. Vonk-Noordegraaf concluded that electrocautery was an effective treatment for patients with intraluminal microinvasive radiologically occult lung cancer, in which there was a visible distal margin using autoflourescent bronchoscopy.

ND:YAG LASER

Light energy can be generated to increase the temperature of endobronchial tumors, resulting in vaporization or coagulation with hemostasis.[63] Nd:YAG laser therapy (light amplification by stimulated emission of radiation) is the form of laser therapy used most frequently. Nd:YAG laser penetrates to a depth of approximately 5 mm. Nd:YAG laser utilizes a laser beam at 1064 nm that can be transmitted by a flexible quartz fiber placed into the bronchial lumen by flexible or rigid bronchoscopy. Rigid bronchoscopy is usually the preferred approach since it allows simultaneous suctioning and laser use. To minimize the risk of airway perforation Cavaliere et al[64] recommend constant movement of the light source tangential to the bronchial surface.

Results of Nd:YAG laser therapy are summarized in Table 17.7.[64,65] Cavaliere et al reported the results of Nd:YAG laser therapy as definitive treatment for 17 patients with 23 in-situ carcinomas in the lung.[64] Local control at an unspecified length of follow-up was 100%. It is not possible to abstract information regarding the median survival or the complications in the subset of patients with early disease. However the incidence of major complications and deaths in the total population of over 1800 patients, most with locally advanced or recurrent cancers, was very small. There were 60 major non-fatal complications and 12 fatal complications.

Table 17.7 Nd:YAG laser					
Author	Number of patients	Tumor extent	Complications	Local control	Survival
Cavaliere 1996[64]	17 (23 tumors)	CIS	NS	100%*	NS
Nakamura 2001[65]	3	RO, <2.5 cm maximum diameter, CIS or invasion, confined to bronchial wall, cN0	NS	2/3 CR#	NS

*Median length of follow-up not stated.
#Complete response assessed by surgery that followed Nd:YAG.
RO, radiographically occult; CIS, carcinoma in situ; NS, not stated.

PHOTODYNAMIC THERAPY

Photodynamic therapy (PDT) involves the intravenous administration of hematoporphyrins that are either preferentially retained in tumor tissue or have selective toxicity for tumor vasculature.[63] The photosensitizing drugs are activated by light of an appropriate wavelength utilizing an argon or eximer laser source, resulting in the production of singlet oxygen. This results in direct tumor cell death or indirect tumor cell death due to damage to the tumor vasculature. PDT is generally done under direct visualization of the lesion, and most reports of PDT are of lesions in the subsegmental or larger airways. Porfimer sodium (Photofrin) is the hematoporphyrin used most frequently. Photofrin is activated by 630 nm light. Nd:YAG is generally performed 48 hours after injection given that this is when the maximum concentration of Photofrin within tumor relative to the concentration within normal tissues occurs. The treatment is given according to a power density measured in mW per cm of diffusing fiber.[66] Bronchoscopy must be repeated one to two days after Nd:YAG therapy in order to remove necrotic tissue. PDT can be repeated a month later if necessary to obtain a complete response.

There are limited reports of PDT being performed other than under direct bronchoscopic visualization. Okunaka et al reported the results of nine patients with either early peripheral NSCLC or limited number of metastases treated with CT-guided PDT.[67]

Clinical results of PDT in small NSCLCs are summarized in Table 17.8.[65,66,68–74] Most of the patients in these series had squamous cell carcinoma in keeping with the central nature of these small lung cancers. The local control was 75–100% in those series that included only CIS or small T1 lesions.[66,68,69] Local control was lower, in the range of 41–76%, in studies that included larger T1 lesions.[65,71–74] However, many of these failures following PDT were salvaged using either surgery or other non-surgical techniques such as brachytherapy or external beam radiation. This explains the high survival rates in Table 17.6.[61,62]

Nakamura et al retrospectively reviewed the outcome of 27 patients with radiographically occult endobronchial tumors less than 25 mm in maximum diameter treated with PDT followed by surgical resection.[65] They noted that maximum diameter pre-treatment was predictive of complete histological response to PDT. They concluded that PDT treatment alone, i.e. without surgery, would likely be sufficient for those patients with tumors confined to the bronchial wall and less than 10 mm maximum diameter. Kato et al also found that outcome correlated strongly with maximum diameter pre-PDT.[68] There was 'almost 100% complete response' in patients with CIS 2 cm in diameter or less. Furuse et al also found that maximum lesion diameter was an important factor predictive of complete response and local control rates.[72] Complete response was found in 97.8% of tumors with a longitudinal extent of 1 cm or less, as opposed to a 42.9% complete response for larger lesions. However, Miyazu et al concluded that maximum diameter alone, determined by bronchoscopy or high-resolution CT, did not guarantee confinement to the bronchial wall according to endoscopic ultrasound criteria.[69]

The serious complication rate is low in all series summarized in Table 17.6, likely due to the fact that these were small lesions confined to the bronchial wall.[61,62] Fatal hemoptysis can be a complication of PDT if the lesion is close to major blood vessels, particularly if the lesion has extra-cartilaginous extension. PDT as definitive treatment is therefore only recommended by many investigators for lesions confined to the

Table 17.8 Photodynamic therapy

Author	Number of patients	Tumor extent	Complications	Local control	Survival
Nakamura 2001[65]	27	RO, <2.5 cm maximum diameter, CIS or invasion confined to bronchial wall, cN0	NS	NS (27% CR)	76% 5-yr
Kato 1998[68]	95 (116 tumors)	CIS	NS	75.8%	68.4% 5-yr (94.8% 5-yr lung-cancer-specific)
Miyazu 2002[69]	9	CIS or T1 confined to bronchial wall as determined by EUS	NS	100%	NS
McCaughan 1997[66]	19	T1N0M0 (16 patients) CIS (3 patients)	None serious	100%	93% 5-yr DFS
Sutedja 1996[70]	11	Stage I	NS**	Local control NS** (10/11 CR)	NS**
Cortese 1997[71]	21 (23 tumors)	RO, 'early stage', clinically N0	None serious	52% 1-yr	72% 5-yr overall survival
Furuse 1993[72]	54 (64 tumors)	CIS (17 patients), T1 (44 patients). All N0	None serious	76% with minimum FU of 6 months	82% survival with median follow-up 20 months (range 7–42 months)

Table 17.8 continued

Author	Number of patients	Tumor extent	Complications	Local control	Survival
Imamura 1994[73]	29 (39 tumors)	CIS (12 patients), T1 (17 patients), RO. All N0.	Mild–moderate skin reaction (41%). Nonfatal anaphylactic reaction (3%). Life-threatening airway obstruction (3%). 'Most' patients temporary non-life-threatening symptoms of airway obstruction	41%	2 yrs 93%, 3 yrs 72% (only 1 death due to lung cancer). Median DFS 38 months
Patelli 1999[74]	23 (26 tumors)	0.5–2.0 cm maximum diameter. All N0	NS	58%	NS

RO, radiographically occult; NS, not stated; CR, complete response; EUS, endoscopic ultrasound; CIS, carcinoma in situ; DFS, disease-free survival.
**NS for 11 early patients. For total group of 26 patients (combination of stage I and III patients) median survival 7 months, local control 62% at 1 year.

bronchial wall. Confinement to the bronchial wall, i.e. within the mucosa or submucosa, is determined prior to treatment, sometimes with the aid of endoscopic ultrasound.[69] Photosensitivity, with a sunburn appearance of varying severity, is one of the most common side effects of PDT.[73] Future research with PDT is evaluating new sensitizers that may be more efficacious or have less associated photosensitivity.[75,76]

CONCLUSION

There are clearly multiple non-surgical techniques that have been applied to the treatment of NSCLC when it is detected at an early stage such as carcinoma in situ or T1. When local control is not achieved with one of these treatments, another is often subsequently utilized. Conventional external beam radiation therapy, even to higher than conventional doses, has yet to show local control rates that are comparable to surgery.[15,19] Early reports of local control and survival following stereotactic radiation therapy for T1 tumors appear promising.[23] The Radiation Therapy Oncology Group will soon launch a study to evaluate the efficacy of this treatment in the multi-center cooperative group setting.

Endobronchial brachytherapy can effectively treat submucosal and peribronchial lesions but tumor regression is often delayed as compared to Nd:Yag, electrocautery or PDT. Careful attention to endobronchial brachytherapy technique and dose is required due to the rise of fistula formation and pulmonary artery erosion. Endobronchial brachytherapy has not been evaluated in CIS. Interstitial brachytherapy has been utilized as an effective prophylactic treatment following sublobar resection of early NSCLC.[46]

The results of radiofrequency ablation in early NSCLC are too preliminary to draw conclusions regarding efficacy. However, RFA can be done percutaneously, representing one of the few non-surgical treatments for peripherally located small tumors.

There are several reasonable alternatives for the treatment of carcinoma in-situ or lesions measuring less than 1 cm in maximum diameter without extrabronchial involvement.[61,65] Electrocautery, cryotherapy, Nd-YAG laser therapy and PDT have all been utilized with good results in terms of local control.[58,61,62,65,68,69,72,73,77] The experience with PDT for the treatment of CIS or early NSCLC is more extensive than that of electrocautery, RFA, Nd:YAG laser or cryotherapy.[65,68,69,72,73,77] Proponents of PDT argue that it is much more selective and less likely to result in damage outside of the bronchial wall as compared to Nd:YAG laser.[78] The results of PDT are delayed and there is a necessity for multiple bronchoscopies for debridement and possibly retreatment. Toxicity, primarily photosensitivity, is a problem. The high costs of electrocautery, PDT, brachytherapy and Nd-YAG laser have also been emphasized.[58] Cryotherapy is apparently less expensive and may be technically easier to deliver for bronchoscopists without experience in the other non-surgical treatments. The impression of bronchoscopists who have experience with several alternative treatments is that electrocautery results in less scarring and subepithelial fibrosis than either PDT or Nd:YAG laser.[61,62]

There are no published prospective randomized studies comparing non-surgical treatments in early NSCLC. In 1994, a prospective study in Japan was ongoing to ascertain whether new forms of treatment are superior to the standard treatment of radiographically occult NSCLC.[73] The protocol called for patients with 'early' cancers to be treated with PDT and then undergo further therapy according to their response to PDT. Patients with a complete response were to be observed. Those without a complete response were to be randomized to either external beam radiation or resection. The results have yet to be reported. Studies such as this are needed to clarify the role of non-surgical treatments for early radiographically occult NSCLC.

REFERENCES

1. Shennib H, Bogart JA, Herndon J, et al, Thoracoscopic wedge resection and radiotherapy for T1N0 non-small cell lung cancer (NSCLC) in high risk patients: Preliminary analysis of a cancer and leukemia group B and Eastern Cooperative Oncology Group phase II trial. Int J Radiat Oncol Bio Phys 2000; 48(Suppl 3), Abstract 240.

2. Cooper JD, Pearson G, Todd TR, et al, Radiotherapy alone for patients with operable carcinoma of the lung. Chest 1985; 87:289–92.

3. Coy P, Kennelly GM, The role of curative radiotherapy in the treatment of lung cancer. Cancer 1980; 45:698–702.

4. Dosoretz DE, Galmarini D, Rubenstein JH, et al, Local control in medically inoperable lung cancer: an analysis of its importance in outcome and factors determining the probability of tumor eradication. Int J Radiat Oncol Biol Phys 1993; 27:507–16.

5. Graham PH, Gebski VJ, Langlands AO, et al, Radical radiotherapy for early nonsmall cell lung cancer. Int J Radiat Oncol Biol Phys 1995; 31: 261–6.

6. Haffty BG, Goldberg NB, Gerstley J, et al, Results of radical radiotherapy in clinical stage I, technically operable non-small cell lung cancer. Int J Radiat Oncol Biol Phys 1988; 15:69–73.

7. Harpole DH, Herndon JE, Young WG, et al, Stage I nonsmall cell lung cancer: A multivariate analysis of treatment methods and patterns of recurrence. Cancer 1995; 76:787–96.

8. Noordijk EM, Poest CE, Hermans J, et al, Radiotherapy as an alternative to surgery in elderly patients with resectable lung cancer. Radiotherapy Oncology 1988; 13:83–9.

9. Talton BM, Constable WC, Kersh CR, Curative radiotherapy in non-small cell carcinoma of the lung. Int J Radiat Oncol Biol Phys 1990; 19: 15–21.

10. Zang HX, Yin WB, Zang LJ, et al, Curative radiotherapy of early operable non-small cell lung cancer. Radiotherapy Oncology 1989; 14: 89–94.

11. Roswell NP, Williams CJ, Radical radiotherapy for stage I/II non-small cell lung cancer in patients not sufficiently fit for or declining surgery (medically inoperable): a systematic review. Thorax 2001; 56:628–38.

12. Sibley GS, Jamieson TA, Marks LB, et al, Radiotherapy alone for medically inoperable stage I non-small-cell lung cancer: the Duke experience. Int J Radiat Oncol Biol Phys 1998; 40(1):149–54.

13. Lagerwaard FJ, Senan S, Van Meerbeeck JP, et al, Has 3-D conformal radiotherapy (3D CRT) improved local tumour control for stage I non-small cell lung cancer? Radiotherapy Oncology 2002; 63:151–7.

14. Cheung PC, Mackillop WJ, Dixon P, et al, Involved-field radiotherapy alone for early-stage non-small cell lung cancer. Radiat Oncol Biol Phys 2000; 48(3):703–10.

15. Robertson JM, Ten Haken RK, Hazuka MB, et al, Dose escalation for non-small cell lung cancer using conformal radiation therapy. Int J Radiat Oncol Biol Phys 1997; 37(5):1079–85.

16. Bradley JD, Wahab S, Lockett MA, et al, Elective nodal failures are uncommon in medically inoperable patients with stage I non-small-cell lung carcinoma treated with limited radiotherapy fields. International Journal of Radiation Oncology, Biology, Physics 2003; 56(2):342–7.

17. Martini N, Bains MS, Burt ME, et al, Incidence of local recurrence and second primary tumors in resected stage I lung cancer. J Thorac Cardiovasc Surg 1995; 109:120–9.

18. Okada M, Nishio W, Sakamoto T, et al, Long-term survival and prognostic factors of five-year

survivors with complete resection of non-small cell lung carcinoma. J Thorac Cardiovasc Surg 2003; 126:558–62.

19. Rosenzweig KE, Mychalczak B, Fuks Z, et al, Final report of the 70.2-Gy and 75.6 Gy dose levels of a phase I dose escalation study using three-dimensional conformal radiotherapy in the treatment of inoperable non-small cell lung cancer. Cancer J 2000; 6:82–7.

20. Lax I, Blomgren H, Naslund I, et al, Stereotactic radiotherapy of malignancies in the abdomen. Methodological aspects. Acta Oncol 1994; 33: 677–83.

21. Blomgren H, Lax I, Naslund I, et al, Stereotactic high dose fraction radiation therapy of extra-cranial tumors using an accelerator. Clinical experience of the first thirty-one patients. Acta Oncologica 1995; 34(6):861–70.

22. Saunders M, Dische S, Barrett A, et al, Continuous, hyperfractionated, accelerated radiotherapy (CHART) versus conventional radiotherapy in non-small cell lung cancer: mature data from the randomised multicentre trial. Radiotherapy Oncology 1999; 52:137–48.

23. Timmerman R, Papiez L, McGarry R, et al, Extracranial stereotactic radioablation. Results of a phase I study in medically inoperable stage I non-small cell lung cancer. Chest 2003; 124:1946–55.

24. Uematsu M, Shioda A, Suda A, et al, Computed tomography-guided frameless stereotactic radiotherapy for stage I non-small-cell lung cancer: a 5 year experience. Int J Radiat Oncol Biol Phys 2001; 51(3):666–70.

25. Harada T, Shirato H, Ogura S, et al, Real-time tumor-tracking radiation therapy for lung carcinoma by the aid of insertion of a gold marker using bronchofiberscopy. Cancer 2002; 95:1720–7.

26. Wong JW, Sharpe MB, Jaffey DA, et al, The use of active breathing control (ABC) to reduce margin for breathing motion. Int J Radiat Oncol Biol Phys 1999; 44:911–19.

27. Ohara K, Okumura T, Akisada M, et al, Irradiation synchronized with respiration gate. Int J Radiat Oncol Biol Phys 1989; 17:853–7.

28. Nakagawa K, Aoki Y, Tago M, et al, Megavoltage CT-assisted stereotactic radiosurgery for thoracic tumors: original research in the treatment of thoracic neoplasms. Int J Radiat Oncol Biol Phys 2000; 48(2):449–57.

29. Blomgren H, Lax I, Goranson H, et al, Radiosurgery for tumors in the body: clinical experience using a new method. J Radiosurg 1998; 1(1):63–74.

30. Wulf J, Hadinger U, Oppitz U, et al, Stereotactic radiotherapy of targets in the lung and liver. Strahlenther Onkol 2001; 177(12):645–55.

31. Fukumoto S, Shirato H, Shimzu S, et al, Small-volume image-guided radiotherapy using hypofractionated, coplanar and noncoplanar multiple fields for patients with inoperable stage I nonsmall cell lung carcinomas. Cancer 2002; 95:1546–53.

32. Hof H, Herfarth KK, Munter M, et al, Stereotactic single-dose radiotherapy of stage I non-small-cell lung cancer (NSCLC). Int J Radiat Oncol Biol Phys 2003; 56(2):335–41.

33. Miller JI, Phillips TW, Neodymium:YAG laser and brachytherapy in the management of inoperative bronchogenic carcinoma. Ann Thorac Surg 1990; 50:190–6.

34. Khanavkar B, Stern P, Alberti W, et al, Complications associated with brachytherapy alone or with laser in lung cancer. Chest 1991; 99:1062–5.

35. Marsiglia H, Baldeyrou P, Lartigau E, et al, High-dose-rate brachytherapy as sole modality for early-stage endobronchial carcinoma. Int J Radiat Oncol Biol Phys 2000; 47(3):665–72.

36. Fuwa N, Matsumoto A, Kamata M, External irradiation and intraluminal irradiation using middle-dose-rate iridium in patients with roentgenographically occult lung cancer. Int J Radiat Oncol Biol Phys 2001; 49(4):965–71.

37. Saito M, Yokoyama A, Kurita Y, et al, Treatment of roentgenographically occult endobronchial carcinoma with external beam radiotherapy and intraluminal low dose rate brachytherapy. Int J Radiat Oncol Biol Phys 1996; 34(5):1029–35.

38. Tredaniel J, Hennequin C, Zalcman G, et al, Prolonged survival after high-dose rate endo-

bronchial radiation for malignant airway obstruction. Chest 1994; 105(3):767–72.

39. Perol M, Caliandro R, Pommier P, et al, Curative irradiation of limited endobronchial carcinomas with high-dose rate brachytherapy. Results of a pilot study. Chest 1997; 111(5):1417–23.

40. Lorchel F, Spaeth D, Scheid P, et al, High dose rate brachytherapy: a potentially curative treatment for small invasive T1N0 endobronchial carcinoma and carcinoma in situ. Rev Mal Respir 2003; 20(4):515–20.

41. Taulelle M, Chauvet B, Vincent P, et al, High dose rate endobronchial brachytherapy: results and complications in 189 patients. Eur Respir J 1998; 11(1):162–8.

42. Nag S, Kelly JF, Horton JL, Komaki R, Mori D, Brachytherapy for carcinoma of the lung. Oncology (Huntingt) 2001; 15(3):371–81.

43. Lagerwaard FJ, Voet PW, Van Meerbeeck JP, et al, Curative radiotherapy for a second primary lung cancer arising after pneumonectomy – techniques and results. Radiother Oncol 2002; 62(1):21–5.

44. Senan S, Lagerwaard FJ, de Pan C, et al, A CT-assisted method of dosimetry in brachytherapy of lung cancer. Radiother Oncol 2000; 55(1):75–80.

45. Nori D, Bains M, Hilaris BS, et al, New intraoperative brachytherapy techniques for positive or close surgical margins. J Surg Oncol 1989; 42:54–9.

46. Chen A, Galloway M, Landreneau R, et al, Intraoperative 125I brachytherapy for high-risk stage I non-small cell lung carcinoma. Int J Radiat Oncol Biol Phys 1999; 44(5):1057–63.

47. Santos R, Colonias A, Pardas D, et al, Comparison between sublobar resection and 125 iodine brachytherapy after sublobar resection in high-risk patients with stage I non-small-cell lung cancer. Surgery 2003; 134(4):691–7.

48. Lee W, Daly BD, DiPetrillo TA, et al, Limited resection for non-small cell lung cancer: observed local control with implantation of I-125 brachytherapy seeds. Ann Thorac Surg 2003; 75(1):237–42.

49. Kobayashi T, Kaneko M, Sumi M, et al, CT-assisted transbronchial brachytherapy for small peripheral lung cancer. Jpn J Clin Oncol 2000; 30(2):109–12.

50. Mittal BB, Nemcek AA Jr, Sider L, Malignant tumors invading chest wall: treatment with CT-directed implantation of radioactive seeds. Radiology 1993; 186(3):901–3.

51. Dupuy DE, Zagoria RJ, Akerley W, et al, Percutaneous radiofrequency ablation of malignancies in the lung. Am J Roentgenol 2000; 174(1):57–9.

52. Cavaliere R, Ciocatto EC, Giovanella BC, et al, Selective heat sensitivity of cancer cells: biochemical and clinical studies. Cancer 1967; 20:1351–81.

53. Ruers T, Bleichrodt RP, Treatment of liver metastases, an update on the possibilities and results. Eur J Cancer 2002; 38:1023–33.

54. Livraghi T, Goldberg SN, Lazzaroni S, et al, Hepatocellular carcinoma: radio-frequency ablation of medium and large lesions. Radiology 2000; 214:761–8.

55. Curley SA, Izzo F, Delrio P, et al, Radiofrequency ablation of unresectable primary and metastic hepatic malignancies: results in 123 patients. Ann Surg 1999; 230:1–8.

56. Herrera LJ, Fernando HC, Perry Y, et al, Radiofrequency ablation of pulmonary malignant tumors in nonsurgical candidates. J Thorac Cardiovasc Surg 2003; 125(4):929–37.

57. Steinke K, Glenn D, King J, et al, Percutaneous pulmonary radiofrequency ablation: difficulty achieving complete ablations in big lung lesions. Br J Radiol 2003; 76:742–5.

58. Deygas N, Froudarakis M, Ozenne G, et al, Cryotherapy in early superficial bronchogenic carcinoma. Chest 2001; 120(1):26–31.

59. Thurer RJ, Cryotherapy in early lung cancer. Chest 2001; 120(1):3–5.

60. Mathur PN, Edell E, Sutedja T, et al, Treatment of early state non-small cell lung cancer. Chest 2003; 123(1 Suppl):176S–80S.

61. Vonk-Noordegraaf A, Postmus PE, Sutedja TG, Bronchoscopic treatment of patients with intraluminal microinvasive radiographically occult

lung cancer not eligible for surgical resection: a follow-up study. Lung Cancer 2003; 39(1): 49–53.

62. Van Boxem AJ, Venmans BJ, Schramel FM, et al, Radiographically occult lung cancer treated with fibreoptic bronchoscopic electrocautery: a pilot study of a simple and inexpensive technique. Eur Respir J 1998; 11(1):169–72.

63. Chan AL, Yoneda KY, Allen RP, et al, Advances in the management of endobronchial lung malignancies. Curr Opin Pulm Med 2003; 9(4): 301–8.

64. Cavaliere S, Venuta F, Foccoli P, et al, Endoscopic treatment of malignant airway obstructions in 2,008 patients (published erratum of serious dosage error appears in Chest 1997; 111(5):1476) Chest 1996; 110:1536–42.

65. Nakamura H, Kawasaki N, Hagiwara M, et al, Endoscopic evaluation of centrally located early squamous cell carcinoma of the lung. Cancer 2001; 91(6):1142–7.

66. McCaughan JS, Williams TE, Photodynamic therapy for endobronchial malignant disease: a prospective fourteen-year study. J Thorac Cardiovasc Surg 1997; 114(6):940–6.

67. Okunaka T, Kato H, Tsutsui H, et al, Photodynamic therapy for peripheral lung cancer. Lung Cancer 2004; 43(1):77–82.

68. Kato H, Photodynamic therapy for lung cancer – a review of 19 years' experience. J Photochem Photobiol B 1998; 42(2):96–9.

69. Miyazu Y, Miyazawa T, Kurimoto N, et al, Endobronchial ultrasonography in the assessment of centrally located early-stage lung cancer before photodynamic therapy. Am J Respir Crit Care Med 2002; 165(6):832–7.

70. Sutedja T, Baas P, Stewart F, et al, A pilot study of photodynamic therapy in patients with inoperable non-small cell lung cancer. Eur J Cancer 1992; 28A(8–9):1370–3.

71. Cortese DA, Edell ES, Kinsey JH, Photodynamic therapy for early stage squamous cell carcinoma of the lung. Mayo Clin Proc 1997; 72(7): 595–602.

72. Furuse K, Fukuoka M, Kato H, et al, A prospective phase II study on photodynamic therapy with photofrin II for centrally located early stage lung cancer. The Japan Lung Cancer Photodynamic Therapy Study Group. J Clin Oncol 1993; 11(10):1852–7.

73. Imamura S, Kusunoki Y, Takifuji N, et al, Photodynamic therapy and/or external beam radiation therapy for roentgenologically occult lung cancer. Cancer 1994; 73(6):1608–14.

74. Patelli M, Lazzari A, Poletti V, et al, Photodynamic laser therapy for the treatment of early-stage bronchogenic carcinoma. Monaldi Arch Chest Dis 1999; 54(4):315–18.

75. Maier A, Tomaselli F, Matzi V, et al, Comparison of 5-aminolaevulinic acid and porphyrin photosensitization for photodynamic therapy of malignant bronchial stenosis: a clinical pilot study. Lasers Surg Med 2002; 30(1):12–17.

76. Kato H, Furukawa K, Sato M, et al, Phase II clinical study of photodynamic therapy using mono-L-aspartyl chlorin e6 and diode laser for early superficial squamous cell carcinoma of the lung. Lung Cancer 2003; 42(1):103–11.

77. Cavaliere S, Venuta F, Foccoli P, et al, Endoscopic treatment of malignant airway obstructions in 2,008 patients. Chest 1996; 110(6): 1536–42.

78. Barr H, Tralau CJ, Boulos PB, et al, The contrasting mechanism of colonic collagen damage between photodynamic therapy and thermal injury. Photochem Photobiol 1987; 46:795–800.

18 Economic evaluation of lung cancer screening

Deborah Marshall, Kirsten Hall Long

Contents   Introduction • Overview of economic evaluation • Economic evaluations of lung cancer screening • Special issues in economic evaluation of lung cancer screening • Summary and areas for further research

INTRODUCTION

The previous failure in the 1970s and 1980s of lung cancer screening trials (comparing chest radiography alone or in combination with sputum cytology)[1–5] to demonstrate a mortality reduction benefit led to a consensus that screening for lung cancer was not warranted.[6–8] More recently, detailed re-examination of these trial data identified serious flaws and limitations in the study design, so that the conclusions have been questioned.[9–12] In addition, prospective cohort studies have demonstrated the potential benefits of lung cancer screening with low-dose spiral computed tomography (LDSCT).[13–17] Interest in LC screening may be fueled by high levels of public interest and enthusiasm for screening in general.[18]

It has yet to be determined, however, whether true-positive findings from lung cancer screening will translate into improved mortality or gains in quality-adjusted life expectancy. A number of large-scale randomized controlled trials are currently in progress in the USA, France and the Netherlands, or have been proposed to address this current knowledge gap, but results are not expected for some time.[19–22] In the interim, experts continue to debate whether lung cancer screening is appropriate in practice, often highlighting the economic as well

as clinical implications associated with rapid technology dissemination.[22–30]

Costs associated with screening and nodule follow-up are of particular concern. Screening CT costs alone have been estimated at more than $12 billion if all current smokers in the United States were screened.[31] Furthermore, high observed rates of indeterminate nodule detection and suggested clinical follow-up highlight that costs associated with nodule management may also be considerable.[15,17,32] In a world of rising healthcare costs and fixed budgets, economic evaluation plays an increasingly important role in technology assessment and payment decisions.[33–35] In addition to the standard prerequisites for a screening program to be justified[36] (for example, significant disease burden and available treatment) there are additional economic parameters (such as costs and estimated cost-effectiveness) that must be considered in evaluating the potential trade-off of benefits and risks (see Table 18.1).[24] This chapter will provide a brief overview of economic analysis and a summary of research to date assessing the cost-effectiveness of alternative lung cancer screening programs. Specific issues relevant to economic evaluation of lung cancer screening will be explored along with a discussion of areas warranting further research.

Table 18.1 Parameters to consider in the evaluation of helical CT lung cancer screening	
Disease	Prevalence of disease
	Probability of disease in selected population at high risk
	Annual incidence of disease
	Natural history of disease
Screening test	Sensitivity and specificity of screening examination
	Radiation-associated risk
	Loss in quality of life due to screening test and possible follow-up
	Complication rate of further diagnostic follow-up
	Proportion of non-adherence to screening program
	Alternative screening test
Treatment	Available therapy
	Proportion of diagnosed patients that are treatable
	Benefit from early treatment, curability, efficacy, quality of life
	Complication rate of treatment
RCTs	Size
	Screening program
	Duration of follow-up
	Mortality and morbidity reduction
Costs and cost-effectiveness	Costs of screening test and follow-up
	Costs of treatment and follow-up medical care, risk factor modification, lifestyle changes
	Costs of informal caregiving, travel and time costs, lost productivity
	Evaluation of different screening programs and alternatives to screening
	Perspective (societal perspective preferred)
	Effectiveness gained: composite measure that integrates risks, benefits, and quality of life
	Incremental costs of screening program
	Trade-off of costs and effectiveness: incremental costs per effectiveness gained

From Hunink MGM and Gazelle GS.[24] By permission of the American Society for Clinical Investigation.

OVERVIEW OF ECONOMIC EVALUATION

A full economic evaluation in health care applies formal, quantitative methods to identify, measure, and valuate alternative health care interventions in terms of both resource use and expected outcomes.[37–39] Formal quantification of both costs and effects supports explicit policy decision-making conducive to accountability.

Approaches to economic evaluation

There are three main approaches for a full health economic evaluation; cost–benefit analysis (CBA), cost-effectiveness analysis (CEA) and cost–utility analysis (CUA) (Table 18.2). These approaches differ in how effectiveness is measured and whether effectiveness is valued in monetary terms. CEA is the most widely used method in published medical literature, although published guidelines currently consider CUA a more comprehensive approach.[35,39–42]

Cost–benefit analysis (CBA)

In CBA, health benefits associated with an intervention are valued in monetary units (for example, US dollars or Euros). Interventions with positive net benefits are preferred whereas those with negative net benefits are not (net benefits are defined as health outcomes converted to monetary equivalent minus inter-vention costs). Although used routinely in the evaluation of transportation or environmental programs, CBA has not been widely applied in health care. This is likely due in large part to ethical concerns as well as technical issues surrounding the validity of methods used to value outcomes in monetary terms.[43,44] To date, no cost–benefit analysis of lung cancer screening has been reported.

Cost-effectiveness analysis (CEA) and cost–utility analysis (CUA)

In contrast to CBA, CEA and CUA are used to determine the most efficient way of allocating limited healthcare resources, given a fixed budget. A key feature of CEA is that health effects are measured in natural units such as the number of cancer cases detected or a more downstream outcome measure such as years of life (survival). CUA, on the other hand, combines duration of life and health-related quality of life into a single measure of effectiveness commonly expressed as quality-adjusted life years (QALYs). A variety of methods can be used to obtain the quality weights associated with health states for CUA including direct preference-based methods (for example, standard gamble, time-trade off, and visual analog scale), and indirect methods using multi-attribute health status classification systems (such as the

Table 18.2 Approaches to economic evaluation		
Approach	**Costs**	**Benefits**
Cost–benefit analysis (CBA)	Money (e.g. dollars)	Money (e.g. dollars)
Cost-effectiveness analysis (CEA)	Money (e.g. dollars)	Natural units (e.g. life years)
Cost–utility analysis (CUA)	Money (e.g. dollars)	Combine quantity and quality of life (e.g. QALYs)

Adapted from Drummond MF et al.[37]

Health Utility Index, EuroQol and Quality of Well-Being).[37,39,45–51] For example, in their recent CUA comparing lung cancer screening with spiral CT to no screening, Mahadevia et al[52] consider the quality of life implications of disease using published results of EuroQol assessment among patients with non-small-cell lung cancer. The authors assumed in their base case analysis that quality of life is reduced by 33% with advanced-stage lung cancer compared with patients without detected disease.

Life years or QALYs are the preferred metrics by health economists since they allow for direct comparison between interventions for different diseases. For example, life years saved, or survival is a long-term, downstream measure of outcomes that can be used to compare lung cancer screening to colorectal cancer screening. In both CEA and CUA, the measure of interest is the ratio of costs to health effects. For CEA, the result could be reported as cost per lung cancer case detected or costs per life year gained. For CUA, the result could be reported as cost per quality-adjusted life year gained, or cost per healthy year equivalent.[53,54] In any case, the underlying calculation for the incremental cost-effectiveness ratio (ICER) comparing alternatives is the same:

$$\text{ICER} = \frac{\text{Cost}_{\text{intervention A}} - \text{Cost}_{\text{intervention B}}}{\text{Effect}_{\text{intervention A}} - \text{Effect}_{\text{intervention B}}}$$

Published economic evaluations of lung cancer screening to date are summarized for chest radiography and low-dose spiral computed tomography (LDSCT) in Tables 18.3 and 18.4, respectively. Most of these are CEAs, reporting cost per life saved, cost per case of LC detected, or cost per life year gained.[52,55–63] Two have undertaken CUA, and both report cost per QALY.[52,63]

Elements of a high-quality economic evaluation

Now that the basic approaches to economic evaluation (CBA, CEA, CUA) have been reviewed, the key elements required for a high-quality economic evaluation are identified and discussed using the lung cancer screening studies from Tables 18.3 and 18.4. Although there is no definite consensus on a single best approach to economic evaluation, there are important criteria to assess methodological quality that have been emphasized for a high-quality economic evaluation.[37,39,42,64–67] These broadly cover the (1) study design, (2) data collection, and (3) analysis and interpretation of the results of an economic evaluation (Table 18.5).

Study design

A well-designed economic evaluation has a clearly defined research objective that considers both costs and outcomes associated with intervention. The choice of alternatives being compared should be justified along with a detailed description of the target population, study perspective and time horizon considered in evaluation. The type of economic evaluation used (CBA, CEA or CUA) should be stated along with the measure of effectiveness (for example, cancer case detection rates or quality-adjusted life expectancy) and method of health outcome valuation if CUA approach is used (for example, standard gamble or time trade off method).

For example, a question such as 'Is lung cancer screening worth it?' is not sufficient because it does not specify that both costs and effects will be measured, does not identify the alternatives to be compared, nor does it describe the study population or perspective. The objective of the cost-effectiveness analysis by Marshall et al[63] is stated as 'What is the cost-effectiveness of annual lung cancer screening with LDSCT compared to no screening in terms

Table 18.3 Summary of cost-effectiveness lung cancer screening studies: chest X-ray vs. no screening

Author	Comparators	Perspective	Time horizon	Cohort description	Key results*	Special issues in economic evaluation of screening		
						Lead time bias	Overdiagnosis bias	False/positive[†]
Baba 1998[55]	NS vs. CXR	Health care payer	Compare CXR mass screening (1991 to 1994) to NS; 5-year follow-up	General population aged 40–80 years	10.8 million yen/LS; ($93 000/LS)	Not considered	Not considered	Considered
Okamoto 2000[56]	NS vs. CXR	Health care payer	Compare CXR mass screening (1983 and 1993) to NS; length of follow-up unclear	General population aged 40–85 years	4.5 million yen/LYS; ($32 250/LYS)	Not considered	Not considered	Considered
Caro 2000[57]	NS vs. CXR	Health care payer	Lifetime	Former, light, and heavy smokers aged 45–80 years	$19874/LYS; 1998 constant dollars	Not considered	Not considered	Considered

*Results of Baba 1998 and Okamoto 2000 were converted to US dollars based on conversion rates as presented in text. Price year of presented costs was not explicitly stated. [†]Diagnostic follow-up and biopsy costs included in estimates.
CEA, cost-effectiveness analysis; CXR, chest X-ray; LS, life saved; LYS, life year saved; NS, no screening.

Table 18.4 Summary of cost-effectiveness lung cancer screening studies: spiral CT vs other comparators

Author	Comparators	Perspective	Time horizon	Cohort description	Key results*	Special issues in economic evaluation of screening		
						Lead time bias	Overdiagnosis bias	False/positive†
Cost-effectiveness analysis								
Iinuma 1994 (abstract)[58]	CXR vs. LDSCT	Not clear	Not clear	Population with lung cancer incidence of 0.02 persons per year and life expectancy of 30 years	146 000 yen to save one person year with CXR and 203 000 yen to save one person year with LDSCT	Not clear	Not clear	Not clear
Kaneko 1996[59]	CXR and SC vs. CXR, SC and LDSCT	Member of Anti-Lung Cancer Association (ALCA), Japan	Compare twice yearly CXR and SC (1975 to 1993) to CXR, SC and LDSCT (1993 to 1995)	Men 50 years or older with >20 pack years smoking	10.7 million yen per case of LC detected for CXR and SC vs 5.4 million yen per case of LC detected for CXR, SC and LDSCT	Not considered	Not considered	Considered False positives indirectly accounted for in ALCA member fees
Marshall 2001[60]	NS vs. LDSCT (one-time)	Health care payer (Medicare), US	Lifetime	60–74 years with median of 45 pack years smoking	US$6500 per LYG	Sensitivity analysis examined lead time bias as 1-year decrease in survival benefit	Sensitivity analysis examined overdiagnosis as 1-year decrease in survival benefit	Considered

Table 18.4 continued

Author	Comparators	Perspective	Time horizon	Cohort description	Key results*	Special issues in economic evaluation of screening		
						Lead time bias	Overdiagnosis bias	False/positive†
Chirikos 2002[61]	NS vs. LDSCT (annually for 5 years)	National health care payer, US	15 years	45–74 years	US$48000 per LYG under assumptions of highest cost and lowest yield (base case)	Not considered	Not considered	Considered
Wisnivesky 2003[62]	NS vs. LDSCT (one-time)	Health care payer, US	One year for costs; lifetime for outcomes	60 years or older at high risk (at least a 10-pack-year history of smoking)	US$2500 per LYG (restricted to costs incurred in first year after lung cancer diagnosis)	Lead time added as a period of time to the life expectancy of the unscreened individuals and in sensitivity analysis	Sensitivity analysis examined overdiagnosis as varying proportion of screen-detected cancers	Considered
Cost-utility analysis								
Marshall 2001[63]	NS vs. LDSCT (annual)	Health care payer (Medicare), US	5 years	60–74 years with median of 45 pack-years history of smoking	US$19500 per QALY	Sensitivity analysis examined lead time bias as 1-year decrease in survival benefit	Sensitivity analysis examined overdiagnosis as 1-year decrease in survival benefit	Considered

continued

Table 18.4 continued

Author	Comparators	Perspective	Time horizon	Cohort description	Key results*	Special issues in economic evaluation of screening		
						Lead time bias	Overdiagnosis bias	False/positive[†]
Mahadevia 2003[52]	NS vs. LDSCT (annual)	Societal perspective	20-year screening duration with follow up to age 100 years	60 years with over 20 pack-years history of smoking	US$116 000 per QALY for current smokers; $559 000 per QALY for quitting smokers; $2 323 000 per QALY for former smokers	Average 1-year lead time for screen-detected cancers; also varied degree of stage shift in sensitivity analysis	Not considered separately from lead-time bias	Considered Also included disutility from screening, follow up, and treatment

*Follow up HRCT and biopsy costs included in estimates.
[†]Diagnostic follow-up and biopsy costs included in estimates.
CXR, chest X-ray; HRCT, high-resolution computed tomography; LDSCT, low-dose spiral computed tomography; NS, no screening; QALY, quality-adjusted-life-year; SC, sputum cytology.

Table 18.5 Criteria list for the assessment of methodological quality of economic evaluations of lung cancer screening

Study design
- Was a well-defined economic research question defined, examining both costs and outcomes of lung cancer screening in the context of alternatives with a clearly defined target population, viewpoint and time horizon?

Data collection
- Were both costs and effectiveness of the alternative approaches to lung cancer screening identified, measured and valued appropriately?
- Were the data sources provided and documented for both costs and effectiveness of lung cancer screening?
- Were resource use and costs for lung cancer screening reported separately?

Analysis and interpretation of results
- Were both costs and outcomes for lung cancer screening adjusted for differential timing?
- Was allowance made for uncertainty in the estimates of costs and outcomes for lung cancer screening using sensitivity analysis?
- Did the discussion of study results address study limitations and their potential impact on the conclusions?

---

of survival and costs over a time horizon of 5 years in individuals between the ages of 60 and 74 years and at high risk of lung cancer?' The research question is clearly defined and meets this methodologic criterion.

Two other dimensions should be considered in the design of an economic analysis in addition to the type of analysis: the perspective or point of view of the analysis, and the types of costs and benefits that are included.[68,69] These dimensions can be represented as three axes of a cube (Figure 18.1).[70] There are multiple perspectives (patient, payer, provider and society) that may be adopted in an economic analysis, which will largely dictate the types of costs and benefits (direct medical, direct non-medical, indirect and intangible) that are included. The societal perspective is the broadest and most

relevant for an economic evaluation, but seldom used.[37] The cost-effectiveness analysis by Mahadevia et al[52] approximates a societal perspective because it includes direct non-medical costs (such as costs for patient travel time for screening and follow-up visits), costs of informal caregiving, in addition to the direct medical care costs associated with lung cancer diagnosis and treatment (such as high-resolution CT scanning, surgery, hospitalization, clinic visits, medications). The analysis also includes a measure of 'intangible' costs of pain and suffering through a decrement in utility for invasive diagnostic testing, surgical postoperative recovery, radiation or chemotherapy. Nonetheless, indirect costs such as productivity costs from lost work were not included, which should be part of an analysis adopting the societal perspective.

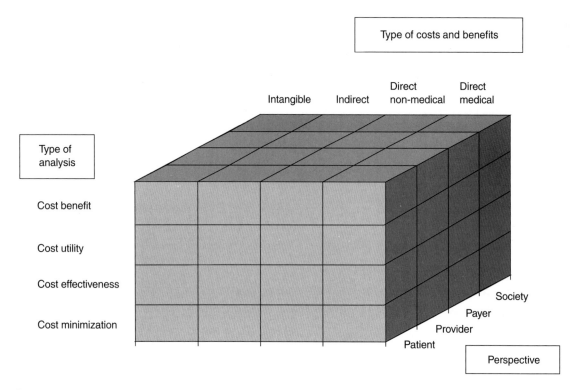

Figure 18.1
The three dimensions of an economic evaluation (adapted from Schulman et al[70]).

Data collection

A full economic evaluation requires data on both the effectiveness and associated costs of the alternatives being assessed. Data on effectiveness can come from a variety of sources (such as clinical trials, observational studies and systematic reviews). A high-quality economic evaluation should clearly describe all sources of effectiveness data in enough detail for readers to assess potential bias and generalizability of results. Furthermore, all relevant costs associated with intervention should be identified, measured accurately and valued in a credible manner. Resource use should be reported separately from costs and details on these data sources provided. Researchers need to provide justification for any modeling techniques used (for instance, decision analytic model, epidemi-

ologic model, regression model) along with enough details to ensure transparency.

For example, Chirikos et al[61] used a variety of sources to estimate the cost-effectiveness of lung cancer screening with LDSCT compared to no screening. The estimates of outcomes were based on published survival data from the Surveillance, Epidemiology and End Results (SEER) cancer registry by stage, age and sex for individuals with lung cancer, and general population survival data from the US population life tables for individuals without lung cancer. Lung cancer prevalence incidence, and the effectiveness of lung cancer screening was based on cancer yields reported by the Early Lung Cancer Action Project cohort study and modeled as a 'down-staging' of detected cancers (i.e. the stage distribution of cancers in the screened cohort is lower (earlier stage disease) than in the unscreened cohort). Professional costs associated with screening and diagnostic CT procedures were based on Medicare reimbursement rates. Lung cancer treatment costs were based on linked Medicare/SEER records for each stage of lung cancer. Details of all data sources were identified and documented, and results for resource use (number of prevalence screens, follow-up CT scans per abnormal screen, biopsy ratio, etc.), costs, and effectiveness were presented separately in addition to the final calculation of cost-effectiveness.

Analysis and interpretation of results

An economic evaluation estimates the incremental cost and incremental effects of an intervention and reports this as the incremental cost-effectiveness ratio (ICER). For example, consider the cost-effectiveness of lung cancer screening with LDSCT compared to no screening in a high-risk cohort reported by Marshall et al.[63] The ICER was calculated as:

$$\frac{Cost_{LDSCT} - Cost_{No\ screening}}{Effect_{LDSCT} - Effect_{No\ screening}}$$

$$= \frac{\$2814 - \$2718}{419\,020 - 413\,984}$$

$$= \frac{\$96\ million}{5036\ life\ years}$$

$$= \$18\,968\ per\ life\ year\ saved$$

It would be incorrect to compare the ratio of cost to outcomes for LDSCT and no screening (i.e. $\$2814/419\,020 = \$6716$ per life year for LDSCT and $\$2718/413\,984 = \$6566$ per life year for no screening). This would be the average cost-effectiveness ratio, and is not relevant for economic evaluation.

As with the example of LDSCT for lung cancer screening above, most new technologies are more effective than the alternative, but also more costly. The results of an economic evaluation will depend on whether the new intervention is more costly or less costly than the alternative, and whether it is more effective or less effective than the alternative. This can be illustrated as four quadrants in a diagram referred to as the 'cost-effectiveness plane'.[71] For example, in Figure 18.2, the horizontal axis represents the effect difference in QALYs between LDSCT and no screening, and the vertical axis represents the cost difference in US dollars between LDSCT and no screening. 'No screening' is considered to lie at the intersection of both axes.

In the northwest quadrant, LDSCT would be less effective and more costly than no screening. If all other things were equal, LDSCT would be rejected. In the southeast quadrant, LDSCT would be more effective and less costly than no screening. In this case, LDSCT would be accepted. In the southwest and northeast quadrants, there is no obvious decision, and other factors would need to be considered. In the southwest quadrant, LDSCT is less effective and less costly than no screening. The cost–utility analysis results of LDSCT screening by Mahadevia et al[52] for different groups of smokers all fall in the northeast quadrant of the cost-effectiveness plane. In the northeast quadrant, LDSCT is more effective and more costly than no screening. In this case, a decision about whether or not LDSCT screening should be adopted depends on what a society considers an acceptable price to pay for an additional quality-adjusted year of life. Based on the results by Mahadevia, if $\$100\,000$ per QALY is used as a threshold, then LDSCT might be considered for adoption for current smokers (line A Figure 18.2), but not for quitting or former smokers.

A high-quality economic evaluation adopts a time horizon long enough to capture all major

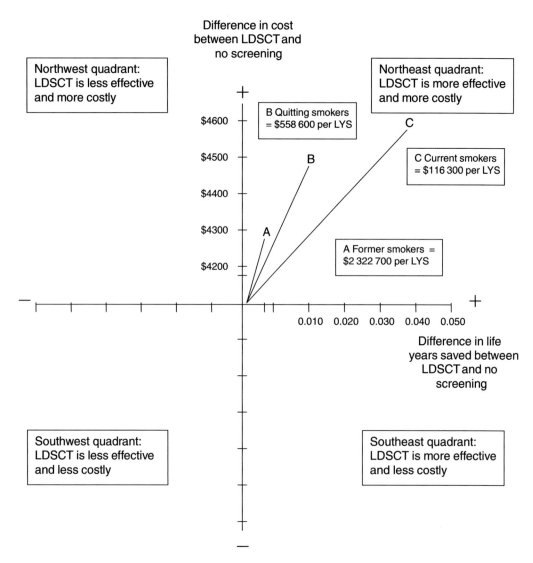

Figure 18.2
The cost-effectiveness plane (adapted from Black[71]).

economic and health outcomes of the intervention and relevant alternatives. Study results, therefore, should be adjusted for differences in the timing of the costs and consequences of intervention; most recommendations suggest an annual discount rate between 3–6%.[34,35,37,39] Uncertainty should be carefully addressed through estimation of confidence intervals around data inputs or surrounding the ICER for trial-based economic evaluation. Model-based economic evaluations need to address methodological, and/or modeling structure uncertainty by performing sensitivity analyses such as univariate or multivariate analyses or best case/worst case scenarios.[64–67,72] Probabilistic sensitivity analysis by Monte Carlo simulation methods is also gaining acceptance as the appropriate method of capturing the joint uncertainty of multiple parameter inputs.[73–76] Results should be presented in a manner that answers all study objectives with all major outcomes presented in disaggregated as well as aggregated (i.e. single index or ratio) form. Conclusions should be consistent with reported results and authors should discuss study limitations and their potential impact on conclusions. Comparisons with other economic evaluations should be made with caution unless it can be demonstrated that study methods and settings are similar.

Strong analytic methods and interpretation of results can be seen in Mahadevia et al[52] who modeled the costs and effects associated with 20 years of screening along with follow-up to 100 years of age for occurrence of clinical events. All costs and effects were discounted 3% annually. Detailed sensitivity analyses were performed (univariate as well as best case/worst case analyses) to assess strength of results to changing assumptions such as the degree of stage shift, age at first screening, and length of follow-up. The authors also acknowledge study limitations including the fact that their model did not consider incidental diagnoses from screening or include costs associated with disability or lost productivity.

ECONOMIC EVALUATIONS OF LUNG CANCER SCREENING

Ten full health economic evaluations of lung cancer screening having been conducted since 1994 (Tables 18.3 and 18.4). Three of these analyses focus on estimating the relative cost-effectiveness of screening with traditional radiography compared with no screening[55–57]; the remaining seven studies have a primary objec-tive of assessing the incremental cost-effectiveness of screening with helical CT compared with a no screening option.[52,58–63]

Both CEA and CUA can be conducted along-side randomized controlled trials of medical interventions with direct identification, measurement, and valuation of patient-specific costs and outcomes.[70,77,78] More often, however, CEA and CUA are based on models that synthesize secondary data sources to estimate clinical and economic outcomes associated with interventions. This is especially true in the economic evaluation of lung cancer screening programs. In the absence of randomized controlled trials comparing screening alternatives, studies to date rely on modeling techniques to compare relevant strategies (traditional radiography, helical CT or no screening option) and to translate cancer detection rates (as observed in cohort studies) to estimated survival and quality-adjusted survival.

Cost-effectiveness of screening with traditional radiography

Since 1987, lung cancer screening has been conducted on a voluntary basis in several Japanese communities using chest X-ray and sputum cytodiagnosis until the introduction of CT screening in the 1990s. Early reported economic analyses of lung cancer screening focus on assessing the relative cost-effectiveness of this Japanese mass screening program with chest X-ray compared with no screening.[55,56] The first economic analysis of lung cancer screening from the US healthcare perspective was reported by Caro et al.[57] A summary of study characteristics and primary results can be seen in Table 18.3.

The analyses of Baba et al[55] and Okamoto et al[56] use survival data among lung cancer patients detected by mass screening compared with survival among patients with incidentally found disease in combination with assumed costs of care (including screening, detailed follow-up examination, and cancer treatment costs), to estimate the costs per life saved with chest X-ray screening. Using age- and gender-specific life expectancy data, Okamoto[56] extends this analysis to also estimate the costs per life year saved with mass screening. Lack of published details on study methods and choice of endpoints make interpretation of results difficult. However, these early Japanese studies clearly highlight the trade-off that exists between costs and clinical benefits associated with screening. Furthermore, their results suggest that the estimated cost-effectiveness of screening with chest X-ray may improve with target population screening focused on older individuals.

Caro et al[57] developed an economic model to assess the potential impact of a chest X-ray screening program among male smokers aged 45–80 years should it be considered in the United States. These authors assume an annual mortality reduction of 18% with screening and include all direct costs associated with an ongoing yearly screening program including costs associated with diagnostic work-ups and consultations with a positive chest X-ray. Costs and benefits were discounted at 3% per annum and detailed sensitivity analyses were performed to assess uncertainty in model assumptions and parameters.

Base case results suggest an estimated incremental cost-effectiveness of less than $20 000 per life year saved for chest radiography compared to no screening. Estimated cost-effectiveness ratios ranged from $21 091 to $59 621 per life year saved in sensitivity analyses – amounts considered an efficient use of health care resources by many.[79,80] However, the quality-of-life implications associated with false-positive findings (for example anxiety and discomfort

with unnecessary biopsies) were not considered in their model suggesting that the authors may have overestimated the clinical benefits associated with screening.

Cost-effectiveness of screening with low-dose spiral CT

The earliest publications reporting cost-effectiveness of spiral CT CEA were also from Japan[58,59] and are limited to a macro-economic analysis. Total costs for a large cohort of health care plan members are calculated and the total number of lung cancer cases detected is identified for each screening program alternative. Subsequent studies examining LDSCT are all US-based.

A summary of these economic evaluations of lung cancer screening with LDSCT in Table 18.4 indicates that to date, only two are cost–utility analyses[52,63] and the rest are cost-effectiveness analyses measuring cost per life year gained. Since no mortality-based trials are available for LDSCT, estimates of the effectiveness and cost-effectiveness of lung cancer screening with LDSCT are based on decision analytic models that make a number of assumptions. As noted previously in this discussion, a long-term time horizon, with a lifetime perspective preferred, is critical to correctly evaluate the cost-effectiveness of a screening program. Only Mahadevia,[52] Marshall[63] and Chirokos[61] (20 years) have attempted to capture the lifetime consequences of screening.

Furthermore, only Mahadevia[52] used a pooled estimate from multiple data sources for estimating the rate of nodule detection. All the other models were based on the findings reported by the Early Lung Cancer Action Project (ELCAP) cohort analysis.[13,14] This may explain, at least in part, the substantially higher cost-effectiveness estimate by Mahadevia[52] ($119 000 per QALY in the base case for current smokers) compared to previous analyses (ranging from $2500 per life year gained to $48 000 per life year gained). Certainly part of the reason for the higher estimate obtained by Mahadevia is that the QALY estimate incorporates the disutility associated with false positive findings and the subsequent workup as a consequence of lung cancer screening. In addition, Mahadevia assumed a 30-day mortality rate of 4.5% after surgical resection; more positive postoperative mortality rates (less than 1%) have been reported in current clinical practice.[81]

The wide range of cost-effectiveness estimates for lung cancer screening with LDSCT likely reflects differences in assumptions and parameter estimates used in these models. This highlights the importance of testing model robustness under alternative assumptions through sensitivity analyses. All published models to date assess uncertainty through sensitivity analyses. In general, assumptions regarding potential screening biases, costs for screening and nodule management, adherence with screening and follow-up, as well as quality-of-life decrements associated with disease and nodule 'anxiety' are influential parameters on the estimate of cost-effectiveness. Future studies should also consider the use of probabilistic approaches to sensitivity analysis. Probabilistic modeling has emerged as the preferred method of jointly capturing the uncertainty of multiple parameter inputs.[73–76]

SPECIAL ISSUES IN ECONOMIC EVALUATION OF LUNG CANCER SCREENING

Models versus trial-based economic evaluation in lung cancer screening

In the absence of direct evidence from a well-designed appropriately powered lung cancer screening trial that incorporates current LDSCT technology, has appropriate comparators, and includes both clinical and economic outcome measures, there is still a need to make informed decisions about care. Thus, decision analytic modeling is sometimes referred to as an 'unavoidable fact of life'.[82] Models provide an alternative to trial-based economic evaluation.[70,77,78,83] This explains why cost-effectiveness analyses of lung cancer screening to date have relied on decision analysis modeling techniques to compare relevant strategies (traditional radiography, helical CT, or no screening option) and to translate cancer detection rates (as observed in cohort studies) to estimated survival and quality-adjusted survival.

Models necessarily incorporate data from diverse sources and require a number of assumptions to be made about disease progression and relationships between risk factors and clinical outcomes.[83] For example, in the decision analysis by Mahadevia et al,[52] data are combined from four cohort studies in the US and Japan over different time periods, using different follow-up protocols to estimate the rate of nodule detection and LDSCT screening performance. Annual survival probabilities for each cancer stage were obtained from the Surveillance, Epidemiology and End Results (SEER) cancer registry database. Costs and utilities were obtained from a variety of published literature. There are a number of valid concerns about the use of models,[84–87] and many feel that unequivocal proof of lung cancer mortality reduction through screening is required before general recommendations can be made for population screening, even in selected subgroups.[19,22,30]

Screening trials such as the National Lung Screening Trial (NLST) in the United States promise to provide this proof.[19,20] However, trials that compare screening strategies require large sample sizes, and long follow-up periods in order to measure differences in outcomes and costs. Launched in 2002, the NLST enrolled 50 000 patients over the course of 18 months randomized to LDSCT or standard chest X-ray and will collect and analyze the data for 8 years to examine the comparative risks and benefits. It is powered to determine if there is a 20% or greater drop in lung cancer mortality from using spiral CT compared to chest X-ray. Some argued that trial enrolment would be a challenge, and that it was too late to initiate a trial of lung cancer screening because the promising results from the cohort studies had pushed us past the point of equipoise, where a rational, informed person has no preference between the alternatives, and it is ethically sound to randomize.[88] Furthermore, no single trial can provide all the necessary information for an economic evaluation. By the time the trial is complete, the technology will have changed and the relevant alternatives to be compared may have changed. Further, it will not be possible to evaluate the impact of various screening intervals and follow-up regimens. Thus, model-based economic evaluation of lung cancer screening programs may continue to play an important role in clinical and health policy decision-making even if ongoing large-scale trials demonstrate a mortality benefit associated with screening.

Complexity of lung cancer screening and diagnostic follow-up

Economic evaluation of screening programs is particularly challenging because of the complexity and hierarchical nature of screening, diagnostic follow-up and subsequent treatment.[89,90] Screening for lung cancer is a complex series of decisions that begins with the screening test, such as the LDSCT scan. The performance characteristics (sensitivity and specificity) of the screening test as well as the profile of the target population in terms of the prevalence and incidence of lung cancer, will determine the diagnostic accuracy of the screening test.[24] As a result, some patients will be correctly diagnosed – either having lung cancer or not – and some patients will be incorrectly diagnosed – either falsely identified as having lung cancer (false positives) or falsely identified as not having lung cancer (false negatives). One of the key barriers to cost-effective LDSCT screening is the observed high incidence of false-positive findings that have important cost and quality of life implications.[15,17,32,91] In the absence of RCTs with long-term follow-up, and verification by autopsy at death, it is not possible to define with certainty the sensitivity and specificity of LDSCT scanning for lung cancer. Estimates from the two cohorts in the US[13,14,91] and two cohorts in Japan[92,93] range from 55–94% for sensitivity, and 49–89% for specificity. This means that in some instances, approximately 50% of nodules are initially identified as potentially cancerous and then found to be benign after follow-up tests.

Furthermore, clinical outcomes depend critically on subsequent treatment, for which there are multiple alternatives. A widely recognized problem in evaluating screening programs is accurately capturing this whole chain of clinical events, resource use and outcomes that arise from the initial screening intervention. Costs in an economic evaluation of lung cancer screening need to include all downstream expenses associated with subsequent diagnostic procedures, cancer treatment, patient care and complications resulting from testing and treatment. Estimating these downstream outcomes and costs almost always requires some kind of decision analytic modeling. Virtually all of the cost-effectiveness analyses of lung cancer screening in Tables 18.3 and 18.4 made some attempt to capture the costs and outcomes from follow-up diagnostic testing. Most, in fact, assume patients undergo detailed clinical follow-up once nodules are found with screening.

As CT technology improved with thin sections that can be acquired rapidly and reconstructed in three dimensions, there has been a marked increase in the detectability of small nodules that may be false positives and require further work-up.[94] Optimal strategies to investigate small nodules have been evaluated, including CT-guided needle biopsy, positron emission tomography, video-assisted thoracoscopic surgery and fiberoptic bronchoscopy.[95,96] Others have suggested that some smaller nodules do not justify immediate work-up, but only annual repeat screening to determine whether interim growth has occurred.[97] The success of efficient, non-invasive case work-up would have an important impact on the estimate of the cost-effectiveness of lung cancer screening.[96,97] Future cost-effectiveness studies should consider both the increased frequency of nodule detection with new LDSCT technology, and alternative strategies for diagnostic work-up of nodules detected on screening.

Adjusting for screening biases

Survival from the time of diagnosis is commonly reported in screening trials, however, it is not an appropriate outcome measure for screening tests because of potential screening biases, such as lead-time bias and overdiagnosis bias.[68,98] Lead time bias may occur if screening allows for earlier diagnosis, but does not actually alter the time of death. The consequence is that survival appears longer, but mortality is the same. Overdiagnosis bias may occur if screening detects a case of cancer that would not have led to death during the lifetime of the individual. The consequence is that a stage shift may be observed in detection of cancer, and survival improves, but mortality is the same.

There has been considerable controversy over the results of the early lung cancer screening trials about the use of survival as a measure of outcome because of these potential screening biases.[5,9,10,12,27,99–101] In a re-analysis of the Mayo Lung Project data,[10] it was observed that the screened group had better overall survival than the control group, if measured from randomization instead of the time of diagnosis. Measuring from the time of randomization presumably removes the potential lead-time bias. In an extended follow-up of the Mayo Lung Project, Marcus et al[12] reported better overall survival in the screened group compared to the control group, but there was no difference in lung cancer mortality. This discrepancy between survival and mortality was attributed by the authors to overdiagnosis bias, but others disagree.[10,27]

In any case, such biases clearly complicate the analysis and interpretation of these study results, and pose considerable challenges to economic evaluation of lung cancer screening. The majority of cost-effectiveness analyses of lung cancer screening have not explicitly accounted for possible lead-time or overdiagnosis bias. The cost-effectiveness models by Marshall et al,[60,63] Wisnivesky et al,[62] and Mahadevia et al[52] made at least some attempt to consider these screening biases in sensitivity analyses by incorporating a 1-year decrease in survival, or a stage shift for detection. The models demonstrated that lead time bias and overdiagnosis bias were highly influential parameters on the estimates of the cost-effectiveness of lung cancer screening.

SUMMARY AND AREAS FOR FURTHER RESEARCH

This chapter provides a brief overview of approaches and dimensions of economic evaluation, and summarizes the cost-effectiveness studies of lung cancer screening to date. It was observed that virtually all the studies are model-based evaluations, owing to the fact that direct evidence from well-designed and appropriately powered lung cancer screening trials that apply current LDSCT technology, appropriate comparators, and include both clinical and economic outcome measures, is lacking. A wide range of estimates have been reported, from a few thousand US dollars per life year saved to over $100 000 US dollars per life year saved, reflecting a variety of underlying assumptions and parameter estimates used in these models.

Finally, some of the special methodologic challenges associated with economic evaluation of lung cancer screening are discussed: the complexity and hierarchial nature of screening, diagnostic follow-up and treatment, the potential impact of misdiagnosis (false positives and false negatives), and screening biases (lead-time and overdiagnosis biases). These are areas warranting further research to provide better data that can inform decisions about the adoption and implementation of lung cancer screening programs. The use of advanced decision analysis simulation techniques to estimate the value of information may be helpful in prioritizing this research by identifying the most important data parameters that influence the estimated cost-effectiveness of lung cancer screening.[77,102–105]

To date, it remains unproven that lung cancer screening is cost-effective. Although some cost-effectiveness models are more optimistic, lung cancer screening with spiral CT seems unlikely to be highly cost-effective without a substantial reduction in mortality, lower false-positive results, lower follow-up costs and minimal screening biases.

REFERENCES

1. Melamed MR, Flehinger BJ, Zaman MB, et al, Screening for early lung cancer: Results of the Memorial Sloan-Kettering Study in New York. Chest 1984; 86(1):44–53.
2. Tockman MS, Survival and mortality from lung cancer in a screened population. Chest 1986; 89:324S–5S.
3. Fontana R, Sanderson D, Woolner L, et al, Lung Cancer Screening: The Mayo Program. J Occup Med 1986; 28:746–50.
4. Kubik A, Parkin D, Khlat M, et al, Lack of benefit from semi-annual screening for cancer of the lung: follow-up report of a randomized controlled trial, on a population of high-risk males in Czechoslovakia. Int J Cancer 1990; 45:26–33.
5. Manser RL, Irving LB, Byrnes G, et al, Screening for lung cancer: a systematic review and meta-analysis of controlled trials. Thorax 2003; 58:784–9.
6. Eddy DM, Screening for lung cancer. Ann Int Med 1989; 111:232–7.
7. US Preventive Services Task Force, US Task Force on Preventive Services: Screening for lung cancer, second edition, 1996.
8. Smith RJ, Eschenback AC, Wender R, et al, American Cancer Society guidelines for the early detection of cancer: update of early detection guidelines for prostate, colorectal, and endometrial cancers. CA Cancer J Clin 2001; 51:38–75.
9. Strauss GM, Gleason RE, Sugarbaker DJ, Screening for lung cancer. Another look: A different view. Chest 1997; 111(3):754–68.
10. Strauss GM, The Mayo Lung Cohort: A regression analysis focusing on lung cancer incidence and mortality. J Clin Oncol 2002; 20:1973–83.
11. Fontana RS, Sanderson DR, Woolner LB, et al, Screening for lung cancer: critique of the Mayo Lung Project. Cancer 1991; 67:1155–64.
12. Marcus PM, Bergstralh RJ, Fagerstrom RM, et al, Lung cancer mortality in the Mayo Lung Project: Impact of extended follow-up. J Natl Cancer Inst 2000; 92(16):1308–16.

13. Henschke CI, McCauley DI, Yankelovitz D, Early Lung Cancer Action Project: Overall design and findings from baseline screening. Lancet 1999; 354(9173):99–105.

14. Henschke CI, Naidich DP, Yankelevitz DF, et al, Early Lung Cancer Action Project: Initial findings on repeat screening. Cancer 2001; 92(1):153–9.

15. Swensen SJ, Jett JR, Hartman TE, et al, Lung cancer screening with CT: Mayo Clinic experience. Radiology 2003; 226(3):756–61.

16. Pastorino U, Bellomi M, Landoni C, et al, Early lung-cancer detection with spiral CT and positron emission tomography in heavy smokers: 2-year results. Lancet 2003; 362: 593–7.

17. Diederich S, Wormanns D, Semik M, et al, Screening for early lung cancer with low-dose spiral CT: Prevalence in 817 asymptomatic smokers. Radiology 2002; 222(3):773–81.

18. Schwartz LM, Woloshin S, Fowler Jr F, Welch H, Enthusiasm for cancer screening in the United States. JAMA 2004; 291(1):71–8.

19. Diederich S, Wormanns D, Heindel W, Lung cancer screening with low-dose CT. Eur J Radiol 2003; 45:2–7.

20. Aberle DR, Black WC, Goldin JG, Patz E, Gareen I, National Lung Screening Trial (NLST). A research study for smokers and ex-smokers, 2004.

21. Blanchon T, Lukasiewicz-Hajage E, Lemarie E, et al, DEPISCAN – a pilot study to evaluate low dose spiral CT scanning as a screening method for bronchial carcinoma [French]. Rev Mal Respir 2002; 19:701–5.

22. Canadian Coordinating Office for Health Technology Assessment, Multi-slice/helical computed tomography for lung cancer screening. Canadian Coordinating Office for Health Technology Assessment (CCOHTA). Issues in Emerging Health Technologies, Issue 48, 2003.

23. Casarella WJ, A patient's viewpoint on a current controversy [letter]. Radiology 2002; 224(3):927–34.

24. Hunink MGM, Gazelle GS, CT screening: a trade-off of risks, benefits, and costs. J Clin Invest 2003; 111(11):1612–19.

25. Swensen SJ, Jett JR, Midthun DE, Hartman TE, Computed tomographic screening for lung cancer: Home run or foul ball? Mayo Clin Proc 2003; 78:1187–8.

26. Frame P, Routine screening for lung cancer? Maybe someday, but not yet. JAMA 2000; 284(15):1980–3.

27. Jett JR, Screening for lung cancer: no longer a taboo subject. J Clin Oncol 2002; 20(8): 1959–61.

28. Miettinen O, Screening for lung cancer: can it be cost-effective? Can Med Assoc J 2000; 162(10):1431–6.

29. Health Technology Advisory Committee (HTAC), Helical computed tomography (CT) for lung cancer screening for asymptomatic patients. Minnesota Department of Health, 2000. (Available at http://www.health.state. mn.us/htac/ctdr.htm).

30. Swedish Council on Technology Assessment in Health Care, Swedish Council on Technology Assessment in Health Care. Helical computed tomography (CT) for lung cancer screening for asymptomatic patients. Early Assessment of New Health Technologies, May 27, 2003.

31. Mott FE, Early lung cancer action project (letter). Lancet 1999; 354:1205–6.

32. McWilliams A, Mayo J, MacDonald S, et al, Lung cancer screening. A different paradigm. Am J Respir Crit Care Med 2003; 168: 1167–73.

33. Hjelmgren J, Berggren F, Andresson F, Health economic guidelines – similarities, differences and some implications. Value in Health 2001; 4(3):225–50.

34. NICE, Guidance for Manufacturers and Sponsors. London, 2001.

35. Canadian Coordinating Office for Health Technology Assessment, Guidelines for economic evaluation of pharmaceuticals: Canada, second edition. Ottawa, Canadian Coordinating Office for Health Technology Assessment, 1997.

36. Wilson JMG, Jungner G, Principles and practice of screening for disease. Geneva, World Health Organization, 1968.

37. Drummond MF, O'Brien BJ, Stoddart GL, Torrance GW, Methods for Economic Evaluation of Health Care Programmes, 2nd edition. Oxford, Oxford University Press, 1997.

38. O'Brien BJ, Heyland D, Richardson WS, Levine M, Drummond MF, Users' guides to the medical literature. XIII. How to use an article on economic analysis of clinical practice. B. What are the results and will they help me in caring for my patients? JAMA 1997; 277(22): 1802–6.

39. Gold MR, Siegel JE, Russell LB, Weinstein MC, Cost-effectiveness in Health and Medicine. Oxford, Oxford University Press, 1996.

40. Elixhauser A, Luce BR, Taylor WR, Reblando J, Health care CBA/CEA: an update in the growth and composition of the literature. Med Care 1993; 31(suppl 7):js1–js19.

41. Elixhauser A, Halperin M, Schmier J, Luce BR, Health care CBA and CEA from 1991 to 1996: an updated bibliography. Med Care 1998; 36(5):MS1–MS9.

42. Drummond M, Jefferson TO, Guidelines for authors and peer reviewers of economic submissions to the BMJ. BMJ 1996; 313:275–83.

43. Hunink MG, Glasziou P, Siegel J, et al, Decision Making in Health and Medicine: Integrating Evidence and Values. Cambridge, Cambridge University Press, 2001.

44. Pauly MV, Valuing health care benefits in money terms. In: Sloan FA (ed.) Valuing Health Care. Cambridge, Cambridge University Press, 1995.

45. Spilker B, Quality of life and pharmacoeconomics in clinical trials, 2nd edn. Philadelphia, Lippincott-Raven, 1996.

46. Feeny D, Furlong W, Boyle M, Torrance GW, Multi-attribute health status classification systems: Health Utilities Index. Pharmacoeconomics 1995; 7:490–502.

47. Feeny D, Torrance GW, Labelle R, Integrating economic evaluations and quality of life assessments. Quality of life and pharmacoeconomics in clinical trials. Philadelphia, Lippencott-Raven, 1996; 85–95.

48. Torrance GW, Furlong W, Feeny D, Boyle KF, Multi-attribute preference functions: Health Utilities Index. Pharmacoeconomics 1995; 7: 503–20.

49. Kind P, The EuroQol instrument: an index of health-related quality of life. Quality of Life and pharmacoeconomics in clinical trials. Philadelphia, Lippincott-Raven, 1996, 191–201.

50. Kaplan RM, Anderson JP, The general health policy model: an integrated approach. Quality of life and pharmacoeconomics in clinical trials. Philadelphia, Lippincott-Raven, 1996; 309–22.

51. Kaplan RM, Anderson JP, A general health policy model: update and applications. Health Serv Res 1988; 23:203–35.

52. Mahadevia PJ, Fleisher LA, Frick KD, et al, Lung cancer screening with helical computed tomography in older adult smokers. A decision and cost effectiveness analysis. JAMA 2003; 289(3):313–22.

53. Mehrez A, Gafni A, Quality-adjusted life years, utility theory and healthy-year equivalents. Med Decis Making 1989; 9:142–9.

54. Mehrez A, Gafni A, Preference based outcome measures for economic evaluation of drug interventions: quality adjusted life years (QALYs) versus health years equivalents (HYEs). Pharmacoeconomics 1992; 1:338–45.

55. Baba Y, Takahaski M, Takizawa T, et al, Cost-effectiveness decision analysis of mass screening for lung cancer. Acad Radiol 1998; 5(Suppl 2): S344–6.

56. Okamoto N, Cost-effectiveness of lung cancer screening in Japan. Cancer 2000; 89(11): 2489–93.

57. Caro JJ, Klittich WS, Strauss G, Could chest X-ray screening for lung cancer be cost-effective? Cancer 2000; 89(11):2502–5.

58. Iinuma T, Tateno Y, Matsumoto T, Comparison of two types of mass screening of lung cancer in terms of cost-effectiveness: Indirect

chest X-ray vs. lung cancer screening CT. Nippon Acta Radiol 1994; 54(10):943–9.

59. Kaneko M, Eguchi K, Ohmatsu H, Kakinuma R, Naruke T, Peripheral lung cancer: screening and detection with low-dose spiral CT versus radiography. Radiology 1996; 201(3):798–802.

60. Marshall D, Simpson KN, Earle CC, Chu C, Potential cost-effectiveness of one-time screening for lung cancer (LC) in a high risk cohort. Lung Cancer 2001; 32(3):227–36.

61. Chirikos TN, Hazelton T, Tockman M, Clark R, Screening for lung cancer with CT. Chest 2002; 121(5):1507–14.

62. Wisnivesky JP, Mushlin AI, Sicherman N, Henschke C, The cost-effectiveness of low-dose CT screening for lung cancer. A preliminary cost effectiveness analysis. Chest 2003; 124(2):614–21.

63. Marshall D, Simpson KN, Earle CC, Chu CW, Economic decision analysis model of screening for lung cancer. Eur J Cancer 2001; 37(14):1759–67.

64. Sculpher M, Fenwick E, Claxton K, Assessing quality in decision analytic cost-effectiveness models: A suggested framework and example. Pharmacoeconomics 2000; 17:461–77.

65. Hay J, Jackson J, Luce B, et al, Methodological issues in conducting pharmacoeconomic evaluations – modeling studies. Value in Health 1999; 2:78–81.

66. Akehurst R, Anderson P, Brazier J, et al, Decision analytic modelling in the economic evaluation of health technologies. A consensus statement. Pharmacoeconomics 2000; 17(5):443–4.

67. Weinstein M, Hornberger J, Jackson J, et al, Principles of good practice of decision analytic modeling in health care evaluation: Report of the ISPOR Task Force on Good Research Practices – Modeling Studies. A Draft for Discussion. Value in Health 2003; 6(1):9–17.

68. Sackett DL, Haynes RB, Tugwell P, Clinical epidemiology: a basic science for clinical medicine. Boston, Little, Brown and Company, 1992.

69. Guyatt GH, Tugwell P, Feeny D, Haynes RB, Drummond M. A framework for clinical evaluation of diagnostic technologies. Can Med Assoc J 1986; 134:587–94.

70. Schulman KA, Glick HA, Yabroff R, Eisenberg JM, Introduction to clinical economics: Assessment of cancer therapies. Journal of the National Cancer Institute Monographs 1995; 19:1–9.

71. Black WC, A graphic representation of cost-effectiveness. Med Decis Making 1990; 10:212–14.

72. Briggs AH, Sculpher M, Buxton M, Uncertainty in the economic evaluation of health care technologies: the role of sensitivity analysis. Health Econ 1994; 3(20):95–104.

73. Doubilet P, Begg CB, Weinstein MC, Braun P, McNeil BJ, Probabilistic sensitivity analysis using Monte Carlo simulation. A practical approach. Med Decis Making 1985; 5(2):157–77.

74. Briggs AH, Handling uncertainty in economic evaluation. Br Med J 1999; 319:120.

75. Briggs AH, Mooney CZ, Wonderling DE, Constructing confidence intervals around cost-effectiveness ratios: an evaluation of parametric and non-parametric methods using Monte Carlo simulation. Stat Med 1999; 18:3245–62.

76. Claxton K, The irrelevance of inference: a decision-making approach to the stochastic evaluation of health care technologies. J Health Econ 1999; 18(3):341–64.

77. Glick HA, Polsky D, Schulman KA, Trial-based economic evaluations: an overview of design and analysis. In: Drummond M, McGuire A (eds) Economic evaluation in health care: merging theory with practice. New York, Oxford University Press, 2001, 113–40.

78. O'Brien BJ, Economic evaluation of pharmaceuticals: Frankenstein's monster or vampire of trials? Med Care 1996; 34(12 suppl):DS99–108.

79. Laupacis A, Feeny D, Detsky AS, Tugwell P, How attractive does a new technology have to be to warrant adoption and utilization? Tentative guidelines for using clinical and economic

evaluations. Can Med Assoc J 1992; 146: 473–81.

80. Garber AM, Phelps CE, Economic foundations of cost-effectiveness analysis. J Health Econ 1997; 16:1–31.

81. Watanabe S, Asamura H, Suzuki K, Tusuchiya R, Recent results for postoperative mortality for surgical resections in lung cancer. Ann Thorac Surg 2004; 78:999–1002.

82. Buxton MJ, Drummond MF, van Hout BA, et al, Modelling in economic evaluation: an unavoidable fact of life. Health Econ 1997; 6(3):217–27.

83. Kuntz KM, Weinstein MC, Modelling in economic evaluation. In: Drummond M, McGuire A (eds) Economic Evaluation in Health Care. Merging Theory with Practice. Oxford, Oxford University Press, 2001, 141–71.

84. Bloom B, Buxton M, Drummond M, Luce B, Sheldon T, The Pros and Cons of Modelling in Economic Evaluation, 33. 1997, OHE Briefing.

85. Drummond M, Economic analysis alongside clinical trials: problems and potential. J Rheumatol 1995; 22(7):1403–7.

86. Drummond M, Economic analysis alongside clinical trials: practical considerations. J Rheumatol 1995; 22(7):1418–19.

87. Drummond MF, Davies LM, Economic analysis alongside clinical trials: revisiting the methodological issues. Int J Technol Assess Health Care 1991; 7:561–73.

88. Chard JA, Lilford RJ, The use of equipoise in clinical trials. Soc Sci Med 1998; 47(7): 891–8.

89. Sassi F, McKee M, Roberts JA, Economic evaluation of diagnostic technology. Methodological challenges and viable solutions. Int J Technol Assess Health Care 1997; 13(4):613–30.

90. Mushlin AI, Ruchlin HS, Callahan MA, Cost effectiveness of diagnostic tests. Lancet 2001; 358:1353–5.

91. Swensen SJ, Jett JR, Sloan JA, et al, Screening for lung cancer with low-dose spiral computed tomography. Am J Respir Crit Care Med 2001; 165:508–13.

92. Sone S, Z-G Yang FL, Honda T, et al, Results of three-year mass screening programme for lung cancer using mobile low-dose spiral computed tomography scanner. Br J Cancer 2001; 84(1): 25–32.

93. Sobue T, Moriyama N, Kaneko M, et al, Screening for lung cancer with low-dose helical computed tomography: Anti-Lung Cancer Association Project. J Clin Oncol 2002; 20(4): 911–20.

94. Kostis WJ, Yankelevitz DF, Reeves AP, Fluture SC, Henschke CI, Small pulmonary nodules: reproducibility of three-dimensional volumetric measurement and estimation of time to follow-up CT. Radiology 2004; 231:446–52.

95. Tsushima Y, Endo K, Analysis models to assess cost effectiveness of the four strategies for the work-up of solitary pulmonary nodules. Med Sci Mon 2004; 10(5):MT65–72.

96. Libby DM, Smith JP, Altorki NK, et al, Managing the small pulmonary nodule discovered by CT. Chest 2004; 125:1522–9.

97. Henschke CI, Yankelevitz DF, Nzidich DP, et al, CT screening for lung cancer: suspiciousness of nodules according to size on baseline scans. Radiology 2004; 231:164–8.

98. Last JM (ed.), A Dictionary of Epidemiology. New York, Oxford University Press, 2000.

99. Strauss GM, Measuring effectiveness of lung cancer screening: from consensus to controversy and back. Chest 1997; 112(Suppl 4): 216S–28S.

100. Strauss GM, Screening for lung cancer: an evidence-based synthesis. Surg Oncol Clin N Am 1999; 8(4):747–74.

101. Patz EF, Goodman PC, Bepler G, Screening for lung cancer. N Engl J Med 2000; 343(22): 1627–33.

102. Claxton K, Posnett J, An economic approach to clinical trial design and research-priority setting. Health Econ 1996; 5:513–24.

103. Claxton K, Sculpher M, Drummond M, A rational framework for decision making by the National Institute For Clinical Excellence (NICE). Lancet 2002; 360:711–15.

104. Claxton K, Bayesian approaches to the value of information: implications for the regulation of new pharmaceuticals. Health Econ 1999; 8:269–74.

105. Claxton K, Neumann P, Araki S, Weinstein MC, Bayesian value-of-information analysis. An application to a policy model of Alzheimer's disease. Int J Technol Assess Health Care 2001; 17(1):38–55.

19 Chemoprevention

Nico van Zandwijk, James L Mulshine

Contents Introduction • Early diagnosis • Multistep carcinogenesis and field cancerization (check cancerization) • Lung cancer susceptibility: genetics, diet and gender • Different chemoprevention strategies • Specific chemopreventive agents • Other agents and so-called targeted approaches • Intermediate markers • Conclusions

INTRODUCTION

Lung cancer is the leading cause of cancer death worldwide accounting for over 1 million victims annually.[1] Despite all efforts in conventional treatment of lung cancer by surgery, radiotherapy and chemotherapy, the survival of lung cancer has seen only minor improvements over the last 25 years. The main reason for this lack of progress is related to the fact that lung cancer is a conglomerate of diseases that elicit symptoms in a relatively late stage. Thus in most cases the diagnosis is being made when the disease has significantly advanced and is beyond the stage of cure.

The dominant public health response for lung cancer has been focused on tobacco control.[2] Preventing people from starting smoking is a major aim in many countries and there is good epidemiological evidence that smoking cessation even into the middle age is associated with a major reduction of lung cancer incidence.[3,4]

However, even if all goals of national anti-smoking efforts are met, a large number of former smokers will remain at risk of dying from lung cancer for a significant number of years as is shown in the US where former smokers account for about half of the new cases of lung cancers.[5,6] In addition there is an alarming increase of tobacco consumption in developing countries and lung cancer will remain an important picture of hospital care for decades to come. Therefore it is clear that apart from eliminating or reducing the environmental exposure to known carcinogens emphasis should be laid on early diagnosis and treatment of preneoplastic or preinvasive lesions including chemoprevention. Chemoprevention has been defined as pharmacologic intervention with natural or synthetic agents to suppress or reverse carcinogenesis and to prevent the development of invasive cancer.[7]

EARLY DIAGNOSIS

Spiral computer tomography (CT) is acknowledged as the most sensitive diagnostic method for the detection of small intrapulmonary nodules.[8,9] This technique has the potential to routinely detect much smaller-volume primary lung cancers and allow an evolution in management focus from late to early disease. A growing number of observational studies in subjects at risk suggest that in excess of 80% of lung cancers can be detected as stage IA cancers in a program of annual screening.[10] In light of these developments, there is a critical research need to define the most efficient and safest way to identify lung cancers cased in the subset of individuals identified in lung cancer screening as having suspicious pulmonary nodules.[11] Similarly, in light of widely disparate outcomes with thoracic surgery, it is critical to ensure that the definitive thoracic resection is done at a specialized thoracic center which performs a large number of thoracic surgical resections with a low surgical complication rate. Additional issues include follow-up studies of completely resected non-small-cell lung cancer (NSCLC) patients are essential to find the second cancers which occur on the order of 1–3% per year or 10–30% over a decade.[12] This tendency to develop multiple independent cancers in the aerodigestive tract of persons chronically exposed to the carcinogens from tobacco smoke has been termed 'field cancerization'.[13] It reflects the clonal emergence of independent foci of carcinogen-induced cancer cells from different areas of the respiratory tract and underlines the rationale to combine screening and chemoprevention research. With the growing number of large trials evaluating spiral CT lung cancer screening underway, there is a complementary opportunity emerging to conduct chemoprevention research in these same cohorts since so many individuals with field cancerization will be identified. Clearly, success with lung cancer early-detection efforts will increase the need for successful lung cancer chemopreventive approaches so coupling these research efforts makes strategic sense. Improved lung cancer imaging is stimulating research at multiple levels in defining the optimal approaches to the clinical management of early lung cancers.

Examination of sputum from high-risk persons has been another active area for early lung cancer detection research. Hypermethylation of p16, occurring early in lung tumorigenesis along with other molecular targets has been detected in the bronchial epithelium of chronic smokers.[14,15] As p16 methylation status can be detected with high sensitivity in exfoliated cells this is considered a potentially valuable tool for early detection.[16] In other reports morphometric and proteomic changes in sputum from high-risk individuals have been proposed as markers for early detection.[17,18] Additionally, the definition of high-risk individuals has been refined. In work from the University of Colorado Lung SPORE (Specialized Program of Research Excellence) COPD, adding the selection criteria of a FEV_1 <0.75 to a 30+ pack-years smoking history in a cohort of 1798 persons, resulted in a high lung cancer incidence of 4.6%.[19] Establishing a precise risk probability of developing lung cancer may improve over using smoking history alone with the addition of molecular analyses of sputum or blood in the near future. While a growing fraction of new lung cancers are being detected in the peripheral airways the growing capabilities of specialized endoscopic techniques such as fluorescence bronchoscopy, endobronchial ultrasound and optical coherence tomography are still expected to provide useful new information in the evaluation of the central airways.[20]

MULTISTEP CARCINOGENESIS AND FIELD CANCERIZATION

While we have already discussed the implication of chemoprevention development in light of the principles of field cancerization, the concept of multi-step carcinogenesis is also fundament to the development of more successful chemoprevention approaches. We now understand that there is a series of molecular steps in the development of a cancer including the accumulation of progressive changes from pre-invasive histological changes to an invasive neoplastic process.[21] The earliest events of this process are thought to be the mutations, deletions or polysomy in the chromosomes of epithelial cells chronically exposed to carcinogens. It is not clear that these genetic modifications initially translate into morphological changes.[22] Additional types of molecular events are necessary to induce the full malignant phenotype including uncontrolled cellular proliferation as well as competence to invade a basement membrane and then to establish as an autonomous metastatic clone. It has been proposed that multiple (10–20 or more) genetic events may be essential for the development of a fully invasive lung cancer.[23]

The original description of 'field cancerization' by Slaughter and co-workers suggested that multiple foci of epithelial hyperplasia hyperkeratinization, atypia and also carcinoma in situ occur in otherwise normal-appearing epithelium adjacent to cancers of the oropharynx and suggested that the carcinogen exposure has widespread effects throughout the entire epithelial surface of the organ.[13] These diffuse histological changes suggested that the development of malignancy in the proximal aerodigestive tract is not random but rather a predictable consequence of the dose of carcinogen impacting on different cell populations as a function of anatomy and the properties of the carcinogen (typically particulate tobacco combustion residue). The same pattern of heterogeneous, multi-focal histological changes of the bronchial epithelium in relation to tobacco smoke was exhaustively catalogued in reports by Auerbach and colleagues.[24] Field cancerization can thus be seen as a concept to describe the diffuse damage elicited by chronic exposure to carcinogens. This concept forms the basis for understanding the observation that patients who survive a first cancer in this region are subsequently susceptible to the development of a second primary tumor.[25,26]

The most common chromosomal abnormalities in lung cancer are allelic deletions or loss of heterozygosity of tumor suppressor gene sites. For example, it has been shown that highly specific deletions in the short arm of chromosome 3 occur during hyperplasia, the earliest stage of carcinogenesis recognized so far.[27] Similar evidence exists for deletions of the short arm of chromosome 9 and 17 and the long arm of chromosome 13 (retinoblastoma gene/RB).[28–30] One of the genes on chromosome 3 is the fragile histidine triad (FHIT) gene that is also lost very early in the carcinogenic process.[31] Similarly to the p53 gene on chromosome 17 this gene is thought to have a tumor-suppressor function.[32] Both deletions of chromosome 3 and 9 losses have been associated with smoking and they remain detectable many years after smoking cessation.[31,33] p53 has been called the 'guardian of the genome' and acts as a transcription factor in the control of G1 arrest and apoptosis (programmed cell death). Phosphorylation of the retinoblastoma (RB) gene is reduced by p53, thereby halting the cell cycle at checkpoint G1/S enabling DNA repair or apoptosis. Mutations of p53 are more frequent in small-cell lung cancer (SCLC) (70–100%) than in NSCLC (45–75%) and an increase of p53 mutations has been noted during the carcinogenic process.[29,34–36]

RB protein is the main effector of G1 arrest if DNA is damaged. Expression of RB is lost in 80% of SCLC and only in 15% of NSCLC.[37] However inactivation of RB is also common in NSCLC. This is caused by loss of the CDK inhibitor p16INK4, which negatively controls CDK-cyclin activity by overexpression of cyclin D1. 'Silencing' of this gene may be caused by mutation/deletion or by promoter methylation.[38,39]

Activation of oncogenes can be elicited by a variety of mechanisms including mutation, amplification, chromosomal rearrangement as well as by epigenetic events such as change in

DNA methylation status. Of the large number of oncogenes identified to date in lung carcinogenesis, RAS, c-MYC, epidermal growth factor receptors ErbB1 (EGFR), and ErbB2 (HER2/NEU) exert their effect by tyrosine kinase activity. The RAS family of genes encode 21 kDa proteins that bind to GTP forming a RAS–GTP complex, that act by inducing proliferation signals through a number of transcription factors including c-FOS, c-JUN and c-MYC. K-ras mutations which are preferentially detected in non-squamous lung cancers, are associated with exposure to carcinogens from tobacco smoke.[40,41] c-MYC is important for cellular proliferation and is also involved in the induction of apoptosis in normal cells. In lung cancer, this last pathway is frequently dysregulated. Oncogenic activation of MYC occurs in 20% of SCLC and 10% of NSCLC in association with genetic amplification and is being regarded as an early event in carcinogenesis.[42] EGFR and HER2/NEU are both involved in the transduction of growth signals and are overexpressed in a large percentage of NSCLC. This overexpression is associated with disease progression, metastatic growth and poor survival.[43,44]

As already discussed, there is a growing awareness that lung cancer develops in a stepwise fashion as the result of multiple genetic events. Although the particular events and their sequence(s) leading to the development of lung cancer are not yet fully elucidated, it is hoped that strategic disruption of one or more of these pre-invasive steps may be fundamental to defining successful chemoprevention strategies.

LUNG CANCER SUSCEPTIBILITY: GENETICS, DIET AND GENDER

Carcinogens from tobacco smoke form the unquestionable link between smoking and lung cancer. Epidemiological studies show that not more than 15% of heavy smokers will ultimately develop lung cancer. The fact that 85% of heavy smokers will not develop lung cancer has been cited to suggest that there may be important differences in lung cancer susceptibility in the population. From a broader perspective, it is important to understand that some of the confusion may result from the very significant competing risks that exist for a heavy smoker with cardiovascular disease, chronic obstructive pulmonary disease as well as the other lethal tobacco-related diseases.

According to Sir Richard Peto, every other heavy smoker dies of smoking.[45] On the other hand, more and more evidence is accumulating that genetic and epigenetic factors are responsible for modulating individual susceptibility to lung cancer or other consequences of tobacco exposure.[46] Carcinogens from cigarette smoke such as benzpyrene and 4-(methylnitrosamino)-1-(3-pyridyl)-1-butanone (NNK) require metabolic activation before they can exert carcinogenic effects. The activation pathways are competing with detoxification pathways and the balance between activation and detoxification is assumed to affect the cancer risk. The genes for the cytochrome P-450 carcinogen metabolizing enzymes (activation) and also glutathione transferases (detoxification enzymes) are known to be polymorphic. Approximately 40–50% of the human population has a so-called null genotype, that has a modest association with lung cancer.[47] 'Successful' metabolic activation will lead to the formation of DNA adducts, which are carcinogen metabolites bound covalently to DNA. If DNA adducts escape cellular repair mechanisms and persist, they may cause miscoding, resulting in a permanent mutation (Figure 19.1).[48–50]

Dietary factors may represent one of the most powerful epigenetic factors influencing lung

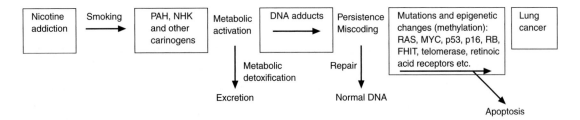

Figure 19.1
Scheme linking nicotine addiction and lung cancer via tobacco smoke carcinogens and their induction of multiple mutations in critical genes. PAH = polycyclic aromatic hydrocarbons; NNK = 4-(methylnitrosamino)-1-(3-pyridyl)-1-butone. Adapted from [50].

cancer susceptibility. In case-control studies defective detoxification and defective repair of genetic damage have been associated with increased individual susceptibility to lung cancer, while certain food constituents seemed to afford a degree of protection to individuals with limitations in their detoxification capacity.[51,52] In the light of these gene–environment and gene–diet interactions it is not surprising that smoking has been found to interact synergistically with a family history of lung cancer.[53,54]

The relationship between diet and lung cancer has been extensively explored in many ecologic and case-control studies and there are many leads to support the association between a high intake of fruits and vegetables and a reduced risk of lung cancer.[55] Much effort has been expended to identify the specific components of these foods that may be responsible for the lower lung cancer risk. In the majority of studies, attention has focused on the pro-vitamin A carotenoids, particularly beta-carotene because of their antioxidant properties and the importance of vitamin A in cell growth and differentiation.

More recently other micronutrients have been identified as having the potential to decrease lung cancer risk, including vitamin E, selenium, isothiocyanates, allyl sulfur compounds and green tea polyphenols. While vitamin E (a term that refers to eight natural compounds, including the tocopherols) failed to lower the lung cancer risk in a large randomized (ATBC) trial, a protective effect of selenium was found in a subset analysis performed on the data from the Skin Cancer Prevention Trial.[56,57]

Isothiocyanates are non-nutrient compounds in cruciferous vegetables that can influence P-450 enzyme levels and enhance detoxification. A recent series of newly diagnosed lung cancer cases had significantly lower isothiocyanate intake when compared with controls. In this study, glutathione-S-transferase (GST) (null) genotype and smoking were associated with increased lung cancer risk, suggesting that smokers with low intake of isothiocyanates and a null GST genotype carry an extra risk.[52] Allyl sulfur compounds present in onions and garlic were able to induce apoptosis suggesting that they may be interesting to evaluate as chemoprevention agents. An increasing number of studies support the premise that green tea polyphenols may be useful as preventive agents for NSCLC.[58–62]

In addition attention has focused on cooking practices. Increased lung cancer risk has been noted as a consequence of high intake of heterocyclic amines, which are produced when meats are cooked at high temperatures.[63]

Overall, the epidemiological data support the hypothesis that a different intake of dietary compounds could modulate the risk of lung cancer. The confirmation of this hypothesis, however, can only be provided by carefully designed prospective trials that balance for smoking behavior and ideally also take diet–gene interactions into account.[52,64]

Finally, it is important to note that a number of cohort studies have suggested that females are more susceptible to the carcinogenic effects of tobacco smoke than men.[65,66] A recent CT screening study also pointed to females as being more susceptible.[67] These observations have been confirmed by the smoking analysis of a large chemoprevention study revealing significantly less exposure to tobacco (pack-years) before occurrence of the lung or head and neck cancer in females in comparison with males.[68] Explanations for this difference may be sought in detoxification capacity and/or hormonal factors.

DIFFERENT CHEMOPREVENTION STRATEGIES

As indicated above, chemoprevention can be defined as pharmacologic intervention with natural or synthetic agents to prevent the development of invasive cancer. Frequently chemoprevention approaches have been based on epidemiologic and basic biological research and translated into clinical chemical interventions to suppress or reverse the process of carcinogenesis. In one classification, three different categories of chemoprevention have been defined. (1) Primary prevention = prevention of cancer in healthy individuals, who are at high risk (e.g., current or former smokers). (2) Secondary prevention = prevention of development of cancer in individuals with precancerous lesions (e.g.,

intraepithelial neoplasia, leukoplakia, dysplasia) and (3) Tertiary prevention to prevent second primary tumors in patients who had a previous cancer.[69]

As mentioned earlier, smoking history as defined by pack years is a relatively rough estimate of lung cancer risk and modified criteria have been proposed for screening studies.[70] To conduct cost-effective chemoprevention studies it is essential to define the optimal risk subset of individuals that share the greatest risk for progression to lung cancer without missing an important fraction of cancers. Strategies combining tobacco exposures with other biological markers, so-called intermediate endpoint markers have been discussed as a strategy to more efficiently conduct screening in high-risk smoking cohorts.[71,72]

SPECIFIC CHEMOPREVENTIVE AGENTS

Hundreds of natural and synthetic agents have shown the potential of chemopreventive activity in experimental systems, but only a handful has been validated in clinical trials. Among the agents studied in clinical trials are NSAIDs, selenium, α-tocopherol, calcium, tamoxifen, N-acetylcysteine, but retinoids/carotenoids have attracted most investigational interest.[58]

Vitamin A
Due to their ability to regulate cell proliferation and differentiation the derivatives of vitamin A or retinoids have been regarded as a potentially useful class of agents from the very beginning of chemoprevention research.[7] In multiple animal model systems at different organ sites and with a variety of inducing carcinogens retinoids were found to be preventive. Retinoids are potent regulators of gene expression and work through an elaborate family of cytoplasmic retinoic acid

binding proteins as well as intranuclear retinoic acid receptors.[73] The family of retinoid nuclear receptors is a member of the corticosteroid superfamily, which includes other members such as thyroid hormone receptors. For the nuclear retinoid receptors, the two main types are RAR and RXR and at least three sub-types: alpha, beta and gamma. The receptors are ligand activated following binding to retinoids and work together to regulate cell growth, differentiation and death. Loss of expression of RAR beta has been noticed in the airways of smokers and there is increasing evidence that RAR beta has tumor-suppressive activity.[74–76] The retinoid receptors do not efficiently bind all the different synthetic retinoids currently available and this has been suggested as an explanation for the lack of effect seen with most retinoids so far.

Chemoprevention studies in humans: retinoids/carotenoids

One of the earliest studies with relevance to lung cancer was a trial in 103 patients with previous head and neck cancer in which the effect of 13-cis retinoic acid (13-cis RA) on recurrence and second primary cancer was studied.[77] The incidence of second primary tumors (SPTs) in the treatment arm receiving 50–100 mg/m^2 of 13-cis-retinoic acid was 4% compared to a response rate of 24% in patients receiving placebo. The second trial involved 307 patients with early-stage lung cancer, randomized after complete surgical resection to receive either a vitamin A precursor (retinyl palmitate) or no further treatment.[78] Also in this study there was a significant difference in the frequency of second primaries (12% versus 21%). Both studies were carried out in populations at risk for SPTs and are considered tertiary chemoprevention trials (Table 19.1).

In contrast with these two first tertiary chemoprevention trials several secondary chemoprevention trials, i.e. controlled studies in individuals with premalignant changes in the bronchial tree (sputum) but otherwise 'healthy' have been negative (Table 19.2).

A significant challenge in conducting and interpreting these trials is whether the endpoint, such as reversal of histological change, can be measured reliably and further whether a change in histological status in fact correlates with a significant reduction in the frequency of cancer progression. These issues have been considered

Table 19.1 Randomized 'tertiary' chemoprevention trials

Number of individuals	Endpoint	Intervention	Effect	Authors	Reference
103	SPT[a]	Isotretinoin (H&N pts)	Yes	Hong et al	77
307	SPT	Retinyl palmitate	Yes	Pastorino et al	88
2592	SPT	Retinyl palmitate NAC[b]	No	Van Zandwijk et al	90
41 161	SPT	Isotretinoin[c]	No	Lippman et al	91

[a]Second primary tumor.
[b]NAC, N-acetylcysteine.
[c]Isotretinoin is synonym for 13-cis retinoic acid (13-cis RA).

Table 19.2 Randomized 'secondary' chemoprevention trials

Number of individuals	Endpoint	Intervention	Effect	Authors	Reference
72	Reversal of metaplasia	Folate/Vitamin B_{12}	Yes/No	Heimburger	79
150	Reversal of atypia	Etretinate	No	Arnold et al	80
152	Reversal of metaplasia	Isotretinoin	No	Lee et al	81
755 (asbestos workers	Reversal of atypia	β-carotene and retinal	No	McLarthy et al	82
139	Reversal of metaplasia	4-HPR[a]	No	Kurie et al	83
57	HTERT expression	4-HPR	Yes	Soria et al	93
41	DNA Adducts, micro-nuclei (mouth floor)	N-Acetylcysteine	Yes	Van Schooten et al	109
101	Reversal of dysplasia	Anethole dithioleethione (ADT)	Yes	Lam et al	112
112	Reversal of dysplasia	Budesonide	No	Lam et al	85

[a]4-HPR, N-(4-hydroxyphenyl) retinamide.

in a review of intraepithelial neoplasia (IEN) as a surrogate for drug effect in evaluating chemo-prevention drugs.[84]

The results of a number of large primary chemoprevention trials with beta carotene, a retinoid precursor in 'healthy' individuals with elevated risk for lung cancer became available in the 1990s. Among these were the Alpha Tocopherol Beta Carotene (ATBC) and the Beta Carotene and Retinol Efficacy (CARET) trials.[57,86] The ATBC trial accrued 29 133 Finnish male smokers and tested the effects of dietary supplementation of beta-carotene and alpha-tocopherol. Against all expectations this trial did not show any protective effect from either alpha-tocopherol or beta-carotene. On the contrary, beta-carotene was associated with a significant increase in lung cancer incidence (18%) and mortality (8%). The detrimental association of beta-carotene was confirmed by the CARET study, involving 18 314 smokers,

former smokers or aerospace workers exposed to asbestos. CARET revealed a 28% higher rate of lung cancer and 17% higher overall death rate in those participants taking beta-carotene (Table 19.3).

The findings of ATBC and CARET have clearly been a shock for the prevention community. On the other hand they also confirmed the unquestionable importance of large-scale controlled (randomized) studies. Since the detrimental effect of beta-carotene had not been observed in the Physicians Health Study involving 22 071 mainly non-smoking physicians,[87] it has been hypothesized that cigarette smoke in the lungs, which is highly oxidizing, may interact with beta-carotene, yielding unstable by-products that could have pro-oxidant activity.[88] An experimental study in ferrets exposed to cigarette smoke and beta-carotene confirmed that a negative interaction existed.[89] Thus the importance of smoking cessation is once more

Table 19.3 Randomized 'primary' chemoprevention trials					
Number of individuals	Endpoint	Intervention	Effect	Authors	Reference
29 133	Lung cancer incidence	Vitamin E, β-carotene	No	ATBC prevention study group	57
18 314	Lung cancer incidence	Vitamin A, β-carotene	No	Omenn et al	86
22 071	Lung cancer incidence	β-carotene	No	Hennekens et al	87

emphasized and smokers should avoid beta-carotene supplementation. In addition, this trial experience demonstrated the obligate need to do the necessary early clinical development including defining a safe chemopreventive dose in a phase I trial as well as to define pharmaco-dynamic efficacy in vivo as part of a phase II trial. On such a foundation, a phase III trial has a much more responsible scientific basis allow-ing for a more predictable drug development process.

The results of EUROSCAN, a large tertiary chemoprevention study designed to assess the effects of retinyl palmitate and the anti-oxidant N-acetylcysteine (NAC) became available in 2000. The early positive experience with retinyl palmitate and the promise of the antioxidant NAC could not be confirmed in a population of almost 2600 patients with early-stage head and neck cancer or lung cancer, who received a 2-year supplementation with retinyl palmitate and/or NAC following treatment with curative intent.[90] No reduction of SPTs or tumor recur-rences was noted. A similar result has been obtained in the US NCI intergroup trial with a daily dose of 25 mg of 13-cis-retinoic acid in 1486 stage I NSCLC patients. 13-cis-retinoic acid did not improve the rate of SPTs or mortal-ity.[91] Subgroup analyses suggested that 13-cis-RA acid might have been associated with a short time to disease progression in individuals who

manifested metastatic disease. The subset of patients belonging to the category of never smokers was associated with a more favorable outcome. However, in contrast to the beta-carotene studies, there was absolutely no evid-ence of any increase in the number of new lung cancers occurring in the overall group or any subgroup that received 13-cis-retinoic acid. From this perspective the results from the beta-carotene studies are very different from the results of the Intergroup trial but neither type of trial suggested a chemopreventive benefit. Both EUROSCAN and the NCI intergroup trial under-line the importance of large confirmatory studies and strengthen the importance of smoking ces-sation, i.e. participants, who had permanently stopped smoking, had a better survival than those who continued smoking. As mentioned above, explanations for the lack of preventive effects of retinoids in these studies are provided by the observation that RAR beta is frequently suppressed in preneoplastic bronchial lesions and the distinct patterns of binding of different retinoids to nuclear receptors.

New retinoids, other ways of prescription

N-(-4-hydroxyphenyl) retinamide (4-HPR), in spite of its inability to bind directly to nuclear receptors, showed some preventive activity in experimental animals and was also active in lung cancer cell lines by inhibiting growth and

These observations led to an in-depth biological analysis of the role of the cyclooxygenase-2 (COX-2) in colorectal carcinogenesis and also prompted further investigations into the potential use of COX-2 and other inhibitors of the eicosanoid pathways in the prevention of other solid tumors that express COX-2, such as lung cancer.[121–123] Manipulation of prostaglandin production distal to cyclooxygenase significantly reduced the tumor incidence elicited by exposure to tobacco smoke in transgenic mice.[124]

Other biological pathways of lung carcinogenesis are also providing attractive targets for chemopreventive purposes. As mentioned above, the Erb B family of receptors has been recognized as a potentially important site to halt carcinogenesis.[125,126] Likewise, activation of the EGFR involves RAS activation. Thus, treatment with small molecule tyrosine kinase inhibitors of the EGF receptor, antibodies against the same receptor and/or blocking the RAS-signaling pathway by farnesyl transferase inhibitors are new avenues in chemoprevention research.[127] As a result of vastly expanded pharmaceutical development capabilities, a large number of candidate drugs for lung cancer will be introduced over the next few years. Most of these compounds will be considered for application in managing early lung cancer. Rather than providing a lengthy list of candidates which would be soon obsolete, it may be more useful to consider some core principles in evaluating new candidates for lung cancer chemoprevention.

Drug targets for chemoprevention should be directed at molecular pathways that appear to be modulated in the process of carcinogenesis relative to normal pathways. Ideally, there should be mechanistic evidence demonstrating that the process of carcinogenesis is causally linked to the function of that mechanism. In addition, early developmental work should demonstrate that the pathway can be abrogated using clinically achievable dose and schedule of the agent. Further clinical trials should establish that such dose and schedule can be routinely administered without incurring unpleasant or dangerous side effects. There is an emerging sense in the research community developing lung cancer chemoprevention agents that more concerted attention to the pharmacology issues in rigorously defining a dose and schedule associated with a robust pharmacodynamic effect is crucial. Many of the early chemoprevention trials proceeded in the absence of any firm understanding of the molecular pharmacology of the candidate agent. In this setting, it is difficult to make progress since firm conclusions about the next steps can not be established. There is an extensive and growing literature about developing new trial structures for chemoprevention development. Much of this literature has been summarized in the American Association of Cancer Research White Paper on the use of intraepithelial neoplasia as a surrogate marker in the development of early cancer drugs.[84] Design of chemoprevention trials will be an ongoing area of dynamic clinical research interest and one of the most critical issues in this regard will be developing an effective approach to designing drug validation trials around the response of disease surrogates.

INTERMEDIATE MARKERS

When the frequency of development of invasive cancer is used as an endpoint, as has been done in many of the aforementioned clinical studies, significant investments in time and money are needed to permit a critical study size and duration to be realized. The disappointing results of chemoprevention studies so far have been a strong stimulus to invest in new approaches based on new technology and better understanding of essential pathways of pulmonary carcinogenesis. One approach to avoid the premature start of large comparative chemoprevention trials with cancer as the primary endpoint is the use of intermediate biological endpoints as surrogates to definitive clinical endpoints. Premalignant lesions are a potential source of intermediate markers and if the disappearance of these lesions correlates with a reduction in cancer incidence, markers of premalignant disease could serve as intermediate endpoints for chemoprevention trials. Another step forward would be the development of better tools to accurately identify individuals at high risk of developing a particular cancer and it will be important to define much more appropriate and efficient populations for chemoprevention trials. A detailed overview of intermediate markers and their validation and related issues is given in Chapter 8.

CONCLUSIONS

The rapidly expanding understanding of the molecular and the biological basis of lung cancer has been a strong stimulus for chemoprevention research. In addition, the promising developments with spiral CT as reviewed elsewhere in this volume are likely to result in a much larger number of early-stage patients being diagnosed with potentially curative lung cancer. A consequence of this is that many more individuals will be brought to clinical attention where concerns about field cancerization and subsequent primary lung cancers will be problematic. This is a population that would need effective chemoprevention drugs but also represents a growing cohort to participate in the research process to develop such drugs.

An increasing number of molecular and genetic lesions considered essential for the final malignant phenotype have been identified and some of these lesions are directly related with exposure to carcinogens from tobacco smoke. At the same time an increasing number of studies have pointed to the wide variation of individual susceptibility to carcinogens from tobacco smoke. Despite an overwhelming number of epidemiological and experimental data no definitive proof for a preventive effect of vitamin A and its analogs against lung cancer has been provided so far. Several explanations for the negative outcomes with retinoids are brought forward and there is consensus that the premature start of large and costly comparative studies with cancer as an endpoint should be avoided and that relatively small comparative studies with surrogate or intermediate endpoint markers should precede.

Potential valuable intermediate endpoint markers have appeared on the horizon and also the target populations for chemoprevention studies are being better defined while several novel agents with chemopreventive potential have been identified.

Thus it is anticipated that after a period with increasing insight into lung carcinogenesis but without appreciable benefits of the chemoprevention approach in randomized trials, the road is now being paved for more successful studies in high-risk individuals. Considering the continuing lung cancer epidemic worldwide it is clear that we must continue our effort to strengthen the fundamental strategy of avoidance of exposure to carcinogens in parallel with the development of additional approaches such as chemoprevention.

REFERENCES

1. Parkin DM, Bray F, Ferlay J, et al, Estimating the world lung cancer burden: Globocan 2000. Int J Cancer 2001; 94:153–6.

2. American Society of Clinical Oncology, Policy Statement Update: Tobacco Control-Reducing Cancer Incidence and Saving Lives. J Clin Oncol 2003; 21:2777–86.

3. Peto R, Darby S, Deo H, et al, Smoking, smoking cessation and lung cancer in the UK since 1950: combination of national statistics with two case-control studies. Br Med J 2000; 321:323–9.

4. Enstrom JE, Heath CW Jr, Smoking cessation and mortality trends among 118,000 Californians, 1960–1997. Epidemiology 1999; 10: 500–12.

5. Tong MR, Spitz MR, Fueger JJ, Amos CA, Lung carcinoma in former smokers. Cancer 1996; 78:1004–10.

6. Strauss G, DeCamp M, Dibiccaro E, et al, Lung cancer diagnosis is being made with increasing frequency in former cigarette smokers! Proc Am Soc Clin Oncol 1995; 14:362.

7. Sporn MB, Dunlop NM, Newton DL, Smith JM, Prevention of chemical carcinogenesis by vitamin A and its synthetic analogs (retinoids). Fed Proc 1976; 35:1332–8.

8. Henschke CI, McCauley DI, Yankelevitz DF, et al, Early lung cancer action project: overall design and findings from baseline screening. Lancet 1999; 354:99–105.

9. Sobue T, Moriyama N, Kaneko M, et al, Screening for lung cancer with low-dose helical computed tomography: Anti-lung Cancer Association project. J Clin Oncol 2002; 20:911–20.

10. Warner EE, Mulshine JL, Surgical considerations with lung cancer screening. J Surg Oncol 2003; 84:1–6.

11. Patz FP, Swensen SJ, Herndon II JE, Estimate of lung cancer mortality from spiral computed tomography screening trials: implications for current mass screening recommendations. J Clin Oncol 2004; 22:2202–6.

12. Tockman MS, Mulshine JL, Piantadosi S, et al, Prospective detection of preclinical lung cancer: results from two studies of heterogeneous nuclear ribonucleoprotein A2/B1 overexpression. Clin Cancer Res 1997; 3:2237–46.

13. Slaughter DP, Southwick HW, Smejkal W, 'Field cancerization' in oral stratified squamous epithelium: Clinical implications of multicentric origin. Cancer 1953; 6:963–8.

14. Belinsky SA, Palmisano WA, Gilliland FD, et al, Aberrant promotor methylation in bronchial epithelium and sputum from current and former smokers. Cancer Res 2002; 62:2370–7.

15. Herman JG, Baylin SB, Gene silencing in cancer in association with promoter hypermethylation. N Engl J Med 2003 20; 349: 2042–54.

16. Belinsky SA, Gene-promoter hypermethylation as a biomarker in lung cancer. Nature Reviews Cancer 2004; 4:707–17.

17. Valle RP, Chavany C, Zhukov TA, Jendoubi M, New approaches for biomarker discovery in lung cancer. Expert Rev Mol Diagn 2003; 3: 55–67.

18. Palcic B, Garner DM, Beveridge J, et al, Increase of sensitivity of sputum cytology using high-resolution image cytometry: field study results. Cytometry 2002; 50:168–76.

19. Prindiville SA, Byers T, Hirsch FR, et al, Sputum cytological atypia as a predictor of incident lung cancer in a cohort of heavy smokers with airflow obstruction. Cancer Epidemiol Biomarkers Prevent 2003; 12:987–93.

20. McWilliams A, MacAulay C, Gazdar AF, Lam S, Innovative molecular and imaging approaches for the detection of lung cancer and its lesions. Oncogene 2002; 21:6949–59.

21. Mao L, Lee JS, Kurie JM, et al, Clonal genetic alterations in the lungs of current and former smokers. J Natl Cancer Inst 1997; 89:857–62.

22. Mao LM, El-Naggar A, Papadimitrakopoulou V, et al, Phenotype and genotype of advanced premalignant lesions after chemopreventive therapy. J Natl Cancer Inst 1998; 90:1545–51.

23. Bartsch H, Petruzzelli S, De Flora S, et al, Carcinogen metabolism in human lung tissues and the effect of tobacco smoking: results from a case-control multicenter study on lung cancer patients. Environ Health Perspect 1992; 98: 119–24.

24. Auerbach O, Gere JB, Foreman JB, et al, Changes in the bronchial epithelium in relation to smoking and cancer of the lung. N Engl J Med 1957; 256:98–104.

25. Boice JD, Fraumeni JF, Second cancer following cancer of the respiratory system in Connecticut, 1935–1982. Natl Cancer Inst Monogr 1985; 68:83–98.

26. De Vries N, Snow GB, Multiple primary tumours in laryngeal cancer. J Laryngol Otol 1986; 100:915–18.

27. Hung J, Kishimoto Y, Sugio K, et al, Allele-specific loss in chromosome 3p deletions occur at an early stage in the pathogenesis of lung cancer. J Am Med Assoc 1995; 273:558–63.

28. Kishimoto Y, Sugio K, Hung JY, et al, Allele-specific loss in chromosome 9p loci in pre-neoplastic lesions accompanying non-small cell lung cancer. J Natl Cancer Inst 1995; 87: 1224–9.

29. Kishimoto Y, Murakami Y, Shiraishi M, et al, Aberrations of the p53 tumor suppressor gene in human non-small cell carcinomas of the lung. Cancer Res 1992; 52:4799–804.

30. Brambilla E, Gazzeri S, Moro D, et al, Alterations of Rb pathway (Rb, p16, Cyclin D1) in preinvasive bronchial lesions. Clin Cancer Res 1999; 5:243–50.

31. Sozzi G, Sard L, de Gregoria L, et al, Association between cigarette smoking and FHIT gene alterations in lung cancer. Cancer Res 1997; 57:5207–12.

32. Mao L, Tumor suppressor genes: does FHIT fit? J Natl Cancer Inst 1998; 90:412–14.

33. Wistuba II, Lam S, Behrens C, et al, Molecular damage in the bronchial epithelium of current and former smokers. J Natl Cancer Inst 1997; 89:1366–73.

34. Levine AJ, P53, the cellular gatekeeper for growth and division. Cell 1997; 88:323–31.

35. Takahashi T, Takahashi T, Suzuki H, et al, The p53 gene is very frequently mutated in small-cell lung cancer with a distinct nucleotide substitution pattern. Oncogene 1991; 6:1775–8.

36. Brambilla E, Gazzeri S, Lantuejoul S, et al, P53 mutant phenotype and deregulation of p53 transcription pathway (Bcl2, Bax, Waf1) in precursor bronchial lesions of lung cancer. Clin Cancer Res 1998; 4:1609–18.

37. Reissmann PT, Koga H, Takahashi R, et al, Inactivation of the retinoblastoma susceptibility gene in non-small-cell lung cancer. The Lung Cancer Study Group. Oncogene 1993; 8:1913–19.

38. Gazzeri S, Gouyer V, Vour'ch C, et al, Mechanisms of p16INK4A inactivation in non small-cell lung cancers. Oncogene 1998; 16: 497–504.

39. Belinsky SA, Nikula KJ, Palmisano WA, et al, Aberrant methylation of P16INK4 is an early event in lung cancer and a potential biomarker for early diagnosis. Proc Natl Acad Sci USA 1998; 95:11891–6.

40. Rodenhuis S, Ras and human tumors. Semin Cancer Biol 1992; 3:241–7.

41. Westra WH, Slebos RJ, Offerhaus, et al, K-ras oncogene activation in lung adenocarcinomas from former smokers. Evidence that K-ras mutations are an early and irreversible event in the development of adenocarcinoma of the lung. Cancer 1993; 72:432–8.

42. Gosney JR, Field JK, Gosney MA, et al, c-myc oncoprotein in bronchial carcinoma: expression in all major morphological types. Anticancer Res 1990; 10:623–8.

43. Hirsch FR, Varella-Garcia M, Bunn PA Jr, et al, Epidermal growth factor receptor in non small cell lung carcinomas: correlation between gene copy number and prot expression and impact on prognosis. J Clin Oncol 2003; 21:4268–9.

44. Meert AP, Martin B, Paesmans M, et al, The role of HER-2/neu expression on the survival of patients with lung cancer: a systematic review of the literature. Br J Cancer 2003; 89: 959–65.

45. Peto, R, Lopez AD, Boreham J, Thun M, Heath C Jr, Mortality from tobacco in developed countries: indirect estimation from national vital statistics. Lancet 1992; 339:1268–78.

46. Xu H, Spitz MR, Amos CI, Shete S, Complex

segregation analysis reveals a multigene model for lung cancer. Hum Genet 2005; 116:121–7.

47. Spivack SD, Fasco MJ, Walker VE, Kaminsky LS, The molecular epidemiology of lung cancer. Crit Rev Toxicol 1997; 27:319–65.

48. Denissenko MF, Preferential formation of benzo(a)pyrene adducts in lung cancer hotspots in p53. Science 1996; 374:430–2.

49. Wei Q, Cheng L, Amos CI, et al, Repair of tobacco carcinogen-induced DNA adducts and lung cancer risk: a molecular epidemiological study. J Natl Cancer Inst 2000, 92:1764–72.

50. Hecht SS, Tobacco smoke carcinogens and lung cancer. J Natl Cancer Inst 1999; 91: 1149–210.

51. Spitz MR, Wu X, Wang Y, et al, Modulation of nucleotide excision repair capacity by XPD polymorphisms in lung cancer patients. Cancer Res 2001; 61:1354–7.

52. Spitz MR, Duphorne CM, Detry MA, et al, Dietary intake of isothiocyanates: evidence of a joint effect with glutathione transferase polymorphisms in lung cancer risk in current smokers. Cancer Epidemiol Biomarkers Prevent 2000; 9:1017–20.

53. Ooi WL, Elston RC, Chen VW, et al, Increased familial risk for lung cancer. J Natl Cancer Inst 1986; 76:217–22.

54. Osann KE, Lung cancer in women: The importance of smoking, family history of cancer, and medical history of respiratory disease. Cancer Res 1991; 51:4893–7.

55. Block G, Patterson B, Subar A, Fruit, vegetables and cancer prevention: a review of the epidemiological evidence. Nutr Cancer 1992; 18:1–41.

56. Clark LC, Combs GF, Turnbull BW, et al, Effects of selenium supplementation for cancer prevention in patients with carcinoma of the skin. JAMA 1996; 276:1957–63.

57. The Alpha-Tocopherol, Beta Carotene Cancer Prevention Study Group, The effect of vitamin E and beta-carotene on the incidence of lung cancer and other cancers in male smokers. N Engl J Med 1994; 330:1029–35.

58. Kelloff GJ, Boone CW (eds), Cancer chemopreventive agents. Drug development status and future prospects. J Cell Biochem suppl 1995; 22:1–262.

59. Hong YS, Ham YA, Choi JH, Kim J, Effects of allyl sulfur compounds and garlic extract on the expression of Bcl-2, Bax, and p53 in non small cell lung cancer cell lines. Exp Mol Med 2000; 32:127–34.

60. Fujiki H, Suganuma M, Okabe S, et al, Cancer prevention with green tea and monitoring by a new biomarker, hnRNPB1. Mutat Res 2001; 480–481:299–304.

61. Schuller HM, Porter B, Riechert A, Walker K, Schmoyer R, Neuroendocrine lung carcinogenesis in hamsters is inhibited by green tea theophylline while the development of adenocarcinomas is promoted: implications for chemoprevention in smokers. Lung Cancer 2004; 45:11–18.

62. Vittal R, Selvanayagam ZE, Sun Y, et al, Gene expression changes induced by green tea polyphenol(−)-epigallocatechin-3-gallate in human bronchial 21BES cells analyzed by DNA microarray. Mol Cancer Ther 2004; 3:1091–9.

63. Sinha R, Kulldorff M, Swanson CA, et al, Dietary heterocyclic amines and the risk of lung cancer among Missouri women. Cancer Res 2000; 60:3753–6.

64. Feskanish D, Ziegler RG, Michaud DS, et al, Prospective study of fruit and vegetable consumption and risk of lung cancer among men and women. J Natl Cancer Inst 2000; 92:1812–23.

65. Risch HA, Howe GR, Jain M, et al, Are female smokers at higher risk for lung cancer than male smokers? A case-control analysis by histologic type. Am J Epidemiol 1993; 138:281–93.

66. Prescott E, Osler M, Hein HO, et al, Gender and smoking related risk of lung cancer: The Copenhagen Center for Prospective Population Studies. Epidemiology 1998; 91:79–83.

67. Henschke CI, Miettinen OS, Women's susceptibility to tobacco carcinogens. Lung Cancer 2004; 43:1–5.

68. Van Zandwijk N, Pastorino U, De Vries N, van

Tinteren H, Smoking analysis of EUROSCAN, the chemoprevention study of the EORTC Head & Neck and Lung Cancer Cooperative groups in patients with cancer of the upper and lower airways. Abstracts 9th World Conference on Lung Cancer, Tokyo, Japan Lung Cancer 2000; 29(suppl):219 # 749.

69. Lippman SM, Spitz MR, Lung cancer chemoprevention: an integrated approach. J Clin Oncol 2001; 19 (suppl 18):74–82.

70. van Klaveren R, de Koning HJ, Mulshine J, et al, Lung cancer screening by spiral CT. What is the optimal target population for screening trials? Lung Cancer 2002; 38:243–52.

71. Lee JS, Lippman SM, Hong WK, et al, Determination of biomarkers for intermediate endpoints in chemoprevention trials. Cancer Res 1992; 52 (suppl 9):2707s–10s.

72. Hirsch FR, Bunn PA Jr, Miller YE, et al, Intermediate biomarker profile for lung cancer and for monitoring chemoprevention trials. Proc Am Soc Clin Oncol 2001; 20:322a.

73. Gudas LJ, Retinoids and vertebrate development. J Biol Chem 1994; 269:399–402.

74. Xu XC, Sozzi G, Lee JS, et al, Suppression of retinoic acid receptor beta in a non small cell lung cancer in vivo: implications for lung cancer development. J Natl Cancer Inst 1997; 89:624–9.

75. Xu XC, Lee JS, Lee JJ, et al, Nuclear retinoid receptor beta in bronchial epithelium of smokers before and during chemoprevention. J Natl Cancer Inst 1999; 91:1317–21.

76. Virmani AK, Rathi A, Zochbauer-Muller S, et al, Promoter methylation and silencing of the retinoic acid receptor beta gene in lung carcinomas. J Natl Cancer Inst 2001; 92:1303–7.

77. Hong WK, Lippman JM, Itri L, et al, Prevention of second primary tumors with isotretinoin in squamous cell carcinoma of the head and neck. N Engl J Med 1990; 323:795–801.

78. Pastorino U, Infante I, Maioli M, et al, Adjuvant treatment of stage I lung cancer with high dose vitamin A. J Clin Oncol 1993; 11: 1216–22.

79. Heimburger DC, Alexander CB, Birch R, et al, Improvement in bronchial squamous metaplasia in smokers treated with folate and vitamin B12. Report of a preliminary randomized, double-blind intervention trial. J Am Med Assoc 1988; 259:1525–30.

80. Arnold AM, Brownman GP, Levine MN, et al, The effect of the synthetic retinoid etrenitate on sputum cytology: results from a randomized trial. Br J Cancer 1992; 65:737–43.

81. Lee JS, Lippman SM, Benner SE, et al, Randomized placebo controlled trial of isotretinoin in chemoprevention of bronchial squamous metaplasia. J Clin Oncol 1994; 12:937–45.

82. McLarthy JW, Holiday DB, Girard WM, et al, Beta-carotene, vitamin A and lung cancer chemoprevention: results of an intermediate endpoint study. Am J Clin Nutr 1995; 62 (6 suppl):1431s–8s.

83. Kurie JM, Lee Js, Khurie FR, et al, N-(4-hydroxyphenyl)retinamide in the chemo prevention of squamous metaplasia and dysplasia of the bronchial epithelium. Clin Cancer Res 2000; 6:2973–6.

84. O'Shaughnessy JA, Kelloff GJ, Gordon GB, et al, Treatment and prevention of intraepithelial neoplasia: an important target for accelerated new agent development. Clin Cancer Res 2002; 8:314–46.

85. Lam S, leRiche JC, McWilliams A, et al, A randomized phase IIb trial of pulmicort turbuhaler (budesonide) in people with dysplasia of the bronchial epithelium. Clin Cancer Res 2004; 10:6502–11.

86. Omenn GS, Goodman GE, Thornquist M, et al, Effects of combination of beta-carotene and vitamin A on lung cancer and cardiovascular disease. N Engl J Med 1996; 334:1150–5.

87. Hennekens CH, Buring JE, Manson JE, et al, Lack of longterm supplementation with beta-carotene on the incidence of malignant neoplasms and cardiovascular disease. N Engl J Med 1996; 334:1145–9.

88. Pastorino U, Beta-carotene and the risk of lung cancer. J Natl Cancer Inst 1997; 89:456–7.

89. Wang XD, Liu C, Bronson RT, et al, Renitoid signaling and activator protein-1 expression in ferrets given beta-carotene supplements and exposed to tobacco smoke. J Natl Cancer Inst 1999; 91:60–6.

90. Van Zandwijk N, Dalesio O, Pastorino U, de Vries N, van Tinteren H, Euroscan, a randomized trial of vitamin A and N-acetylcysteine in patients with head and neck cancer or lung cancer. J Natl Cancer Inst 2000; 92:977–86.

91. Lippman SM, Lee JJ, Karp DD, et al, Randomized phase III intergroup trial of isotretinoin to prevent second primary tumors in stage I non small cell lung cancer. J Natl Cancer Inst 2001; 93:605–18.

92. IARC Working Group on the Evaluation of Cancer Preventive Agents, IARC handbooks of cancer prevention. Retinoids 1999; 4: 331.

93. Soria JC, Moon C, Wang L, et al, Effects of N-(4-hydroxyphenyl)retinamide on hTERT expression in the bronchial epithelium of cigarette smokers. J Natl Cancer Inst 2001; 93: 1257–63.

94. Hail N Jr, Lotan R, Mitochondrial permeability transition is a central coordination event in N-(4-hydroxyphenyl) retinamide-induced apoptosis. Cancer Epidemiol Biomarkers Prev 2000; 9(12):1293–301.

95. Tuma RS, Retinoids and lung cancer: targeting the right population. J Natl Cancer Inst 2002; 94:969–70.

96. Kurie JM, Lotan R, Lee JJ, et al, Randomized, placebo controlled trial of 9-cis retinoic acid (9cRA) versus 13-cis retinoic (13 cis RA) plus alpha tocopherol (AT) in the reversal of biomarkers of bronchial preneoplasia in former smokers. Proc Am Soc Clin Oncol 2002; 21: 295a # 1177.

97. Degos L, Wang ZY, All trans retinoic acid in acute promyelocytic leukemia. Oncogene 2001; 20:7140–5.

98. Khuri FR, Rigas JR, Figlin RA, et al, Multi-institutional phase I/II trial of oral bexarotene in combination with cisplatin and vinorelbine in previously untreated patients with advanced non small cell lung cancer. J Clin Oncol 2001; 19:2626–37.

99. Mulshine JL. Hirsch F, Lung cancer chemoprevention: moving from concept to a reality, Lung Cancer 2003; 41:163–74.

100. Dahl AR, Grossi IM, Houchens DP, et al, Inhaled istretinoin (13 cis retinoic acid) is an effective lung cancer chemopreventive agent in A/J mice at low doses: a pilot study. Clin Cancer Res 2000; 6:3015–24.

101. Wang DL, Marko M, Dahl AR, et al, Topical delivery of 13-cis-retinoic acid by inhalation up-regulates expression of rodent lung but not liver retinoic acid receptors. Clin Cancer Res 2000; 6:3636–45.

102. Brooks AD, Tong W, Benedetti F, et al, Inhaled aerosolization of all-trans-retinoic acid for targeted pulmonary delivery. Cancer Chemother Pharmacol 2000; 46:13–318.

103. Kohlhaufl M, Haussinger K, Stanzel F, et al, Inhalation of aerosolized vitamin A: reversibility of metaplasia and dysplasia of human respiratory epithelia – a prospective pilot study. Eur J Med Res 2002; 7:72–8.

104. Mulshine JL, de Luca LM, Dedrick RL, et al, Considerations in developing successful, population-based molecular screening and prevention of lung cancer. A Can Society, 2000.

105. Wattenberg LW, Wiedmann TS, Estensen RD, Chemoprevention of cancer of the upper respiratory tract of the Syrian golden hamster by aerosol administration of difluoromethylornithine and 5-fluorouracil. Cancer Res 2004; 64:2347–9.

106. Dimery IW, Hong WK, Lee JJ, et al, Phase I trial of alpha-tocopherol effects on 13-cis retinoic acid toxicity. Ann Oncol 1997; 8:85–9.

107. Shin DM, Khuri FR, Murphy B, et al, Combined interferon-alpha, 13-cis retinoic acid and alpha-tocopherol in locally advanced head and neck squamous cell carcinoma: novel bioadjuvant phase II trial. J Clin Oncol 2001; 19: 3010–17.

108. Shamberger RJ, Frost DV, Possible protective effect of selenium against human cancer. Can Med Assoc J 1969; 100:682.

109. Van den Brandt PA, Goldbohm RA, van 't Veer

P, et al, Prospective cohort study on selenium status and the risk of lung cancer. Cancer Res 1993; 53:4860–5.

110. De Flora S, Izotti A, D'Agostini F, Balansky RM, Mechanism of N-acetylcysteine in the prevention of DNA damage and cancer, with special reference to smoking-related endpoints. Carcinogenesis 2001; 22:999–1013.

111. Van Schooten FJ, Nia AB, De Flora S, et al, Effects of oral administration of N-acetyl-L-cysteine: a multi-biomarker study in smokers. Cancer Epidemiol Biomarkers Prevent 2002; 11:167–75.

112. Kennsler TW, Groopman JD, Roebuck BD, Chemoprotection by oltipraz and other dithioleethiones. In: Wattenberg L, Lipkin M, Boone C, Kelloff G (eds) Cancer Chemoprevention. Boca Raton, FL, CRC Press, 1992, pp. 205–25.

113. Pepin P, Bouchard L, Nicole P, Castonguay A, Effects of sulindac and oltipraz on the tumorigenicity of 4-(methylnitrisamino)1-(3 pyridyl)-1-butanone in A/J mouse lung. Carcinogenesis 1992; 13:341–8.

114. Lam S, MacAulay C, le Rich JC, et al, A randomized phase 11b trial of anethole dithioleethione in smokers with bronchial dysplasia. J Natl Cancer Inst 2002; 94:1001–9.

115. Hecht SS, Upadhyaya P, Wang M, et al, Inhibition of lung tumorigenesis in A/J mice by N-acetyl-S-(N-2-phenethylthiocarbamoyl)-L-cysteine and myo-inositol, individually and in combination. Carcinogenesis 2002; 23:1455–61.

116. Wattenberg LK, Wiedmann TS, Estensen RD, et al, Chemoprevention of pulmonary carcinogenesis by brief exposures to aerosolized budesonide or beclomethasone dipropionate and by the combination of aerosolized budesonide and dietary myo-inositol. Carcinogenesis 2000; 21:179–82.

117. Hida T, Yatabe Y, Achiwa H, et al, Increased expression of cyclooxygenase 2 occurs frequently in human lung cancers, specifically in adenocarcinomas. Cancer Res 1998; 58:3761–4.

118. Dannenberg AJ, Alturki NK, Subbaramaiah K, Selective inhibitors of COX-2: New applications in oncology. Educational Book Am Soc Clin Oncol 2001; 21–7.

119. Hastürk S, Kemp B, Kalapurakal S, et al, Expression of cyclooxygenase-2 in bronchial epithelium and non small cell lung carcinoma. Cancer 2002; 94:1023–31.

120. Akhmedkhanov A, Toniola P, Zeleniuch-Jacquotte A, Koenig KL, Shore RE, Aspirin and lung cancer in women. Br J Cancer 2002; 87: 49–53.

121. Schuller HM, Tithof PK, William M, et al, The tobacco specific carcinogen 4-(methulnitrosamino)-1-(3-pyridyl)-1-butanone is a beta-adrenergic agonist and stimulates DNA synthesis in lung adenocarcinoma via beta-adrenergic receptor-mediated release of arachidonic acid. Cancer Res 1999; 59:4510–15.

122. Harris RE, Beebe-Donk J, Schuller HM, Chemoprevention by non-steroidal anti-inflammatory drugs in cigarette smokers. Oncol Rep 2002; 9:693–5.

123. Lee H-Y, Suh Y-A, Kosmeder JW, et al, Deguelin-induced inhibition of cyclooxygenase-2 expression in human bronchial epithelial cells. Clin Cancer Res 2004; 10:1074–9.

124. Keith RL, Miller YE, Hudish TM, et al, Pulmonary prostacyclin synthetase overexpression chemoprevents tobacco smoke lung carcinogenesis in mice. Cancer Res 2004; 64:5897–904.

125. Baselga J, Albanell J, Targeting epidermal growth factor receptor in lung cancer. Curr Oncol Rep 2002; 4:317–24.

126. Franklin WA, Veve R, Hirsch FR, Helfrich BA, Bunn PA, Epidermal growth factor family in lung cancer and premalignancy. Semin Oncol 2002; 29(suppl 4):3–14.

127. Khuri RF, Cohen V, Molecularly targeted approaches to the chemoprevention of lung cancer. Clin Cancer Res 2004; (suppl) 10: 4249s–53s.

20 The selection of the optimal target population for spiral CT screening and chemoprevention trials

Rob J van Klaveren, Fred R Hirsch, Carola A van Iersel, Paul A Bunn Jr

Contents   Introduction • Spiral CT screening • Chemoprevention • Lung cancer epidemiology • Identification of high-risk individuals • Choice of high-risk populations and biomarkers • Selection criteria • Conclusions

INTRODUCTION

Lung cancer is today the most frequent cause of cancer deaths in the Western world. On a global basis it is estimated that 1.2 million people are diagnosed with this disease every year (12.3% of the total number of cancer diagnosed), and about 1.1 million people are dying of this disease yearly (17.8% of the total cancer death).[1] More than two-thirds of these people are diagnosed with locally advanced or metastatic disease, and their poor prognosis is due to late diagnosis and lack of effective treatment of metastatic disease. The 5-year survival is – in best scenario – about 15%, and in several European countries the 5-year survival is far less. Despite the optimal use of therapeutic resources, the overall improvement in survival during recent decades has only been modest, and major reductions in lung cancer mortality can only come from primary prevention, early detection and truly innovative treatments.

Lung cancer prevention covers different areas of experimental and clinical research:

1. Primary prevention: aimed at preventing lung cancer to originate by eliminating the etiological factors, for example:

    •   reducing or eliminating the environmental exposure to known carcinogens, i.e. cigarette smoke;

    •   chemoprevention; the prevention of cancer development in high-risk populations by drugs or natural substances that inhibit carcinogenesis.

2. Secondary prevention: aimed at the early detection of lung cancer in a pre-clinical phase and the treatment of pre-neoplastic or pre-invasive disease, for example:

    •   Spiral CT screening: early detection and treatment of lung cancer by spiral CT;

    •   Chemoprevention; the prevention of progression of known premalignant lesions into cancer, but no frank cancer.

3. Tertiary prevention: prevention of the development of second primary lung cancer, for example:

- Extensive follow up after curative lung cancer treatment;
- Inhibiting the process of carcinogenesis by chemoprevention.

While the target populations for secondary and tertiary chemoprevention are better defined, the populations for primary prevention are not very well defined. This chapter is aimed at focusing on selection of populations for screening and chemoprevention trials and elucidating some of the current limitations in the selection for these programs. Developments in molecular biology will be discussed in relation to their potential use to define the most optimal high-risk populations.

SPIRAL CT SCREENING

Multislice or multidetector low-dose spiral computer tomography (CT) is a relatively new technology that offers great potential as a screening tool because it is fast, potentially very accurate, relatively non-invasive, and exposes people to only a low dose of radiation comparable with two to ten conventional chest X-rays in two directions.[2] Therefore, the technology can be used for high-throughput population screening purposes. The first publications of the use of the spiral CT in the early diagnosis of lung cancer, and especially the report from the Early Lung Cancer Action Program (ELCAP) in 1999, inflated the interest in lung cancer screening by low-dose spiral CT tremendously.[3] In several single-arm cohort studies it has been demonstrated that 60–100% of lung cancers detected by spiral CT screening are at a very early stage (Table 20.1). The potential benefit of lung cancer screening by spiral CT could be enormous if a reduction in lung cancer mortality is truly demonstrated. To clarify the impact

and magnitude of spiral CT screening, several single-armed observational studies have already been initiated in the US, Japan and Europe and several randomized clinical trials have been launched also (Table 20.1).[4-9] Because of the potential enormous impact lung cancer screening might have on the total health care, it is important to make the evaluation as quickly as possible in the most cost-effective way in order to see if spiral CT screening will reduce the lung cancer mortality. This can only be achieved when the lung cancer risk of participants in randomized and non-randomized clinical trials is high, so that the sample size and costs of these large-scale trials can be limited. The identification of the optimal high-risk target population is, therefore, crucial. Only when lung cancer screening is proven to be effective in a confined study population, should extension to lesser-risk groups be considered.

CHEMOPREVENTION

Chemoprevention is a relatively new approach to reducing the incidence of lung cancer and involves the ingestion of naturally occurring or synthetic agents. These must be associated with minimal toxicity because they are applied to an, in principle, 'healthy' non-cancerous population. The proof of principle lies in other disease areas, particularly cardiovascular medicine where the use of aspirin, cholesterol-reducing and antihypertensive agents have proven effective in reducing the long-term burden from heart disease and strokes. The World Health Organization has recognized the importance of focusing on preneoplastic changes, and the current classification scheme for lung cancer includes pre-invasive lesions. Lung cancer is likely to be the final step of a multi-step process of carcinogenesis, from

Table 20.1 Selection criteria and outcomes of lung cancer screening with low-dose spiral computed tomography in different cohort studies

	Age (yrs)	Smoking history PY	Ex-smokers	Screening interval (months)	Screening type	Tests performed	Positive test results (%)	Lung cancer n (%)	Stage I disease %
Henschke et al[3,4]	≥60	≥10 (median 45)	No	6–18	Baseline	1000	237 (24)	31 (3.1)	85
					Incidence	1184	40 (3)	9 (0.9)	67
Sone et al[5]	≥40	≥1 and never smokers	Yes	12	Baseline	5483	279 (5)	22 (0.4)	100
					Incidence	8303	309 (4)	37 (0.6)	86
Diederich et al[7]	≥40	≥20	No	12	Baseline	817	350 (43)	11(1.3)	58
Nawa et al[6]	50–69	≥1 and never smokers	Yes	12	Baseline	2099	7956 (26)	36 (0.4)	86
					Incidence	5568	NR	4 (0.1)	100
Sobue et al[8]	40–79	≥1 and never smokers	Yes	6	Baseline	1611	186 (12)	13 (0.9)	77
					Incidence	7891	721 (9)	19 (0.3)	79
Swensen et al[9]	≥50	≥20	Yes, quit <10yrs	12	Baseline	1520	782 (51)	27 (1.8)	66
					Incidence	2916	336 (12)	11 (0.7)	

varying degrees of dysplasia, to carcinoma in situ, to frankly invasive disease. The primary chemoprevention approach is only useful when there is a long pre-clinical period before the disease becomes manifest. For lung cancer it has been estimated that this pre-clinical period is between 10–20 years, and therefore it offers as such a large window of opportunities for early detection and chemoprevention.

Different levels of chemoprevention can be distinguished: Primary chemoprevention trials have been designed for individuals at high risk of developing lung cancer because of previous heavy exposure to tobacco smoke, asbestos or other carcinogens. The doses selected for preventive agents have been relatively low, in order to avoid any side effects and to obtain high recruitment and compliance rates. A second level of intervention involves subjects affected by pre-cancerous or pre-invasive lesions such as bronchial dysplasia detected by white light or autofluorescent bronchoscopy. The aim is to induce regression of the pre-neoplastic disease to prevent progression to invasive cancer. The third level of intervention focuses on the prevention of second primary tumors in patients cured for lung cancer or head and neck cancer, who could also be enrolled in CT screening trails. The target population for chemoprevention and spiral CT screening trials thus show an overlap to some extent.

LUNG CANCER EPIDEMIOLOGY

Although there has been a decline in the lung cancer incidence rates among men since 1984 in the US and many other countries, there is a continuing increase in incidence among women.[1,10,11] Due to the success of public education and smoking cessation programs, today there are many more former smokers than current smokers among the newly diagnosed lung cancer patients. It is estimated that for the birth cohort 1940–44, more than half of all lung cancer cases will occur in ex-smokers at age of 70 and over.[12,13] In this setting, smoking cessation results in a prompt and significant reduction in the risk of cardiovascular mortality. However, the risk of developing lung cancer is only reduced by 50% 10 years after cessation, and remains twice the risk of a never smoker 15–20 years after cessation.[13] The net effect is that more former smokers live long enough to manifest a lung cancer because cardiovascular disease falls off as a competing risk factor. Therefore, former smokers represent the majority of lung cancer cases by the age of 70. The extent to which young people become cigarette smokers over the next few decades will strongly affect mortality in the middle and second half of the 21st century, but lung cancer mortality in the first half of the 21st century will predominantly be affected by the number of adult smokers who have quit.[14] Therefore, secondary prevention (screening) and chemoprevention strategies aimed at the reduction of the lung cancer mortality in current high-risk or ex-smokers deserves high priority.

IDENTIFICATION OF HIGH-RISK INDIVIDUALS

To be as cost-effective as possible CT screening and chemoprevention strategies should be directed to those individuals who are potentially the most at need. Currently, high-risk individuals are primarily defined on epidemiological parameters. Although 85–90% of all patients with lung cancer have a history of direct exposure to tobacco, only 20% of all smokers develop lung cancer.[10] In addition to the other major causes of tobacco-related mortality including heart and pulmonary disease, the causes of lung cancer are multi-factorial, and may involve more than a simple association with smoking. Several of the most widely accepted risk factors are listed in Table 20.2.[14,15]

It is generally accepted that a further refinement of the risk assessment is needed and a validated 'Molecular-Epidemiological Lung Cancer Risk Assessment Model' be developed. In such a refined model, a number of current complementary approaches need to be integrated. The conceptional model of the biomarker-based lung cancer screening journey cascade was presented for the first time in 2003 at the Third International Lung Cancer Detection Workshop in Liverpool (Figure 20.1). This model constitutes the bases for future strategies to optimize the identification and selection of the high-risk individuals for participation in CT screening and chemoprevention strategies.

Table 20.2 Co-variates and lung cancer risk[14,15]

Relative risk factors for lung cancer

Tobacco exposure	Variable	Gender	Variable
Environmental (Radon)	3	Diet	Variable
Occupational exposure (asbestos)	5	Chronic obstructive lung disease	4.5
Genetic factors	Uncertain	Family history	2.5

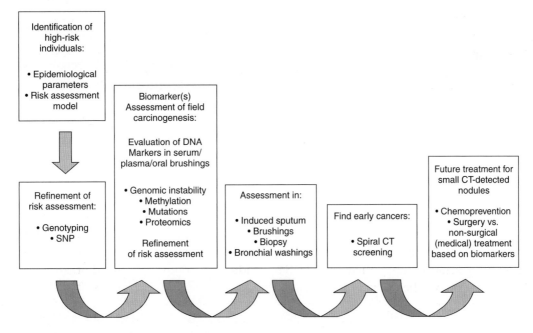

Figure 20.1
Biomarker-based lung cancer screening journey cascade.

CHOICE OF HIGH-RISK POPULATIONS AND BIOMARKERS

Smoking history

Major prospective studies[16-19] and several case-control studies[20-23] have demonstrated a clear dose–response relationship between the development of lung cancer and the degree of exposure to cigarette smoke, as measured by the total number of cigarettes smoked per day, the age at which smoking began, the duration of smoking and the duration of smoking cessation.[16,17,21]

The unit 'pack-years' (PY), defined as the number of packs of cigarettes smoked per day multiplied by the number of years of smoking, is commonly used as an estimate of this lung cancer risk. Despite its widespread use, this unit does not take age and the duration of smoking cessation into account. Moreover, both the number of cigarettes smoked and the duration of smoking receive equal weight in the calculation of the number of pack-years. However, lung cancer incidence increases with a factor of 4.5 based on duration of smoking, compared to 1.5 based on average daily consumption.[24,25] Therefore, we should refrain from PY as a criterion in the selection of lung cancer screening candidates, and select people based on smoking duration, time since cessation and the average number of cigarettes smoked per day. Independent from the duration and the number of cigarettes smoked per day, age alone is also an important risk factor. The data from the Cancer Prevention Study II (CPS-II) showed a 3–4-fold increase in lung cancer risk with 10-year intervals both for males (Table 20.3A) and for females (Table 20.3B).

For calculation of the sample size in chemoprevention and lung cancer screening trials, it is important that the absolute lung cancer risk is taken into account because it provides us with

Table 20.3A Death rates from lung cancer in current male cigarette smokers in different age groups, by amount and duration of smoking. Cancer Prevention Study II (/100 000 person-years)[26]

Cigarettes smoked per day	Age (years)	Smoking duration (years)			
		20–29	30–39	40–49	50+
1–19	50–59	62.5	99.2	173.7	NA
	60–69	170.3	154.6	346.8	330.1
	70–79	227.1	265.5	575.3	842.5
20–39	50–59	73.0	161.7	240.5	292.2
	60–69	355.9	220.3	463.9	859.0
	70–79	676.4	660.9	759.7	1166.3
40+	50–59	127.6	212.6	363.9	1047.7
	60–69	123.7	528.0	648.1	837.3
	70–79	NA	929.8	1453.5	4190.1

NA, not available.

Table 20.3B Death rates from lung cancer in current female cigarette smokers in different age groups, by amount and duration of smoking. Cancer Prevention Study II (/100 000 person-years)[26]

Cigarettes smoked per day	Age (years)	Smoking duration (years)			
		20–29	30–39	40–49	50+
1–19	50–59	28.8	66.6	62.6	NA
	60–69	66.2	132.3	143.8	235.5
	70–79	102.8	124.9	170.3	238.0
20–39	50–59	67.9	123.7	231.3	NA
	60–69	153.8	223.8	292.9	618.5
	70–79	331.5	296.0	545.6	532.3
40+	50–59	108.2	163.7	190.3	NA
	60–69	744.2	258.9	532.4	411.9
	70–79	456.6	277.2	496.9	742.8

NA, not available.

the absolute number of cancer cases that eventually will be found during a certain period of time. An absolute cancer risk with a death rate of at least 300/100 000 person-years might be considered as a high-risk threshold above which people can be enrolled in chemoprevention or lung cancer screening trials, although this is rather arbitrary. Lung cancer incidence and mortality follow with a lag time of 20–30 years after the first exposure to smoking. Since most smokers started smoking by their early 20s a sharp rise in lung cancer incidence is seen above the age of 50, where the 300/100 000 person-years death rate threshold is crossed. This is illustrated in Table 20.4, where the lung cancer incidence above 300/100 000 is indicated by the shaded area.[26]

In light of the increasing incidence of lung cancer among ex-smokers, there is a need to improve prospects for these individuals who have accomplished the difficult task of cessation.[12,27] This constitutes an important high-risk population to consider for participation in lung cancer screening trials for a number of reasons. The question is, however, after how many years of cessation is the risk to develop lung cancer still so high that enrolment in lung cancer screening programs is justified. Peto and Halpern et al argue that the relative risk of lung cancer after smoking cessation decreases at about the same rate as the relative risk of lung cancer increases as people age.[24,28] Therefore, they conclude that the absolute risk of lung cancer remains approximately the same over time, which justifies why in several lung cancer screening trials even ex-smokers of up to 15 years are enrolled. By contrast, Samet and Lubin et al have found an independent risk-reducing effect of quitting smoking, such that longer durations of abstinence are associated with greater reductions in risk.[29,30] The risk of developing lung cancer in ex-smokers is complex, and not only related to the years since smoking cessation, but also to past smoking duration.[28]

Table 20.4 Lung cancer incidence rates by age and amount smoked per day (rates per 100 000 person-years)[26]

Number of cigarettes smoked per day	Age at incidence (Death – 5 years) in years								
	30–34	35–39	40–44	45–49	50–54	55–59	60–64	65–69	70–74
1–9	–	–	–	42	114	258	362	560	725
10–19	–	–	–	101	103	192	360	859	574
20	–	–	43	83	200	297	652	854	1372
21–39	–	–	25	114	218	442	510	1042	1326
40	–	–	57	159	254	507	836	1244	1525
40+	–	53	141	220	335	499	999	1469	4067
Total	6	19	41	115	206	361	582	909	1118

Cancer Prevention Study II (CPS) data.[26]

The younger the age at cessation, the greater the decrease in mortality.[31] Bach et al developed a lung cancer risk model, in analogy to the Gail Model in breast cancer.[32] This model showed that individuals who quit smoking neither undergo a further increase nor show a decrease in the previous increased lung cancer risk compared to never-smokers. The difference in risk between continuing smokers and quitters could be explained almost entirely by differences in duration of smoking between the two groups. These findings are consistent with the findings by Peto and Halpern et al.[24,28] The Bach model is based on the data of 18 172 subjects enrolled in the Carotene and Retinol Efficacy Trial (CARET). It consisted of two populations; 14 254 heavy smokers (men and women, aged 50–69 years) who had at least 20 pack-years of smoking exposure and were either current smokers or had quit within 6 years of enrolment, and 4060 asbestos-exposed men (aged 45–69 years, either current smokers or former smokers who had quit within 15 years of enrolment) who had either radiological evidence of asbestos exposure or a history of asbestos

exposure. The model was validated internally by assessing the extent to which a model estimated on data from five CARET study sites could predict events in the sixth study site. Table 20.5 shows the approximate 10-year risk percentage of developing lung cancer in current or ex-smokers with a smoking history of one or two packs per day according to this Bach model. It is assumed that ex-smokers will continue to abstain for the next 10 years and those who are still smoking will keep smoking the same amount for the next 10 years. Although the model is not yet used in clinical practice, it is a first step towards a more individualized computer-assisted risk prediction.

COPD

Chronic obstructive pulmonary disease (COPD) and lung cancer are both tobacco-related diseases. The diagnosis of obstructive lung disease has traditionally been based on the presence of symptoms such as chronic cough or sputum production. New international guidelines for the diagnosis of obstructive lung disease are almost exclusively based on measured lung

Table 20.5 Approximate 10-year risk percentage of developing lung cancer in current or ex-smokers with a smoking history of one or two packs per day according to the Bach model[32]

Age, years	Duration of smoking					
	25 years		40 years		50 years	
	Ex-smoker	Current smoker	Ex-smoker	Current smoker	Ex-smoker	Current smoker
10-year lung cancer risk in 1 pack per day smokers (%)						
55	<1	1	3	5	NA	NA
65	<1	2	4	7	7	10
75	1	2	5	8	8	11
10-year lung cancer risk in 2 packs per day smokers (%)						
55	<1	2	4	7	NA	NA
65	1	3	6	9	10	14
75	2	3	7	10	11	15

NA, not available.

function to diagnose and classify disease.[33] Most studies of the association of obstructive lung disease and lung cancer in the United States have been performed in smaller populations not necessarily representative of the US population.[34,35] They showed an increased risk of lung cancer with increasing levels of airway obstruction during a follow-up period that ranged from 1 to 25 years. Also a Danish study of 13 946 participants followed up for 10 years found increased lung cancer mortality risks in subjects with an FEV_1 of less than 40% (HR 3.9) or 40–79% (HR 2.1) when compared with subjects with an FEV_1 of at least 80%.[36] In a Scottish study of 15 411 subjects followed up for 15 years, men and women with low lung function (FEV_1 <73% and <75%, respectively) had a higher risk for lung cancer mortality (HR 2.5 and 4.4, respectively).[37] In a study by Mannimo et al a total of 5402 adult smokers or ex-smokers between 25 and 74 years were followed

for 22 years. They were classified as moderate or severe COPD if the ratio FEV_1/FVC was less than 70% or if the FEV_1 was less than 80%. When adjusted for age, sex, race, education, smoking status and the duration and intensity of smoking, the presence of moderate or severe COPD was associated with a higher risk for incident lung cancer (HR 2.8; 95% confidence interval 1.8–4.4).[38] From these studies we may conclude that pulmonary function tests among current and former smokers may help to identify a subgroup of patients in whom lung cancer is more likely to develop and who are more likely to benefit from screening and case detection.

Asbestos

Exposure to carcinogenic agents interacts synergistically with tobacco smoking and concurrent exposures causes a multiplicative increase in the risk of cancer. Exposure to all types of asbestos is associated with a significantly increased risk of lung cancer. The relative risk of lung cancer in asbestos workers in general is approximately 2 (95% CI 1.9–2.1) whereas it is 6 in individuals who develop interstitial and pleural fibrosis known as asbestosis (95% CI 5.0–7.0) as compared with the general population.[39] When smoking is combined with asbestos exposure, the relative risk of lung cancer is multiplicative and has been reported to increase to 50.[40] Most of these data came from people with a high degree of exposure, and there are no data available on the relationship between the amount and duration of the exposure and the risk to develop lung cancer. In general, however, asbestos exposed (ex)-smokers are at high risk to develop lung cancer and belong to the target population for chemoprevention or lung cancer screening trials.

Biomarkers for selection of high-risk individuals

An increasing understanding of the molecular and genetic biology of lung cancer may in the near future provide alternative strategies for early lung cancer detection, or may allow stratification of risk for developing the disease. High-throughput technologies for cDNA microarray analysis, comparative genomic hybridization and proteomics might be of great value, and have already led to the identification of novel potentially useful new biomarkers. At present, however, these emerging tools do not play a part in the general lung cancer screening strategy and the selection of participants for chemoprevention trials. Biomarkers measurable in the peripheral blood have included carbohydrate-rich cell matrix molecules such as carcinoembryonic antigen,[41] cytokeratin-derived intermediate filament molecules such as CYFRA-21.1,[42,43] tissue-specific antigen (TPA)[44] and tissue polypeptide specific antigen (TPS),[45] peptides such as

proGRP,[46] neural markers such as neuron-specific enolase,[47,48] and chromogranin A[49,50] and antibodies to immunogenic molecules such as Hu,[51] calcium channel proteins[52] and p53,[53,54] but so far they show insufficient sensitivity or specificity for routine screening and early detection of cancer. More recent studies have reported the presence of DNA markers in the serum of patients with a variety of cancers, including lung cancers.[55,56] Tests for DNA (polymorphisms, mutations and abnormal DNA methylation) and RNA alterations in plasma have great potential for early detection and follow-up, but much needs to be done for validation of these techniques in larger series.[57] Despite current limitations and lack of specificity, biomarkers for early lung cancer (or for risk assessment) may one day help to refine the population chosen to undergo spiral CT screening or treatment with chemopreventive agents. During recent years, a substantial number of studies have examined the gene profiling of lung cancer. Genes that define, or are highly expressed in specific lung cancer types, have been identified as well as genes associated with specific clinical parameters such as nodal involvement, distant metastasis and patient survival.[58–60] However, before these genes can be used in clinical practice validation at multiple levels is required. Genetic instability at both chromosomal and nucleotide level gives rise to molecular genetic abnormalities present in both pre-neoplastic and overtly cancerous cells. Allele loss, gene up- and down-regulation, and p53 mutations are among the specific genetic abnormalities detected in lung cancer. The molecular alterations involved provide potential targets for early detection. The identification of new candidate biomarkers show great promise for the selection of target populations for lung cancer screening, although the biomarkers that have been identified need to be validated in large prospective studies.[57,61]

Autofluorescence bronchoscopy

Pre-invasive lesions in the bronchial epithelium might be difficult to detect using conventional white light bronchoscopy. Fluorescence bronchoscopy is an emerging technique that has been shown to be a far more sensitive method of detecting preoplastic lesions than conventional white-light bronchoscopy.[62] Given its availability and invasive nature, it is unlikely that fluorescence bronchoscopy will become a screening tool in the general population. However, fluorescence bronchoscopy is useful to detect pre-cancerous lesions in heavy smokers with sputum atypia, which is a high-risk population suitable for chemoprevention trials.

Sputum cytology

Sputum atypia can be used to identify high-risk subjects. In a study performed at the University of Colorado Cancer Center high-risk individuals (>30 pack-years smoking history, $FEV_1 <70\%$) with moderate to severe sputum cytology was found to be an independent risk factor with an adjusted relative risk of 3.18 compared to high-risk individuals with normal sputum cytology (Table 20.6 and Figure 20.2).[63]

Table 20.6 Association between sputum cytology and adjusted risk of lung cancer development (University of Colorado high-risk study cohort, $n = 3400$)[63]

	Relative risk
Normal sputum cytology	1.0
Mild atypia	1.10
Moderate atypia	1.68
Moderate atypia or worse	3.18
Worse than moderate atypia	31.4

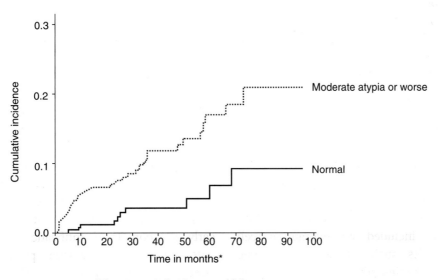

*Time truncated at 8 years of follow-up

Figure 20.2
Time to diagnosis of lung cancer by sputum cytology in the Colorado high-risk cohort.[63]

In a cohort of 2006 individuals 83 incident lung cancer cases were found over 4469 person-years of observation (4% incidence rate). Moderate to severe cytological atypia was associated with continuing cigarette smoking, and with lower levels of fruit and vegetable intake but not with the degree of airflow obstruction, use of vitamin supplements, non-steroidal anti-inflammatory drugs, or metered-dose steroid inhalers.[62]

From a clinical point of view there is no controversy that severe sputum atypia may lead to/or associates to either invasive cancer or carcinoma in situ and mandates further investigation and eventually intervention. The usual work-up in these patients includes bronchoscopy and CT scan. In the presence of severe sputum atypia there is a high likelihood that lung cancer will be imminently diagnosed; in two studies approximately 45% of the subjects with severe atypia developed lung cancer within 2 years.[64,65] The University of Colorado high-risk study (Table 20.6) supports that further investigation and intervention of patients with severe sputum atypia or worse should take place. It is still debatable, however, what the clinical consequences of moderate sputum atypia should be, and very sparse data in the literature are available. Fugita et al reported, in abstract form only, a series of 25 subjects with moderate sputum atypia and negative chest radiography.[66] Of those who underwent bronchoscopy, two were diagnosed with carcinoma. In a recent study from the University of Colorado Cancer Center, of 79 individuals with moderate sputum atypia and normal chest radiographs, five (6.3%) were found to have either invasive cancer (three patients) or carcinoma in situ (two patients) at follow-up bronchoscopy.[67] This surprising high fraction might justify further

investigation in this particular subgroup as well. Ongoing studies include other biomarkers and results from these studies might further refine the group with moderate sputum atypia who will benefit from early bronchoscopy and eventually early intervention. In a nested case-control study of the same high-risk cohort of patients followed at the University of Colorado DNA-methylation of certain genes was studied in sputum as a risk marker for lung cancer development.[63] Preliminary analysis performed on 57 cases and matched controls found that DNA methylation of a panel of eight genes added significantly to the odds ratio for sputum atypia. Combined with sputum atypia (moderate or worse) the risk of developing lung cancer increased with an odds ratio of 7.7 (Table 20.7).

This study is currently being enlarged and includes about 120 cases and controls. Currently it is too early to make any conclusions about whether DNA methylation in sputum can be used as a marker in patient selection for screening or chemoprevention studies, and prospective validation studies are ongoing.

In a pilot study of 33 cases and controls with chronic obstructive lung disease with a history of at least 30 pack-years, DNA aneuploidy in sputum was tested by multi-target DNA fluorescent in situ hybridization (FISH) assay.[68] In the sputum cytology specimens collected within 12 months preceding the diagnosis of lung cancer, the abnormality was more frequent among the 18 lung cancer cases (41%) than in the 17 controls (6%, $P < 0.05$). Aneuploidy had no significant association with cytologic atypia, suggesting that molecular and morphological changes could be independent markers of tumorigenesis, and that a combination of both tests may improve the sensitivity of sputum cytology as a predictive marker of lung cancer.

Table 20.7 DNA methylation and sputum cytology as risk marker for lung cancer development[63]

Marker positive	Odds ratio	
	All samples	Sample closest to diagnosis
Gene 1	1.9	2.2*
Gene 2	1.3	1.3
Gene 3	1.1	1.7
Gene 5	1.5	2.0
Gene 6	1.8	1.8
Gene 7	1.9	1.7
Gene 8	2.8	3.8*
Moderate cytologic atypia or worse	1.8	2.6*
Any methylation marker	3.0*	3.9*
Any biomarker, cytologic or methylated	5.9*	7.7*

*$P < 0.05$.

SELECTION CRITERIA

Age as a selection criterion

Based on the epidemiological data and the current trend of increased teenage smoking, we might conclude that there is no need to set a lower-age cut-off level for spiral CT screening or chemoprevention studies. Once people have reached the high-risk threshold they can be enrolled in these programs, irrespective of the age at which this high-risk level is reached. When a lower age limit is set at 40 years for all participants for example, the lung cancer incidence in the target population will drop considerably, regardless their smoking history and lung cancer risk, as happened in several Japanese lung cancer screening trials (Table 20.1).[5,7,8] An advantage of including younger people is that it might also lead to a larger gain in life years and improvement in the cost-effectiveness ratio of the screening program, although this benefit must be outweighed against the increased radiation risk in young people. Extension of a cancer screening program towards lower age groups might decrease the specificity of the screening test. A mammogram is, for example, more difficult to interpret below the age of 40,[69,70] but there is no evidence that this phenomenon exists in spiral CT screening. It is even more likely that the test characteristics of the spiral CT will be better because the prevalence of benign pulmonary nodules is lower at younger ages.[71] The natural history of cancer is sometimes age dependent, as it is for breast cancer, with a shorter sub-clinical phase and faster tumor progression in women aged 40–49.[69,72] To date, there is no evidence that there is a difference in the biological behaviour of lung cancer detected in younger and older people, neither for symptom-detected cases,[73] nor for chest X-ray- or spiral CT-detected lung cancer. Therefore, there is no contraindication for lung cancer screening in younger people under the condition that they meet the criteria for being a high-risk smoker.

Because only 5–10% of all lung cancer cases are diagnosed below the age of 50,[10,73–75] the lower age cut-off level is often set at the age of 50. To answer the question what the optimal upper age limit for participation in lung cancer screening trials should be, the life expectancy of the target population, the risk of dying from lung cancer without screening and the (cost)-effectiveness of the screening program should be taken into account. The issue of an upper-age cut-off level for (lung) cancer screening is complex[76] and can for lung cancer screening probably not be answered with the currently available data. However, the issue is most important, because 50% of all lung cancer cases occur in patients over 65 years of age.[76–78] Once lung cancer is symptomatic the prognosis for the whole lung cancer population is very poor with a 5-year survival rate of only 15% at best, the potential benefit from spiral CT screening may be high because 60–100% of the screen-detected lung cancers are found in stage I at prevalence screening in pilot studies (5-year survival rates 60–70%) (Table 20.1). However, the favorable difference in survival between symptom-detected and spiral CT-detected lung cancer might be due to lead-time bias. This would occur if the diagnosis is made earlier, but the time of death is unchanged. For chest X-ray screening the lead-time is estimated to be 4–8 years,[79] but for spiral CT screening it would probably be even longer. Therefore, the life expectancy of the population enrolled in screening trials should be at least 10 years, to be able to detect a real gain in life years. This is important because screening interventions can only be cost-effective when real life-years are obtained. The upper age limit is thus dependent of the life expectancy of the target population, which

might vary between the different countries and between males and females. In Western Europe, a quarter of the population is aged over 70 years, and in these countries a 70-year-old women has an average life expectancy of 15 years compared to 8–10 years for a male of the same age.

One of the striking features of the elderly population is its heterogeneity. While many individuals remain quite healthy with advancing age, others develop worsening health and functional impairments that can significantly decrease life expectancy and the benefits-to-harm ratio of screening tests. Many guidelines in ongoing population screening programs now recognize this heterogeneity, recommending that screening decisions should not be based on age alone but should also take into account an older person's health status.[80–83] Many guidelines for breast and cervix cancer screening recommend that the health status should be considered before mammography or Pap smears. Women whose life expectancy is less than 5 years are unlikely to benefit from cancer screening and will probably experience only the potential harms, including the unnecessary test and treatment of clinically insignificant disease and the accompanying psychological distress.[84] The physical functioning and health status of a population can be assessed via the self-rated SF-12 Physical Summary Scale (PCS-12).[85] The PCS-12 is a reasonable predictor of mortality in older adult populations and might, therefore, be useful in selection of populations for screening trials. However, its accuracy in predicting an individual's mortality is not known, and may not be accurate enough to select or exclude individuals from chemoprevention or cancer screening trials.[86] However, clinicians may use several characteristics to identify elderly people with limited life expectancies. End-stage renal disease, severe dementia or severe functional dependence in activities of daily living are examples of characteristics associated with high 5-year mortality rates. Clinicians should consider such characteristics together with clinical judgment and specific co-morbid conditions such as diabetes, COPD, hypertension and heart disease to estimate an individual's potential risk and benefit from chemoprevention or cancer screening, rather than basing these decisions on age alone. Since cancer screening in elderly people will only in a limited number of subjects be of clinical value, especially in these early days of chemoprevention and lung cancer screening, it should not be recommended to enroll people over 75 years of age in these trials.

Gender

The possibility that women are more susceptible than men to developing lung cancer after a similar exposure to cigarette smoke has generated substantial controversy.[87–90] A meta-analysis did not resolve the debate,[91] but most data in this meta-analysis came from case-control studies, and the only prospective study in this meta-analysis did not show a greater risk for women. New prospective data and a review of all six previously published prospective studies (not including the CPS-I study) do not provide any evidence for a greater susceptibility for women with quantitatively similar doses of smoking.[92] Case-control studies typically present only relative risks, i.e. the risk of lung cancer among smokers compared with non-smokers, whereas cohort studies enable absolute incidence of mortality rates to be assessed. The difference between the cohort and case-control studies can also be explained by the recall bias encountered in the case-control interviews. This bias does not occur in the cohort setting where exposure data are obtained prior to disease onset. Also, the Bach's lung cancer model revealed no convincing associ-ation between gender and lung cancer risk, although systematic differences by gender in the ascertainment of other exposures could have masked a small effect.[32] One cohort study, the Cancer Prevention Study II, showed a higher risk for men.

What is not debated is that important differences exist among men and women with lung cancer. Women smokers are more likely to develop adenocarcinoma, women who never smoked are more likely to develop lung cancer than men, and once women have developed lung cancer they experience a survival benefit that is not accounted for solely by a longer life expectancy or imbalance of other prognostic factors.[93] Genetic, metabolic and hormonal factors (estrogen signaling) might all be important to the way women react to carcinogens and develop lung cancer. Given this information, future screening and chemoprevention programs should include at least a proportion of women that reflects the true incidence of lung cancer in women.[94]

Co-morbidity

According to Wilson and Jungner's principles of screening, screening is only meaningful when curative treatment can be offered to test-positive subjects.[95] The current standard of care for small-sized lung cancers is lobectomy and mediastinal lymph node sampling or dissection. Medical inoperability or refusal to undergo surgery will preclude people to benefit from lung cancer screening and they should, therefore, not be exposed to the potential hazards of screening and excluded from participation. Although it could be important, for policy decisions later, to be in the position to know what that proportion of inoperable patients really is, and not to select an atypical group at risk for lung cancer, this potential benefit could be offset by the risk that CT screening trials will be inconclusive or negative just because of this fraction of inoperable subjects with a very poor prognosis. In the Mayo Lung Project, 20% of the detected early-stage lung cancer cases did not undergo surgery,[96] in the Czech study 50% (9/18) of all early-stage lung cancer incidence cases were medically inoperable or refused surgical intervention,[97] and from several large epidemiological studies we know that 5–10% of all heavy smokers (≥20 PY) are inoperable because of poor lung function.[98,99] New developments in chemotherapy (i.e. molecular targeted agents) and radiotherapy (i.e. higher doses and more intensive regimens such as continuous hyperfractionated accelerated and stereotactic radiotherapy) may become alternatives for standard surgery.[100] There is, for example, need for new approaches in the clinical management of the very tiny and sometimes multiple lung cancer lesions. These options have to be validated in prospective randomized clinical trials. Until then, surgery will remain the standard care for stage I lung cancer. As a consequence, people should only be enrolled in lung cancer screening trials when they are fit enough to undergo a thoracic surgical procedure. According to the British Thoracic Society guidelines of 2001, surgery for stage I and II disease can be as effective in patients over 70 years as in younger patients regardless of age.[101] They recommend that age alone is not a contraindication to lobectomy or wedge resection for clinically stage I disease.[100] Because of the impossibility to perform exercise testing in large-scale lung cancer screening programs, the fitness for surgery should be assessed by simple, inexpensive and widely available methods. The first validated method to assess this functional status is by estimating the ability to perform activities of daily life according to the American College of Cardiology and the American Heart Association (ACC/AHA) guidelines for the peri-operative

cardiovascular evaluation for non-cardiac surgery.[102] The functional capacity can be expressed in metabolic equivalent levels (MET). Patients who cannot achieve more than 4 or 5 METs (cannot rake leaves, weed a garden or wash a car), may be at great risk for peri- and postoperative cardiopulmonary events.[94,95] The cardio-pulmonary reserve can also be estimated by symptom-limited stair climbing. People who are able to climb two flight of stairs without rest (one flight is 18 steps) have a good cardiopulmonary reserve, are able to tolerate the cardiopulmonary stress, and have a low probability to develop postoperative complications.[103–106] With increasing age, the effect of co-morbidity becomes more and more important, in terms of the feasibility to perform a curative thoracotomy, postoperative mortality, and an excess of non-lung-cancer-related death. Data on co-morbidity in lung cancer patients are scarce, but Janssen-Heijnen et al investigated this issue in 3864 lung cancer patients registered in the population-based registry of the Comprehensive Cancer Centre South in the Netherlands between 1993–95.[77] It appeared from this study that the prevalence of co-morbidity in lung cancer patients is twice as high as in the general population. The most frequent concomitant diseases were cardiovascular disease (23%), chronic obstructive pulmonary diseases (COPD) (22%) and other malignancies (15%). Although there was a positive correlation between the number of co-morbid diseases and the treatment choice (less surgical resections), this correlation was present for both people below and above 70 years of age. The authors concluded that age alone appeared to be a more important factor in treatment choice than co-morbidity, as was also reported by others.[107,108] This may be explained by the fact that many physicians are reluctant to operate on elderly patients, and in their decision co-morbidity does not appear to play a role. Although these studies give an impression on the prevalence of co-morbid disease in lung cancer patients, they give no insight in the severity of these diseases and in what percentage co-morbidity really formed a contraindication for further thoracic surgical interventions. From the Seven-Countries Study we know that the incidence of COPD in a Dutch cohort of male smokers 40–60 years of age in 1960, was 35% in the period 1960–85.[98] Of the heavy smokers (at least 20 PYs) 10% had a $FEV_1 < 60\%$, $6\% < 50\%$ and $1.7\% < 40\%$ of predicted. Cross-sectional data of 3604 Dutch males and females aged 50–59 in whom a lung function was measured between 1994 and 1997 as part of the Morgen study,[99] revealed that 28% of the (ex)-smokers had COPD. Only 6% of the heavy smokers (at least 20 PYs) had a $FEV_1 < 60\%$, $2\% < 50\%$ and $1.1\% < 40\%$ of predicted. The percentage of severe airway obstruction ($FEV_1 < 50\%$ predicted) in the Lung Health Study conducted in the United States and Canada was 5%,[109] and in a large spirometric screening study in Poland 7% of the smokers over the age of 40 with a smoking history of ≥ 10 PYs had severe COPD.[110] From these data it can be concluded that although the prevalence of COPD among smokers is high (approximately 30%), in only 5–10% of the heavy smokers (≥ 20 PYs) is the disease so severe that it forms an absolute contraindication for thoracic surgical interventions. Because this sub-group has also a very poor prognosis after thoracic surgery (5-year survival rate of 41%),[111] their likelihood to benefit from lung cancer screening is a priori so low that this sub-population should be excluded from lung cancer screening. Over the last decade several approaches such as the Deyo-Charlson[112] and the Romano-Charlson index[113] for identifying patient co-morbidities have been developed to predict a patient's risk of death 1 year after

admission for surgical and non-surgical procedures, but the predictive power of both indices appeared to be low, and its applicability is limited.[114]

Exclusion criteria

People should be excluded from lung cancer screening when they are unable to lie flat, unable to hold their breath for 20 seconds, or when their body weight is above 140 kg, because it is technically impossible to perform a CT scan in these situations. A chest CT scan within 1 year before enrolment should disqualify the patient because the likelihood of detecting lung cancer will be lower and otherwise the population will be a mixture of screened and non-screened participants. A previous history of cancer is in many trials and proposals regarded as a contraindication for lung cancer screening because of the difficulty to differentiate between primary lung cancer and solitary metastases of the previous cancer. However, the relevance and frequency of this clinical problem in the setting of a screening program has not been evaluated prospectively. Presumably, the type of cancer and the corresponding biology and prognosis are probably more important than the fact that cancer has been diagnosed before. Previous lung- and head and neck cancer patients, for example, are usually (ex)smokers with a high annual (second) primary lung cancer rate of 2–3%, which justifies intensive surveillance and participation in lung cancer screening or chemoprevention trials.[115,116] On the other hand, melanoma, breast cancer or hypernephroma may show a very protracted and unpredictable course, and present with metastases even after 5 years, and might not be suitable for enrolment in lung cancer screening or chemoprevention trials. Also people who underwent a pneumonectomy are less likely to benefit from screening because of their limited pulmonary reserve. The exclusion criteria are summarized in Table 20.8.

Target population in ongoing screening trials

In the interpretation of the lung cancer detection rates of several large spiral CT screening trials, the US and European trials should be evaluated apart from the Japanese trials (Table 20.1). The much lower prevalence rates in Japanese trials can be explained by the fact that the underlying incidence rate in Japan is approximately half the incidence rate of the US,[117] that people between 40 and 50 years of age were enrolled as well, and that inclusion was independent of whether they were never smoker, current smoker or ex-smoker. Moreover, many people in the Japanese screening studies had already participated in a mass screening by CXR and sputum cytology conducted in the same area, so that the reported detection rates are not real prevalence data. However, even when the outcomes of the US and Europe screening trials are compared important differences can be found. The detection rates at baseline screening range from 1.3% to 3.1% and between 0.7–0.9% at annual repeat

(Table 20.1) are most likely due to a large variability in lung cancer risk between the target populations, though variations in radiological acquisition and evaluation could also have contributed to these differences. These differences will affect the outcome of these lung cancer screening studies, which needs to be considered in the interpretation of the data.[99] Lower age limits varied from over 40 years of age to 60 years of age and above, and smoking histories ranged between ≥10–≥20 pack-years. Former smokers are enrolled in some trials, but not included in others (Table 20.1). Even within the group of smokers who have a smoking history of at least 20 pack-years, there is a broad range of lung cancer risk and potential reduction in cancer risk for current smokers if they quit. This is illustrated when Bach's lung cancer model is applied to five individual participants of the Mayo Clinic (Table 20.9).[32] A 51-year-old female who smoked one pack per day for 28 years and quit 9 years earlier is in the 5th percentile of risk, while a 68-year-old male current smoker who has smoked two packs per day for 50 years is in the 95th percentile of risk, 15–20 times the risk of the person in the 5th percentile.

Table 20.8 Exclusion criteria for participation in lung cancer screening trials

A functional capacity corresponding with less than four metabolic equivalent levels (ACC/AHA)
The unability to climb two flight of stairs (36 steps) without rest
A previous pneumonectomy
A prior history of breast cancer, melanoma or hypernephroma
Age over 75 years
Body weight over 140 kg
Inability to lie flat
Inability to hold breath for 20 seconds
A chest CT scan within 1 year before enrolment
Unwillingness to undergo a curative treatment if lung cancer is detected

Table 20.9 Predicted lung cancer risk for a sample of participants in the ongoing study of spiral CT screening at the Mayo Clinic according to Bach's lung cancer model[32]

	Percentile of risk in Mayo Clinic Study				
	5th	25th	50th	75th	95th
Age, years	51	52	58	56	68
Sex	Female	Female	Male	Female	Male
Average no. of cigarettes smoked per day	20	20	25	40	40
Duration of smoking, years	28	35	40	44	50
Duration of abstinence, years	9	0	3	0	0
Asbestos exposure	No	No	No	No	No
10-year risk if no further smoking, %	0.80	1.50	4.10	5.60	10.80
10-year risk if continued smoking, %	NA	2.80	NA	8.40	14.90

After Bach et al.[32]
NA, not applicable.

CONCLUSIONS

Despite the limitations in defining high-risk populations, these can nevertheless be identified using epidemiological data. Smoking history, age and COPD are the most important selection criteria, followed by asbestos exposure. Since life gain in elderly people over 75 years of age is often very limited, and very often with the presence of co-morbid conditions, these individuals are not recommended to be enrolled in lung cancer screening or chemoprevention trials. It is expected that new means for selection of individuals at high risk for developing lung cancer will be available for clinical practice in the future, and the selection of high-risk individuals will no longer be based on epidemiological data only. With the emerging role of genomics and proteomics, it will most likely become possible to refine the selection of target populations for lung cancer screening and chemoprevention trials.

REFERENCES

1. Maxwell Parkin D, Global cancer statistics in the year 2000. Lancet Oncology 2001; 2: 533–43.
2. Hetmaniak Y, Bard JJ, Albuisson E, et al, Pulmonary nodules: dosimetric and clinical studies at low dose multidetector CT. J Radiol 2003; 84:399–404.
3. Henschke CI, McCauley DI, Yankelevitz DF, et al, Early lung cancer action project: overall design and findings from baseline screening. Lancet 1999; 354:99–105.
4. Henschke CI, Yankelevitz DF, Libby DM, et al, Early Lung Cancer Action Project: annual screening using single slice helical CT. Ann NY Acad Sci 2001; 952:124–34.
5. Sone S, Li F, Yang ZG, et al, Results of three-year mass screening programme for lung cancer using mobile low-dose spiral computed tomography scanner. Br J Cancer 2001; 84:25–32.
6. Nawa T, Nakagawa T, Kusano S, et al, Lung cancer screening using low-dose spiral CT: results of baseline and 1-year follow-up studies. Chest 2002; 122:15–20.

7. Diederich S, Wormanns D, Semik M, et al, Screening for early lung cancer with low-dose spiral CT: prevalence in 817 asymptomatic smokers. Radiology 2002; 222:773–81.

8. Sobue T, Moriyama N, Kaneko M, et al, Screening for lung cancer with low-dose helical computed tomography: Anti-Lung Cancer Association Project. J Clin Oncol 2002; 15: 911–20.

9. Swensen SJ, Jett JR, Hartman TE, et al, Screening for lung cancer with low-dose spiral computed tomography. Am J Respir Crit Care Med 2002; 165:508–13.

10. Smith RA, Glynn TJ, Epidemiology of lung cancer. Radiol Clin North Am 2000; 38: 453–70.

11. Skuladottir H, Olsen JH, Hirsch FR, Incidence of lung cancer in Denmark: historical and actual status. Lung Cancer 2000; 27:107–18.

12. Jemal A, Chu KC, Tarone RE, Recent trends in lung cancer mortality in the United States. J Natl Cancer Inst 2001; 93:277–83.

13. Burns DM, Primary prevention, smoking and smoking cessation. Implications for future trends in lung cancer prevention. Cancer 2000; 89:2506–9.

14. Samet JM, The epidemiology of lung cancer. Chest 1993; 103(suppl):20S–9S.

15. Beckett WS, Epidemiology and etiology of lung cancer. Clin Chest Med 1993; 14:1–15.

16. Hammond EC, Smoking in relation to the death of one million men and women. Natl Cancer Inst Monogr 1966; 19:127–204.

17. Doll R, Peto R, Mortality in relation to smoking: 20 years observation on male British doctors. BMJ 1976; 2:1525–36.

18. Rogot E, Murray JL, Smoking and causes of death among US veterans: 16 years of observation. Public Health Rep 1980; 95:213–222.

19. Cederlof R, Friberg L, Hrubec Z, The relationship of smoking and smoke: social co-variables to mortality and cancer morbidity – a ten year follow-up in probability sample of 55000 Swedish subjects age 18 to 69 (Part 1 and 2). Stockholm, Sweden, Department of Environ-mental Hygiene, The Karolinska Institute, 1975.

20. Damber LA, Larsson LG, Smoking and lung cancer with special regard to type of smoking and type of cancer: a case-control study in north Sweden. Br J Cancer 1986; 53:673–81.

21. Samet JM, Wiggins CL, Humble CG, Pathak DR, Cigarette smoking and lung cancer in New Mexico. Am Rev Respir Dis 1988; 137: 1110–13.

22. Weiss W, Boucot KR, Seidman H, Carnahan WJ, Risk of lung cancer according to histologic type and cigarette dosage. JAMA 1972; 222:799–801.

23. Rylander R, Axelsson G, Andersson L, Lilje-quist T, Bergman B, Lung cancer, smoking and diet among Swedish men. Lung Cancer 1996; 14:s75–s83.

24. Peto R, Influence of dose and duration of smoking on lung cancer rates. In: Zaridge D, Peto R (eds) Tobacco: a major International Health Hazard. Lyon, France, International Agency for Research on Cancer, 1986, pp. 23–33.

25. Haldorsen T, Grimsrud TK, Cohort analysis of cigarette smoking and lung cancer incidence among Norwegian women. Int J Epidemiol 1999; 28:1032–6.

26. Centers for Disease Control, Public Health Service, US Department of Health and Human Services, The health benefits of smoking cessation. Washington DC, US Gov Printing Office, 1990.

27. Tong L, Spitz MR, Fueger JJ, Amos CA, Lung carcinoma in former smokers. Cancer 1996; 78:1004–10.

28. Halpern MT, Gillespe BW, Warner KE, Patterns of absolute risk of lung cancer mortality in former smokers. J Natl Cancer Inst 1993; 85:457–64.

29. Samet JM, The health benefits of smoking cessation. Med Clin North Am 1992; 76: 399–414.

30. Lubin JH, Blot WJ, Berrino F, et al, Modifying risk for developing lung cancer by changing

habits of cigarette smoking. Br Med J 1984; 288:1953–6.

31. Wakai K, Seki N, Tamakoshi A, et al, Decrease in risk of lung cancer death in males after smoking cessation by age at quitting: findings from the JACC study. Jpn J Cancer Res 2001; 92:821–8.

32. Bach PB, Kattan MW, Thornquist MD, et al, Variations in lung cancer risk among smokers. J Natl Cancer Inst 2003; 95:470–8.

33. Pauwels RA, Buis SA, Calverley PM, Jenkins CR, Hurd SS, Global strategy for the diagnosis, management and prevention of chronic obstructive pulmonary disease: NHLBI/WHO Global Initiative for Chronic Obstructive Disease (GOLD) Workshop summary. Am J Respir Crit Care Med 2001; 163:1256–76.

34. Tockman MS, Anthonisen NR, Wright EC, Donithan MG, Airways obstruction and the risk for lung cancer. Ann Int Med 1987; 106: 512–18.

35. Lange P, Nyboe J, Appleyard M, Jensen G, Schnohr P, Ventilatory function and chronic mucus hypersecretion as predictors of death from lung cancer. Am J Respir Crit Care Med 1990; 141:613–17.

36. Islam SS, Schottenfeld D, Declining FEV_1 and chronic productive cough in cigarette smokers: a 25-year prospective study of lung cancer incidence in Tecumseh, Michigan. Cancer Epidemiol Biomarkers and Prevention 1994; 3: 289–98.

37. Hole DJ, Watt GC, Davey-Smith G, et al, Impaired lung function and mortality risk in men and women: findings from the Renfrew and Paisley prospective population study. BMJ 1996; 313:711–15.

38. Mannino DM, Aguayo SM, Petty TL, Redd SC, Low lung function and incident lung cancer in the United States. Arch Intern Med 2003; 163: 1475–80.

39. Steenland K, Loomis D, Shy C, Review of occupational lung carcinogens. Am J Ind Med 1996; 29:474–90.

40. Steenland K, Thun M, Interaction between tobacco smoking and occupational exposures in the causation of lung cancer. J Occup Med 1986; 28:110–18.

41. Buccheri GF, Violante B, Sartoris AM, et al, Clinical value of a multiple biomarker assay in patients with bronchogenic carcinoma. Cancer 1986; 57:2389–96.

42. Pujol JL, Boher JM, Grenier J, Quantin X, Cyfra 21-1, neuron specific enolase and prognosis of non-small cell lung cancer: prospective study in 621 patients. Lung Cancer 2001; 31:221–31.

43. Pujol JL, Grenier J, Daures JP, et al, Serum fragment of cytokeratin subunit 19 measured by CYFRA 21-1 immunoradiometric assay as a marker of lung cancer. Cancer Res 1993; 53: 61–6.

44. Buccheri G, Ferrigno D, The tissue polypeptide antigen serum test in the preoperative evaluation of non-small cell lung cancer. Diagnostic yield and comparison with conventional staging methods. Chest 1995; 107:471–6.

45. Pujol JL, Grenier J, Parrat E, et al, Cytokeratins as serum markers in lung cancer: a comparison of CYFRA 21-1 and TPS. Am J Resp Crit Care Med 1996; 154:725–33.

46. Holst JJ, Hansen M, Bork R, Schwartz TW, Elevated plasma concentrations of C-flanking gastrin-releasing peptide in small-cell lung cancer. J Clin Oncol 1989; 7:1831–8.

47. Jorgensen LG, Osterlind K, Hansen HH, Cooper EH, Serum neuron specific enolase in progressive small-cell lung cancer (SCLC). Br J Cancer 1994; 70:759–61.

48. Bonner JA, Sloan JA, Rowland KM, et al, Significance of neuron-specific enolase levels before and during therapy for small cell lung cancer. Clin Cancer Res 2000; 6:597–601.

49. Nobels FR, Kwekkeboom DJ, Coopmans W, et al, Chromografin A as serum marker for neuroendocrine neoplasia: comparison with neuron specific enolase and the alpha-subunit of glycoprotein hormones. J Clin Endocrinol Metab 1997; 82:2622–8.

50. Lamy P, Grenier J, Kramar A, Pujol JL, Pro-gastrin-releasing peptide, neuron-specific

enolase and chromogranin A as serum markers for small cell lung cancer. Lung Cancer 2000; 29:197–203.

51. Graus F, Dalmou J, Rene R, et al, Anti-Hu antibodies in patients with small-cell lung cancer: association with complete response to therapy and improved survival. J Clin Oncol 1997; 15:2866–72.

52. Lemon VA, Kryzer TJ, Griesmann GE, et al, Calcium-channel antibodies in the Lambert-Eaton syndrome and other paraneoplastic syndromes. N Engl J Med 1995; 332:1467–74.

53. Winter SF, Minna JD, Johnson BE, et al, Development of antibodies against p53 in lung cancer patients appears to be dependent on the type of p53 mutation. Cancer Res 1992; 52:4168–74.

54. Winter SF, Sekio Y, Minna JD, et al, Antibodies against autologous tumor cell proteins in patients with small-cell lung cancer association of improved survival. J Nat Cancer Inst 1993; 85:2012–18.

55. Sozzi G, Conte D, Leon M, et al, Quantification of free circulating DNA as a diagnostic marker in lung cancer. J Clin Oncol 2003; 21:3902–8.

56. Sugita M, Geraci M, Gao B, et al, Combined use of oligonucleotide and tissue microarrays identifies cancer/testis antigens as biomarkers in lung carcinoma. Cancer Res 2002; 62: 3971–9.

57. Bunn PA Jr, Early detection of lung cancer using serum RNA or DNA markers: ready for prime time or for validation? J Clin Oncol 2003; 21:3891–3.

58. Beer DG, Kardia SL, Huang CG, et al, Gene expression profiles predict survival of patients with lung adenocarcinoma. Nat Med 2002; 8: 816–24.

59. Wigle D, Jurisica I, Radulovich N, et al, Molecular profiling of non-small cell lung cancer and correlation with disease-free survival. Cancer Res 2002; 62:3005–8.

60. Blackhall FH, Wigle DA, Jurisca I, et al, Validating the prognostic value of marker genes derived from a non-small cell lung cancer microarray study. Lung Cancer 2004; 46: 197–204.

61. Hirsch FR, Franklin WA, Gazdar AF, Bunn PA, Early detection of lung cancer: clinical perspective of recent advances in biology and radiology. Clin Cancer Res 2001; 7:5–22.

62. Hirsch FR, Prindiville SA, Miller YE, et al, Fluorescence versus white-light bronchoscopy for detection of preneoplastic lesions: a randomized study. J Natl Cancer Inst 2001; 93:1385–91.

63. Prindiville SA, Byers T, Hirsch FR, et al, Sputum cytological atypia as a predictor of incident lung cancer in a cohort of heavy smokers with airflow obstruction. Cancer Epidemiol Biomarkers Prev 2003; 12:987–93.

64. Risse EK, Vooijs GP, van't Hof MA, Diagnostic significance of 'severe dysplasia' in sputum cytology. Acta Cytologica 1988; 32:629–34.

65. Tockman MS, Gupta PR, Myers JD, et al, Sensitive and specific monoclonal antibody recognition of human cancer antigen on preserved sputum cells: a new approach to early lung cancer detection. J Clin Oncol 1988; 6: 1685–93.

66. Fugita Lung Cancer 1994.

67. Kennedy TC, Franklin WA, Prindiville SA, et al, High prevalence of endobronchial malignancy in high risk patients with moderate dysplasia in sputum. Chest 2004; 125(5 suppl): 109S.

68. Varella-Garcia M, Kittelson J, Schulte AP, et al, Multi-target interphase fluorescence in situ hybridization assay increases sensitivity of sputum cytology as a predictor of lung cancer. Cancer Detect Prevent 2004; 28:244–51.

69. Morrone D, Ambrogetti D, Bravetti P, et al, Diagnostic errors in mammography. I. False negative results. Radiol Med 1991; 82:212–17.

70. Swedish Cancer Society and the Swedish National Board of Health and Welfare, Breast-cancer screening with mammography in women aged 40–49 years. Int J Cancer 1996; 68:693–9.

71. Midthun DE, Swensen SJ, Jett JR, Clinical strategies for solitary pulmonary nodule. Annu Rev Med 1992; 43:195–208.

72. Moskowitz M, Breast cancer: age-specific growth rates and screening strategies. Radiology 1986; 161:37–41.

73. Maruyama R, Yoshino I, Yohena T, et al, Lung cancer in patients younger than 40 years of age. J Surg Oncol 2001; 77:208–12.

74. Minami H, Yoshimura M, Matsuoka H, Toshihiko S, Tsubota N, Lung cancer treated surgically in patients <50 years of age. Chest 2001; 120:32–6.

75. Radzikowska E, Roszkowski K, Glaz P, Lung cancer in patients under 50 years old. Lung Cancer 2001; 33:203–11.

76. Kreeger KY, Cancer screening in older patients: making decisions about age cut-offs. J Natl Cancer Inst 2001; 93:1198–9.

77. Janssen-Heijnen MLG, Schipper RM, Razenberg PPA, Crommelin MA, Coebergh J-WW, Prevalence of co-morbidity in lung cancer patients and its relationship with treatment: a population-based study. Lung Cancer 1998: 21:105–13.

78. Fry WA, Menck HR, Winchester DP, The National Cancer Data Base report on lung cancer. Cancer 1996; 77:1947–55.

79. Walter SD, Kubic A, Parkin DM, et al, The natural history of lung cancer estimated from the results of a randomized trial of screening. Cancer Causes Control 1992; 3:115–23.

80. Humphrey LL, Helfand, M, Chan BK, Woolf SH, Breast cancer screening; a summary of the evidence for the US Preventive task force. Ann Intern Med 2002; 137:347–60.

81. AGS, Health screening decisions for older adults. AGS positions paper. J Am Geriatr Soc 2003; 51:270–1.

82. Smith RA, Saslow D, Swayer KA, et al, American Cancer Society guidelines for breast cancer screening; update 2003. CA Cancer J Clin 2003; 53:141–69.

83. Walter LC, Eng C, Covinsky KE, Screening mammography for frail older women: what are the burdens? J Gen Intern Med 2001; 16: 779–84.

84. Sawaya GF, Grady D, Kerlikowske K, et al, The positive predictive value of cervical smears in previously screened post-menopausal women: the Heart and Estrogen/progestin Replacement Study (HERS). Ann Intern Med 2000; 133: 942–50.

85. Ware J Jr, Kosinski M, Keller SD, A 12-Item Short Form Health Survey: construction of scales and preliminary tests of reliability and validity. Med Care 1996; 34:220–33.

86. Riddle DL, Lee KT, Stratford PW, Use of SF-36 and SF-12 health status measures: a quantitative comparison for groups versus individual patients. Med Care 2001; 39:867–78.

87. Zang EA, Wynder EL, Differences in lung cancer risk between men and women: examination of the evidence. J Natl Cancer Inst 1996; 88:183–92.

88. Perneger TV, Sex, smoking and cancer: a reappraisal. J Natl Cancer Inst 2001; 93:1600–2.

89. Thun MJ, Henley SJ, Calle EE, Tobacco use and cancer: an epidemiologic perspective for geneticists. Oncogene 2002; 21:7307–25.

90. Henschke CI, Miettinen OS, Women's susceptibility to tobacco carcinogens. Lung Cancer 2004; 43:1–5.

91. Khunder SA, Effect of cigarette smoking on major histologic types of lung cancer: a meta-analysis. Lung Cancer 2001; 31:139–48.

92. Bain C, Feskanich D, Speizer FE, et al, Lung cancer rates in men and women with comparable histories of smoking. J Natl Cancer Inst 2004; 96:826–34.

93. Blot WJ, McLaughlin JK, Are women more susceptible to lung cancer? Editorial. J Natl Cancer Inst 2004; 96:812–13.

94. Patel JD, Bach PB, Kris MG, Lung cancer in US women. A contemporary epidemic. JAMA 2004; 291:1763–7.

95. Wilson JMP, Jungner G, Principles and practice of screening for disease. Public Health Papers, WHO, Geneva, 1968, number 39.

96. Marcus PM, Bergstralh EJ, Fagerstrom RM, et al, Lung cancer mortality in the Mayo Lung Project: Impact of extended follow-up. J Natl Cancer Inst 2000; 92:1308–16.

97. Kubik A, Polak J, Lung cancer detection. Results of a randomized prospective study in Czechoslovakia. Cancer 1986; 57:2427–37.

98. Jacobs DR, Adachi H, Mulder I, et al, Cigarette smoking and mortality risk. Twenty-five-years follow-up of the Seven Countries Study. Arch Int Med 1999; 159:733–40.

99. Tabak C, Arts IC, Smit HA, Heederik D, Kromhout D, Chronic obstructive pulmonary disease and intake of catechins, flavonols, and flavones: the MORGEN study. Am J Respir Crit Care Med 2001; 164:61–4.

100. Rowell NP, Williams CJ, Radical radiotherapy for stage I/II non-small lung cancer in patients not sufficiently fit for or declining surgery (medically inoperable): a systematic review. Thorax 2001; 56:628–38.

101. British Thoracic Society; Society of Cardiothoracic Surgeons of Great Britain and Ireland Working Party. BTS guidelines: Guidelines on the selection of patients with lung cancer for surgery. Thorax 2001: 56:89–108.

102. ACC/AHA guidelines for peri-operative cardiovascular evaluation for non-cardiac surgery. Circulation 1996; 93:1280–317.

103. Teplick R, Preoperative cardiac assessment of the thoracic surgical patient. Anaesthesia 1997; 7:655–96.

104. Girish M, Trayner E, Dammann O, Pinto-Plata V, Celli B, Symptom-limited stair climbing as a predictor of postoperative cardiopulmonary complications after high-risk surgery. Chest 2001; 120:1147–51.

105. Kinasewitz GT, Welch MH, A simple method to assess postoperative risk. Chest 2001; 120: 1057–8.

106. Pollock M, Roa J, Benditt J, Celli B, Estimation of ventilatory reserve by stair climbing. A study in patients with chronic airflow obstruction. Chest 1993; 104:1378–83.

107. De Rijke JM, Schouten LJ, Schouten HC, et al, Age-specific differences in the diagnosis and treatment of cancer patients aged 50 years and older in the province of Limburg, the Netherlands. Ann Oncol 1996; 7:677–85.

108. Goodwin JS, Hunt WC, Samet JM, Determinants of cancer therapy in elderly patients. Cancer 1993; 71:524–9.

109. Connett JE, Bjornson-Benson WM, Daniels K, Recruitment of participants in the Lung Health Study II. Assessment of recruiting strategies: Lung Health Study Research Group. Control Clin Trials 1993; 14:38s–51s.

110. Zielinski J, Bednarek M, Early detection of COPD in a high-risk population using spirometric screening. Chest 2001; 119:731–6.

111. Sahn SA, Nett LM, Petty TL, Ten year follow-up of a comprehensive rehabilitation program for severe COPD. Chest 1980; 77(suppl):311–14.

112. Charlson ME, Pompei P, Ales KL, MacKenzie CR, A new method of classifying prognostic comorbidity in longitudinal studies: developments and validation. J Chron Dis 1987; 40: 373–83.

113. Romano PS, Roos LL, Jollis JG, Adapting a clinical comorbidity index for use of a clinical comorbidity index with ICD-9-CM administrative data. J Clin Epidemiology 1993; 46: 1085–90.

114. Cleves MA, Sanchez N, Draheim M, Evaluation of two competing methods for calculating Charlson's comorbidity index when analysing short-term mortality using administrative data. J Clin Epidemiol 1997; 50:903–8.

115. Van Zandwijk N, Dalesio O, Pastorino U, de Vries N, EUROSCAN, a randomized trial of vitamin A and N-acetylcysteine in patients with head and neck cancer or lung cancer. J Natl Cancer Inst 2000; 92:977–86.

116. Younes RN, Gross JL, Deheinzelin D, Follow-up in lung cancer. How often and for what purpose? Chest 1999; 115:1494–9.

117. Marugame T, Mizuno S, mortality trend of lung cancer in Japan: 1960–2000. Jpn J Clin Oncol 2003; 33:148–9.

Index